3/2003

SHOULDER MAGNETIC RESONANCE IMAGING

Shoulder Magnetic Resonance Imaging

EDITORS

Lynne S. Steinbach, M.D.
Professor
Chief, Musculoskeletal Radiology
Department of Radiology
University of California, San Francisco
San Francisco, California

Phillip F.J. Tirman, M.D.
Assistant Clinical Professor
Department of Radiology; and
Medical Director
San Francisco Magnetic Resonance Center–
St. Francis Memorial Hospital
University of California, San Francisco
San Francisco, California

Charles G. Peterfy, M.D., Ph.D.
Assistant Professor
Department of Radiology
University of California, San Francisco; and
Director
Arthritis and MRI Research
Osteoporosis & Arthritis Research Group
San Francisco, California

John F. Feller, M.D.
Assistant Clinical Professor
Department of Radiology
Stanford University School of Medicine
Stanford, California; and
Co-Director
Desert Medical Imaging
Indian Wells, California

ILLUSTRATIONS BY

Gilbert M. Gardner, M.A., C.M.I.
60th Medical Group/AMC
Department of the Air Force
Travis Air Force Base, California

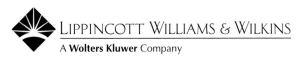

LIPPINCOTT WILLIAMS & WILKINS
A **Wolters Kluwer** Company
Philadelphia · Baltimore · New York · London
Buenos Aires · Hong Kong · Sydney · Tokyo

Acquisitions Editor: James Ryan
Developmental Editor: Lesa E. Ramsey
Manufacturing Manager: Tim Reynolds
Production Manager: Kathleen Bubbeo
Production Editor: Jeffrey Gruenglas
Cover Designer: Karen Quigley
Indexer: Linda Van Pelt
Compositor: Maryland Composition

Printed and bound in China

9 8 7 6 5 4 3 2

Library of Congress Cataloging-in-Publication Data
Shoulder magnetic resonance imaging/editors, Lynne S. Steinbach . . .
    [et al.]; illustrations by Gilbert M. Gardner.
        p.   cm.
    Includes bibliographical references and index.
    ISBN 0-397-51468-9 (hc)
    1. Shoulder joint–Magnetic resonance imaging.   I. Steinbach,
Lynne S.
    [DNLM: 1. Shoulder–physiology–atlases. 2. Shoulder Joint-
-physiology–atlases. 3. Magnetic Resonance Imaging–atlases.   WE
17 S559 1998]
    RD557.5.S546 1998
    617.5'7207548–dc21
DNLM/DLC
for Library of Congress   97-49684
                                                              CIP

Care has been taken to confirm the accuracy of the information presented and to describe generally accepted practices. However, the authors, editors, and publisher are not responsible for errors or omissions or for any consequences from application of the information in this book and make no warranty, expressed or implied, with respect to the contents of the publication.

The authors, editors, and publisher have exerted every effort to ensure that drug selection and dosage set forth in this text are in accordance with current recommendations and practice at the time of publication. However, in view of ongoing research, changes in government regulations, and the constant flow of information relating to drug therapy and drug reactions, the reader is urged to check the package insert for each drug for any change in indications and dosage and for added warnings and precautions. This is particularly important when the recommended agent is a new or infrequently employed drug.

Some drugs and medical devices presented in this publication have Food and Drug Administration (FDA) clearance for limited use in restricted research settings. It is the responsibility of the health care provider to ascertain the FDA status of each drug or device planned for use in their clinical practice.

Contents

Contributors

David P. Adkison, M.D. *Chief, Department of Orthopaedic Surgery, National Naval Medical Center, 8901 Wisconsin Avenue, Bethesda, Maryland 20889*

John P. Belzer, M.D. *Assistant Clinical Professor, Department of Orthopaedics, University of California, San Francisco; and Attending Surgeon, California Pacific Orthopaedics and Sports Medicine, 3838 California Street, Suite 715, San Francisco, California 94118*

Louis U. Bigliani, M.D. *Professor of Orthopaedic Surgery, Department of Orthopaedics, Columbia-Presbyterian Medical Center, 161 Fort Washington Avenue, New York, New York 10032*

Frederic W. Bost, M.D. *Assistant Clinical Professor, Department of Orthopaedics, University of California, San Francisco; and Attending Surgeon, California Pacific Orthopaedics and Sports Medicine, 3838 California Street, Suite 715, San Francisco, California 94118*

Antonio Correa, M.D. *Chief, Magnetic Resonance Imaging, Department of Diagnostic Radiology, Mike O'Callaghan Federal Hospital, Nellis Air Force Base, 4700 North Las Vegas Boulevard, Las Vegas, Nevada 89191-6601*

John F. Feller, M.D. *Assistant Clinical Professor, Department of Radiology, Stanford University School of Medicine, 300 Pasteur Drive, Stanford, California 94305; and Co-Director, Desert Medical Imaging, Indian Wells, California 92210*

Tom D. Howey, M.D. *Clinical Assistant Professor, Department of Surgery, University of South Dakota; and Orthopaedic Associates LTD., 1500 West 22nd Street, Suite 102, Sioux Falls, South Dakota 57005*

Van C. Mow, Ph.D. *Professor of Mechanical Engineering and Orthopaedic Bioengineering, Department of Orthopaedic Surgery, Columbia University, 630 West 168th Street, Black Building 14-1412, New York, New York 10032*

Christian H. Neumann, M.D., Ph.D. *Clinical Professor, Department of Radiology, University of California, San Diego, 9500 Gilman Drive, La Jolla, California 92093-0602; and Director, Magnetic Resonance Imaging, Department of Radiology, Desert Hospital, 1150 North Indian Canyon Drive, Palm Springs, California 92262*

Charles G. Peterfy, M.D., Ph.D. *Assistant Professor, Department of Radiology, University of California, San Francisco; and Director, Arthritis and MRI Research, Osteoporosis & Arthritis Research Group, 513 Parnassus Avenue, Box 0628, San Francisco, California 94143-0628*

Brad R. Plaga, M.D. *Assistant Clinical Professor, Department of Surgery, University of South Dakota; and Orthopaedic Associates, LTD., 1500 West 22nd Street, Suite 102, Sioux Falls, South Dakota 57105*

Lynne S. Steinbach, M.D. *Professor, Chief, Musculoskeletal Radiology, Department of Radiology, University of California, San Francisco, 505 Parnassus Avenue, Box 0628, San Francisco, California 94143*

Phillip F.J. Tirman, M.D. *Assistant Clinical Professor, Department of Radiology; and Medical Director, San Francisco Magnetic Resonance Center–St. Francis Memorial Hospital, University of California, San Francisco, 3333 California Street, Room 105, San Francisco, California 94118-1944*

Howard R. Unger, Jr., M.D. *M&S Associates, 730 North Main Street, Suite B-115, San Antonio, Texas 78205*

James H. Welch, M.D. *Chief, Musculoskeletal/Body MRI, Department of Radiology, Keesler Medical Center, Keesler Air Force Base, Mississippi 39532*

Foreword

In an age in which magnetic resonance (MR) is preeminent as an imaging method, and at a moment when shoulder imaging enjoys great interest and popularity, comes a book whose timeliness can hardly be questioned. Edited by four international leaders in the field, with a supporting cast composed of respected scientists in multiple specialities, *Shoulder Magnetic Resonance Imaging* deserves your immediate attention.

A successful book demands, initially, careful organization. This text clearly succeeds in this area. Early chapters emphasize anatomy fundamental to accurate assessment of MR images and technical considerations, including those related to MR arthrography, that ensure the images are of optimal quality, clear, and informative. The function and biomechanics of the shoulder are summarized, and clinical parameters important for reliable assessment of joint dysfunction are detailed. In later chapters, the application of MR imaging (and MR arthrography) to the analysis of each of the most important disorders of the shoulder is emphasized. It is all here—from those of glenohumeral joint instability, bicipital tendon alterations, arthritides, postoperative abnormalities, and other conditions.

A successful book devoted to imaging also requires attention to detail with regard to the choice and preparation of illustrations. Only the best of these are included in this text—each vividly displaying important findings, with meaningful labeling and informative legends. In some chapters, tables are included that summarize data in a manner that can be comprehended easily and, at the end of each chapter, a list of references (including recent publications) allows the interested reader to study any particular subject in even more detail.

Thus, it requires no clairvoyance on my part to predict that this book will be successful. The timeliness of the subject material, the gathering of experts, the superb organization, the complete discussions, and the inclusion of high-quality illustrations and tables and of selected references guarantee this success. Many radiologists, orthopedic surgeons, rheumatologists, and physicians in related fields should—and will—purchase it. What each will discover here, whether he or she reads the book in its entirety or refers only to particular parts of it, is a text that addresses a complex and important subject in a logical and understandable fashion. Simply, this book will not only be successful because of its popularity but will be effective in providing first-rate instruction so that the interpretation of MR imaging studies of the shoulder will be easier, more enjoyable, and clearly more accurate.

Donald Resnick, M.D.
University of California, San Diego
San Diego, California

Foreword

I am honored to have the opportunity to write a foreword for this important and timely textbook on magnetic resonance imaging (MRI) of the shoulder. As a practicing orthopedist dealing exclusively with the shoulder, I have had the opportunity to witness the evolution of imaging technology available for the shoulder joint and related structures during the past two and a half decades. This experience has given me a keen appreciation for the value of today's high-quality imaging as it relates to the evaluation and treatment of shoulder disease.

Initially in my career only crude radiographic studies were available to assist in visually evaluating the shoulder anatomy below the skin. The paucity of soft tissue imaging tools placed great importance on the history and physical examination as the definitive source of information for clinical diagnosis and preoperative planning. In those days, shoulder surgery was equally crude, requiring large incisions and often muscle and tendon releases in an attempt to visualize and repair damaged joints. It is little wonder that early diagnosis and surgical repair was seldom considered acceptable therapy in any but the most obvious traumatic injuries.

The addition of safe contrast materials and later air for the "double contrast" arthrogram helped the radiologist better visualize the interior surfaces of the shoulder as well as some of the more severe injuries to the rotator cuff tendon. It was seldom possible to diagnose partial tears or bursal side cuff problems. Computer-enhanced tomographic studies improved imaging capabilities, especially for labral and bony trauma, loose bodies, and articular irregularities, but the yield for the more demanding diagnostic problems such as cysts or bursal inflammatory diseases was beyond the capabilities of these studies. Certainly, ultrasound and bone scans have helped in specific cases but no single study was capable of displaying a valuable visual rendering of all the important shoulder anatomy in a way that all interested physicians could readily interpret.

During the first 15 years of my career, there had been very few advances in the traditional history or physical examination that significantly improved my ability to diagnose and treat an injured shoulder. Two valuable tools have evolved that together have empowered us to solve our problems: the video arthroscope and MRI. Together these two marvelous technologic advances have given us the unique ability to safely and accurately evaluate the important anatomy under the skin, thereby assisting us in formulating and rendering a successful treatment.

As with all new medical tools, both the arthroscope and the MRI have had their share of problems in the early phases of development. The unfamiliar intraarticular shoulder and bursal anatomy was highly magnified by the arthroscopic lens, often contributing to inaccurate diagnosis and, therefore, improper treatment. There was no textbook of arthroscopic anatomy in the early years, and the surgeon was often without adequate training and tools to repair pathology when it was encountered.

The early MRI images were crude and were often displayed as indistinct grey scale shadows and motion artifact. The early scanners were weaker magnets with poor quality coils and software. Many orthopedic surgeons and their radiologic colleagues were not trained or prepared to interpret the information provided by these new modalities. These problems during the early learning period caused many thoughtful practitioners to dismiss the arthroscope and MRI as "high-tech toys" that were not a significant benefit in the everyday evaluation and treatment of shoulder disease. Even today, there still exist a substantial number of physicians who fail to understand, accept, and, therefore, benefit from the magnificent potential of these wonderful imaging tools.

In a modern shoulder practice, the MRI is frequently vital to ensure the complete evaluation of a persistent complaint. It is incumbent on the physician (whether he or she is an orthopedist, a physiatrist, rheumatologist, or another discipline that may be evaluating recalcitrant shoulder problems) to be skillful with basic shoulder MRI interpretation. It is never acceptable for any specialist to rely solely on the radiologist's reading as the only interpretation for this important test. Imaging studies, like most things in the medical field, are a valuable resource, and the treating physician is charged with the important task of requesting this, or any other test, only when the information is likely to significantly enhance patient care.

The MRI is never a substitute for a comprehensive orthopedic history and physical examination coupled with a review of basic shoulder x-rays. Because the radiologist does not have the benefit of important clinical information, he or she is often at a disadvantage when formulating a complete diagnosis based on the images alone. An important example is found in cases of subacromial "impingement." A competent radiologist may notice a prominent underhanging lip below the acromioclavicular joint, a situation that sometimes may be associated with a clinical picture of impingement syndrome. If the surgeon bases his or her recommended treatment on the MRI report alone, the result will often be an unnecessary operation and an unhappy patient.

The greatest value delivered by the MRI in my practice has been an enhanced understanding of shoulder anatomy and pathology, and as a complement to my arthroscopic evaluation. I am constantly amazed by the exquisite detail that an excellent quality scan will present, and I use those images to sharpen my arthroscopic diagnostic skills. It is important to have the scan in the operating room for continuous reference during all shoulder arthroscopic procedures.

Several specific examples of the value of the MRI in my practice are illustrative. A ganglion cyst compressing the suprascapular nerve may clinically mimic a rotator cuff tear. A good quality MRI not only will make the diagnosis but also often will guide the arthroscopic treatment of the causative degenerative labral tear, thereby avoiding recurrence of the cyst.

An early case of a bursal-sided rotator cuff tear is always suspected when an inordinate amount of fluid is noted in the subacromial space. Realizing this association mandates a careful bursal evaluation from multiple portals to prove or refute the suspected diagnosis.

A biceps tendon anchor injury (SLAP lesion) may be very difficult to confirm with the routine clinical methods. A good quality MRI scan, often enhanced with intraarticular gadolinium, may add valuable support to the diagnosis.

The future of the medical and surgical treatment of the shoulder will certainly be tied to further advancements in MRI. As more physicians learn to use the scan to its maximum potential, its true value to patient care will be realized. This text is an important building block to bridge the learning gap for all of us, and I consider it essential reading for anyone who purports to practice first-class shoulder care.

Stephen J. Snyder, M.D.
Southern California Orthopaedic Institute
Van Nuys, California

Preface

The shoulder is the second most commonly imaged joint after the knee in musculoskeletal magnetic resonance imaging (MRI) practice. It has become apparent that shoulder MRI is an area that can assist as well as confuse radiologists and clinicians. Hence, a unique interest in this topic has arisen. In response, we introduced a refresher course at the Radiological Society of North America (RSNA) three years ago and have presented updates annually. Each year we have been encouraged by our course and fellowship attendees to produce a comprehensive body of literature that will provide them with this useful information which we have assembled. To date, such a reference is not available.

We write this book with the belief that shoulder magnetic resonance imaging can evaluate a much broader spectrum of anatomy and pathology than any other modality. Superior soft tissue contrast, high spatial resolution, and multiplanar capability have contributed to the success of MRI of the shoulder joint. Refinements relating to technique and diagnosis have been made. Yet many pitfalls and caveats must be explored. MR arthrography has also enhanced diagnosis of certain abnormalities. This book will cover these developments using a practical approach that we have developed during the past decade. We emphasize description of the findings with close clinical correlation.

This book is intended for radiologists, orthopedists, rheumatologists, and general practitioners who work with patients presented with shoulder pain. We have assembled leading clinicians and scientists from several specialties to tie together different aspects of shoulder imaging, pathophysiology, biomechanics, clinical examination, and treatment.

The text is divided into 11 chapters. The first chapter discusses anatomic considerations, a topic covered among others by Christian H. Neumann, who has written many of the original articles covering MRI findings of anatomic variants of the shoulder, as well as both the asymptomatic and the symptomatic rotator cuff. Charles G. Peterfy has written a practical summary of technical considerations specifically geared toward shoulder MRI. MR arthrography has increasingly been used because of its unique ability to demonstrate labral tears, capsular pathology, the undersurface of the rotator cuff, and loose bodies. Phillip F.J. Tirman, one of the pioneers of this technique, introduces the reader to shoulder arthrography in the third chapter. David P. Adkison has the distinction of winning the "Excellence in Research" award from the American Orthopedic Society (AOS) for Sports Medicine this year and was chosen to repair President Clinton's ruptured quadriceps tendon. He has graciously taken the time to write an informative chapter on shoulder biomechanics. John P. Belzer, who completed an orthopedic fellowship with Stephen J. Snyder, one of the premier shoulder arthroscopists, is currently in practice and works closely with Frederic W. Bost, who has been a sports physician for several professional teams. Together they have written an excellent overview regarding how to clinically assess the painful shoulder. With this basic foundation, the following chapters cover shoulder pathology as revealed by MRI. Lynne S. Steinbach, who is an author of many shoulder MR articles during the past decade and the recipient of the President's Medal from the International Skeletal Society in 1996, has written a comprehensive chapter on MR imaging of the rotator cuff. In Chapter 7, Dr. Tirman discusses various aspects of imaging glenohumeral instability, incorporating many of the newest concepts in the orthopedic literature. Dr. Steinbach in the following chapter covers the biceps tendon and SLAP lesions. SLAP lesions have received much attention in the radiologic and orthopedic literature during the last few years. John F. Feller, who was a radiology staff member at Travis Air Force Base before moving to a busy radiology practice, has written in Chapter 9 an up-to-date review of the postoperative shoulder. With radiologic and orthopedic colleagues, Brad R. Plaga and Tom D. Howey, he combines information on the reason behind the surgery as well as important technical and imaging features. Arthritis of the shoulder is discussed in Chapter 10 by Dr. Peterfy, Van C. Mow, and Louis Bigliani, all of whom have contributed significantly to research on MRI of joint cartilage. The final chapter, written by Dr. Feller, among others, completes the book with a review of all other areas of shoulder MR imaging not described in the previous chapters.

We are confident that the reader of this book will obtain a broad knowledge of the most practical and up-to-date information regarding shoulder MRI. With this standard, we hope to contribute to improvement in the quality of interpretation of disorders of the shoulder.

Lynne S. Steinbach, M.D.
Phillip F.J. Tirman, M.D.
Charles G. Peterfy, M.D., Ph.D.
John F. Feller, M.D.

Acknowledgment

The authors wish to acknowledge the talent, patience, and commitment of the book's medical illustrator, Gil Gardner.

SHOULDER MAGNETIC RESONANCE IMAGING

Shoulder Magnetic Resonance Imaging,
edited by Lynne S. Steinbach, et al.
Lippincott–Raven Publishers, Philadelphia © 1998.

CHAPTER 1

Normal Anatomy

Christian H. Neumann, Phillip F.J. Tirman, Lynne S. Steinbach,
and Howard R. Unger, Jr.

The clinical evaluation of the injured shoulder can be challenging. Imaging techniques such as arthrography, frequently combined with computed tomography, provide a means of evaluating rotator cuff integrity and may demonstrate findings suggestive of instability. Magnetic resonance imaging (MRI) has widely replaced these diagnostic procedures, providing diagnostic information not readily available with other modalities because of its multiplanar imaging capability and superior soft tissue contrast. The detailed information on state-of-the-art high-resolution MR images challenges the diagnostician to be familiar with shoulder anatomy and its normal variations. This, in addition to an understanding of the use of the diagnostic instrument and clinical experience with the disease processes investigated, provides the basis for diagnostic results similar to those favorably reported in the literature (1–5).

C. H. Neumann: Department of Radiology, University of California, San Diego, California 92093-0602; and Magnetic Resonance Imaging, Department of Radiology, Desert Hospital, Palm Springs, California 92262

P. F.J. Tirman: Department of Radiology; San Francisco Magnetic Resonance Center–St. Francis Memorial Hospital, University of California, San Francisco, San Francisco, California 94118-1944

L. S. Steinbach: Department of Radiology, University of California, San Francisco, San Francisco, California 94143

H. R. Unger, Jr.: M&S Associates, San Antonio, Texas 78205

SEQUENTIAL MAGNETIC RESONANCE IMAGES OF A LEFT SHOULDER IN OBLIQUE SAGITTAL, OBLIQUE CORONAL, AND AXIAL PROJECTIONS

This chapter is an atlas of sequential MR images of a left shoulder in oblique sagittal, oblique-coronal, and axial planes. They are presented in the following order: The oblique sagittal images of a left shoulder (Fig. 1) are shown in sequence from lateral to medial. The oblique coronal images of a left shoulder (Fig. 2) are shown from anterior to posterior and the axial images of a left shoulder (Fig. 3) are displayed cranial to caudal. Modified axial images with the left shoulder in abduction and external rotation are presented in sequence from cranial to caudal (Fig. 4).

GENERAL ANATOMIC OVERVIEW

The glenohumeral joint is a "multiaxial ball and socket" articulation between the humeral head and the shallow glenoid fossa. Static stability is provided by the capsule and glenohumeral ligaments, with dynamic stability largely supplied by the muscles and tendons of the rotator cuff. The glenohumeral joint is surrounded by a complex array of muscles, tendons, bones, and bursae, which serve mechanical, protective, and supportive functions.

Text continues on page 17

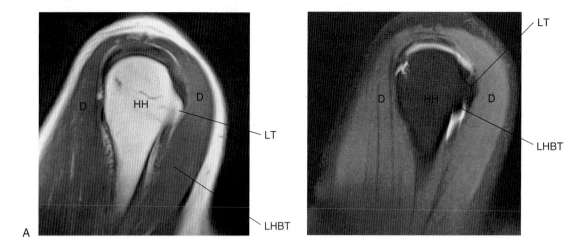

FIG. 1. A: Series of eight anatomically closed matched pairs of oblique sagittal MR images of a left shoulder. T1-weighted images without **(left)** and T1-weighted fat-saturated images after intraarticular application of dilute gadolinium **(right)** from the same volunteer are displayed in sequence from lateral to medial. D, deltoid muscle; HH, humeral head; LHBT, long head biceps tendon; LT, lesser tuberosity.

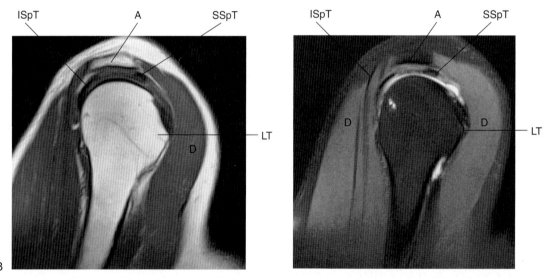

FIG. 1. B: Series of eight anatomically closed matched pairs of oblique sagittal MR images of a left shoulder. T1-weighted images without **(left)** and T1-weighted fat-saturated images after intraarticular application of dilute gadolinium **(right)** from the same volunteer are displayed in sequence from lateral to medial. A, acromion; D, deltoid muscle; LT, lesser tuberosity; ISpT, infraspinatus tendon and/or muscle; SSpT, supraspinatus tendon and/or muscle.

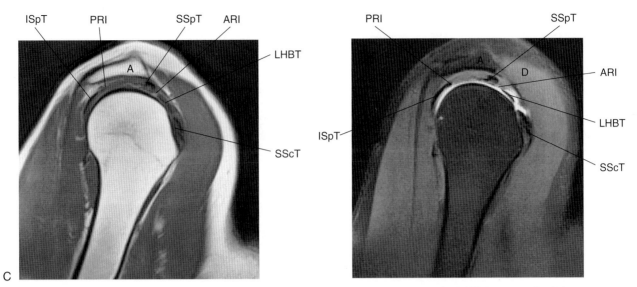

FIG. 1. C: Series of eight anatomically closed matched pairs of oblique sagittal MR images of a left shoulder. T1-weighted images without **(left)** and T1-weighted fat-saturated images after intraarticular application of dilute gadolinium **(right)** from the same volunteer are displayed in sequence from lateral to medial. A, acromion; ARI, anterior rotator interval; D, deltoid muscle; ISpT, infraspinatus tendon and/or muscle; LHBT, long head biceps tendon; PRI, posterior rotator interval; SScT, subscapularis tendon and/or muscle; SSpT, supraspinatus tendon and/or muscle.

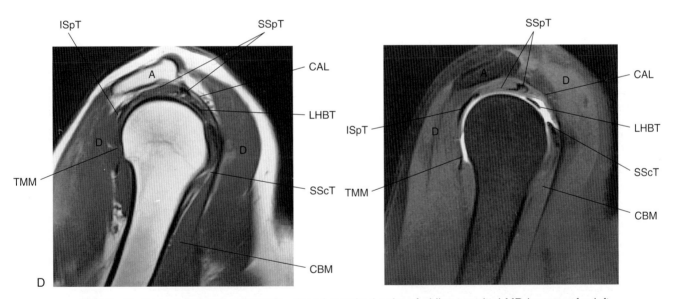

FIG. 1. D: Series of eight anatomically closed matched pairs of oblique sagittal MR images of a left shoulder. T1-weighted images without **(left)** and T1-weighted fat-saturated images after intraarticular application of dilute gadolinium **(right)** from the same volunteer are displayed in sequence from lateral to medial. A, acromion; CAL, coracoacromial ligament; CBM, coracobrachialis muscle; D, deltoid muscle; ISpT, infraspinatus tendon and/or muscle; LHBT, long head biceps tendon; SScT, subscapularis tendon and/or muscle; SSpT, supraspinatus tendon and/or muscle; TMM, teres minor muscle.

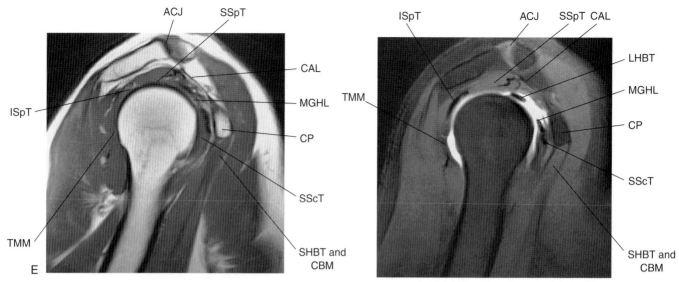

FIG. 1. E: Series of eight anatomically closed matched pairs of oblique sagittal MR images of a left shoulder. T1-weighted images without **(left)** and T1-weighted fat-saturated images after intraarticular application of dilute gadolinium **(right)** from the same volunteer are displayed in sequence from lateral to medial. ACJ, acromioclavicular joint; CAL, coracoacromial ligament; CBM, coracobrachialis muscle; CP, coracoid process; ISpT, infraspinatus tendon and/or muscle; LHBT, long head biceps tendon; MGHL, middle glenohumeral ligament; SHBT, short head biceps tendon; SScT, subscapularis tendon and/or muscle; SSpT, supraspinatus tendon and/or muscle; TMM, teres minor muscle.

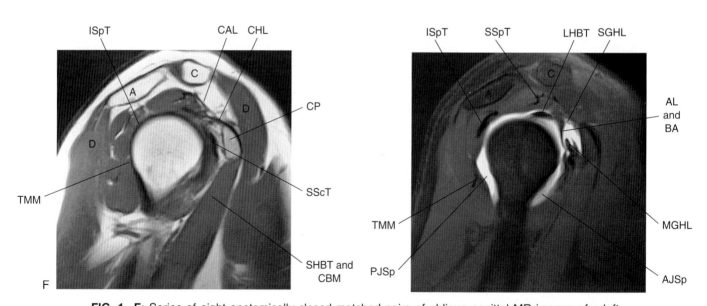

FIG. 1. F: Series of eight anatomically closed matched pairs of oblique sagittal MR images of a left shoulder. T1-weighted images without **(left)** and T1-weighted fat-saturated images after intraarticular application of dilute gadolinium **(right)** from the same volunteer are displayed in sequence from lateral to medial. A, acromion; AJSp, anterior joint space; AL, anterior labrum; BA, biceps anchor; C, clavicle; CAL, coracoacromial ligament; CBM, coracobrachialis muscle; CHL, coracohumeral ligament; CP, coracoid process; D, deltoid muscle; ISpT, infraspinatus tendon and/or muscle; LHBT, long head biceps tendon; MGHL, middle glenohumeral ligament; PJSp, posterior joint space; SGHL, superior glenohumeral ligament; SHBT, short head biceps tendon; SSpT, supraspinatus tendon and/or muscle; TMM, teres minor muscle.

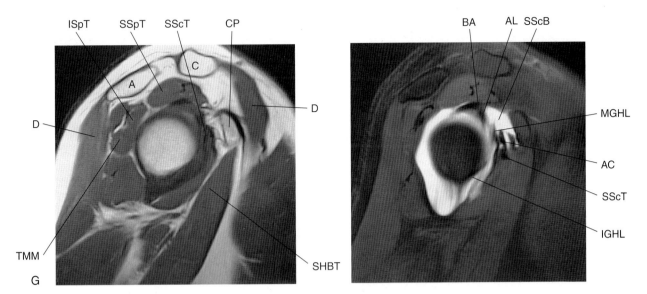

FIG. 1. G: Series of eight anatomically closed matched pairs of oblique sagittal MR images of a left shoulder. T1-weighted images without **(left)** and T1-weighted fat-saturated images after intraarticular application of dilute gadolinium **(right)** from the same volunteer are displayed in sequence from lateral to medial. A, acromion; AC, anterior capsule; AL, anterior labrum; BA, biceps anchor; C, clavicle; CP, coracoid process; D, deltoid muscle; IGHL, inferior glenohumeral ligament; ISpT, infraspinatus tendon and/or muscle; MGHL, middle glenohumeral ligament; SHBT, short head biceps tendon; SScB, subscapularis bursa; SScT, subscapularis tendon and/or muscle; SSpT, supraspinatus tendon and/or muscle; TMM, teres minor muscle.

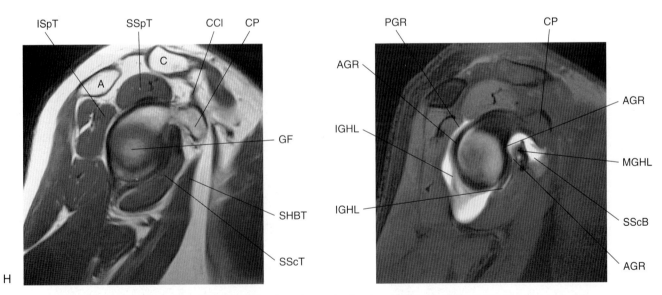

FIG. 1. H: Series of eight anatomically closed matched pairs of oblique sagittal MR images of a left shoulder. T1-weighted images without **(left)** and T1-weighted fat-saturated images after intraarticular application of dilute gadolinium **(right)** from the same volunteer are displayed in sequence from lateral to medial. A, acromion; AGR, anterior glenoid recess; C, clavicle; CCL, coracoclavicular ligament; CP, coracoid process; GF, glenoid fossa; IGHL, inferior glenohumeral ligament; ISpT, infraspinatus tendon and/or muscle; MGHL, middle glenohumeral ligament; PGR, posterior glenoid recess; SHBT, short head biceps tendon; SScB, subscapularis bursa; SScT, subscapularis tendon and/or muscle; SSpT, supraspinatus tendon and/or muscle.

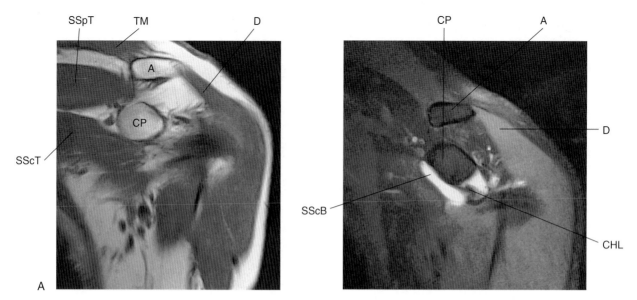

FIG. 2. A: Series of seven oblique coronal MR images of a left shoulder. T1-weighted images without **(left)** and T1-weighted fat-saturated images after intraarticular application of dilute gadolinium **(right)** from the same volunteer are displayed in sequence from anterior to posterior. A, acromion; CHL, coracohumeral ligament; CP, coracoid process; D, deltoid muscle; SScB, subscapularis bursa; SScT, subscapularis tendon and/or muscle; SSpT, supraspinatus tendon and/or muscle; TM, trapezius muscle.

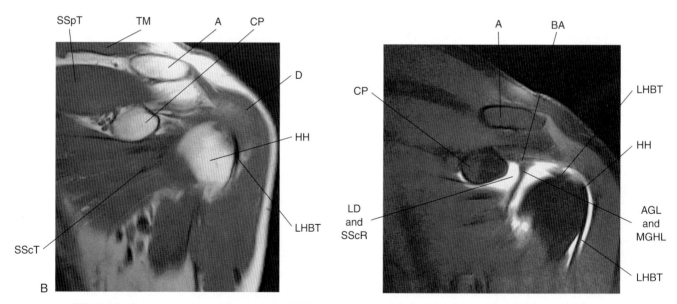

FIG. 2. B: Series of seven oblique coronal MR images of a left shoulder. T1-weighted images without **(left)** and T1-weighted fat-saturated images after intraarticular application of dilute gadolinium **(right)** from the same volunteer are displayed in sequence from anterior to posterior. A, acromion; AGL, anterior glenoid labrum; BA, biceps anchor; CP, coracoid process; D, deltoid muscle; HH, humeral head; LD, labral defect; LHBT, long head biceps tendon; MGHL, middle glenohumeral ligament; SScR, subscapularis recess; SScT, subscapularis tendon and/or muscle; SSpT, supraspinatus tendon and/or muscle; TM, trapezius muscle.

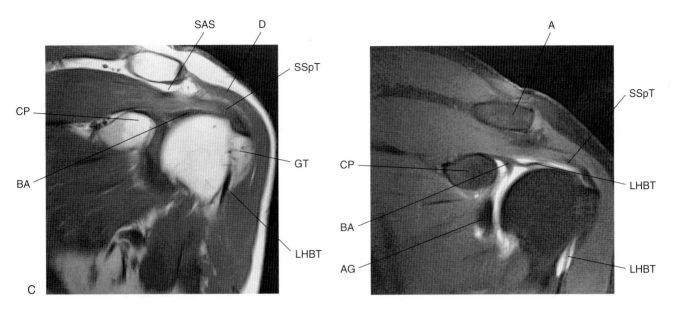

FIG. 2. C: Series of seven oblique coronal MR images of a left shoulder. T1-weighted images without **(left)** and T1-weighted fat-saturated images after intraarticular application of dilute gadolinium **(right)** from the same volunteer are displayed in sequence from anterior to posterior. A, acromion; AG, anterior glenoid; BA, biceps anchor; CP, coracoid process; D, deltoid muscle; GT, greater tuberosity; LHBT, long head biceps tendon; SAS, subacromial/subdeltoid space; SSpT, supraspinatus tendon and/or muscle.

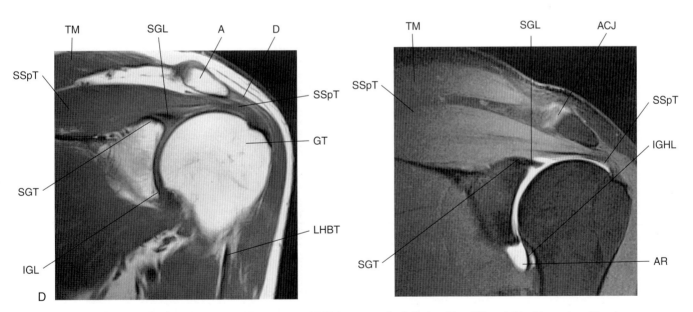

FIG. 2. D: Series of seven oblique coronal MR images of a left shoulder. T1-weighted images without **(left)** and T1-weighted fat-saturated images after intraarticular application of dilute gadolinium **(right)** from the same volunteer are displayed in sequence from anterior to posterior. A, acromion; ACJ, acromioclavicular joint; AR, axillary recess; D, deltoid muscle; GT, greater tuberosity; IGHL, inferior glenohumeral ligament; IGL, inferior glenoid labrum; LHBT, long head biceps tendon; SGL, superior glenoid labrum; SGT, superior glenoid tubercle; SSpT, supraspinatus tendon and/or muscle; TM, trapezius muscle.

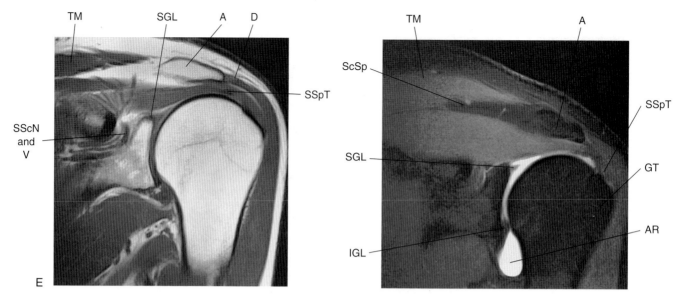

FIG. 2. E: Series of seven oblique coronal MR images of a left shoulder. T1-weighted images without **(left)** and T1-weighted fat-saturated images after intraarticular application of dilute gadolinium **(right)** from the same volunteer are displayed in sequence from anterior to posterior. A, acromion; AR, axillary recess; D, deltoid muscle; GT, greater tuberosity; IGL, inferior glenoid labrum; ScSp, scapular spine; SGL, superior glenoid labrum; SScN and V, suprascapular nerve and vessels; SSpT, supraspinatus tendon and/or muscle; TM, trapezius muscle.

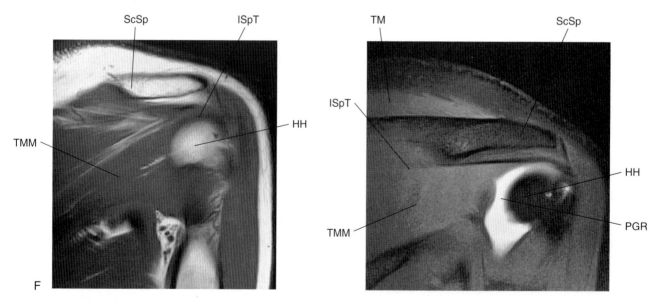

FIG. 2. F: Series of seven oblique coronal MR images of a left shoulder. T1-weighted images without **(left)** and T1-weighted fat-saturated images after intraarticular application of dilute gadolinium **(right)** from the same volunteer are displayed in sequence from anterior to posterior. HH, humeral head; ISpT, infraspinatus tendon and/or muscle; PGR, posterior glenoid recess; ScSp, scapular spine; TM, trapezius muscle; TMM, teres minor muscle.

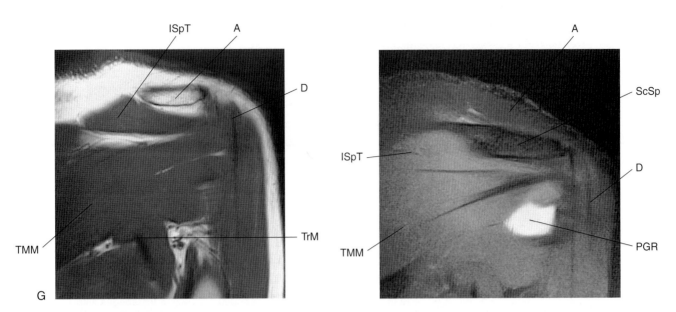

FIG. 2. G: Series of seven oblique coronal MR images of a left shoulder. T1-weighted images without **(left)** and T1-weighted fat-saturated images after intraarticular application of dilute gadolinium **(right)** from the same volunteer are displayed in sequence from anterior to posterior. A, acromion; D, deltoid muscle; ISpT, infraspinatus tendon and/or muscle; PGR, posterior glenoid recess; ScSp, scapular spine; TMM, teres minor muscle; TrM, triceps muscle.

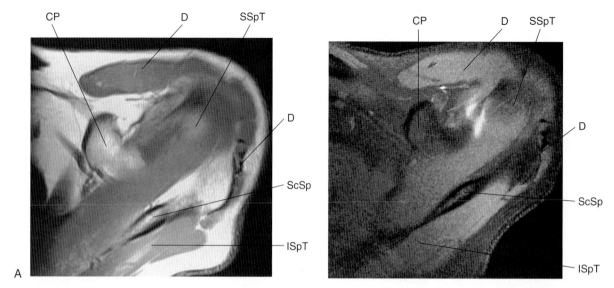

FIG. 3. A: Series of nine matched pairs of axial MR images of a left shoulder. T1-weighted images without **(left)** and T1-weighted fat-saturated images after intraarticular application of dilute gadolinium **(right)** from the same volunteer are displayed in sequence from cranial to caudal. CP, coracoid process; D, deltoid muscle; ISpT, infraspinatus tendon and/or muscle; ScSp, scapular spine; SSpT, supraspinatus tendon and/or muscle.

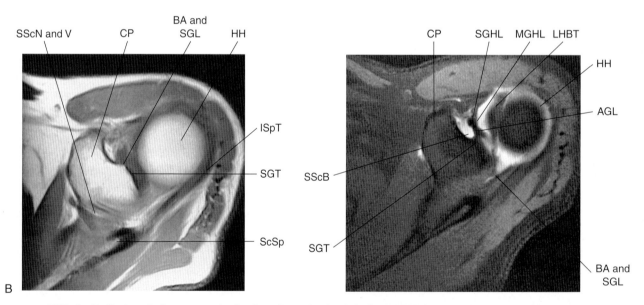

FIG. 3. B: Series of nine anatomically closed matched pairs of axial MR images of a left shoulder. T1-weighted images without **(left)** and T1-weighted fat-saturated images after intraarticular application of dilute gadolinium **(right)** from the same volunteer are displayed in sequence from cranial to caudal. AGL, anterior glenoid labrum; BA, biceps anchor; CP, coracoid process; HH, humeral head; ISpT, infraspinatus tendon and/or muscle; LHBT, long head biceps tendon; MGHL, middle glenohumeral ligament; ScSp, scapular spine; SGHL, superior glenohumeral ligament; SGL, superior glenoid labrum; SGT, superior glenoid tubercle; SScB, subscapularis bursa; SScN and V, suprascapular nerve and vessels.

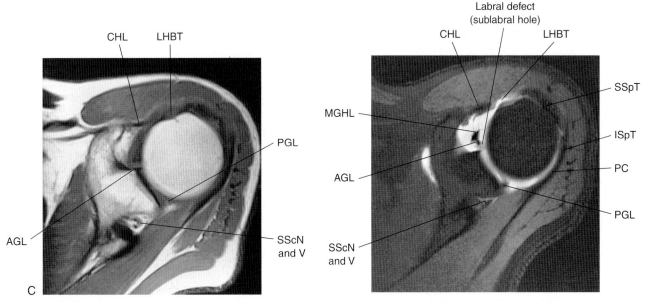

FIG. 3. C: Series of nine anatomically closed matched pairs of axial MR images of a left shoulder. T1-weighted images without **(left)** and T1-weighted fat-saturated images after intraarticular application of dilute gadolinium **(right)** from the same volunteer are displayed in sequence from cranial to caudal. AGL, anterior glenoid labrum; CHL, coracohumeral ligament; ISpT, infraspinatus tendon and/or muscle; LHBT, long head biceps tendon; MGHL, middle glenohumeral ligament; PC, posterior capsule; PGL, posterior glenoid labrum· SScN and V, suprascapular nerve and vessels; SSpT, supraspinatus tendon and/or muscle.

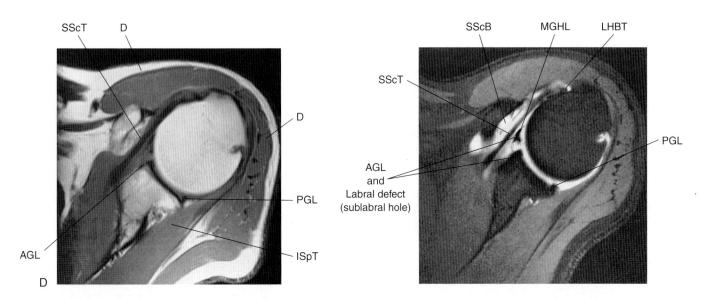

FIG. 3. D: Series of nine anatomically closed matched pairs of axial MR images of a left shoulder. T1-weighted images without **(left)** and T1-weighted fat-saturated images after intraarticular application of dilute gadolinium **(right)** from the same volunteer are displayed in sequence from cranial to caudal. AGL, anterior glenoid labrum; D, deltoid muscle; ISpT, infraspinatus tendon and/or muscle; LHBT, long head biceps tendon; MGHL, middle glenohumeral ligament; PGL, posterior glenoid labrum; SScB, subscapularis bursa; SScT, subscapularis tendon and/or muscle.

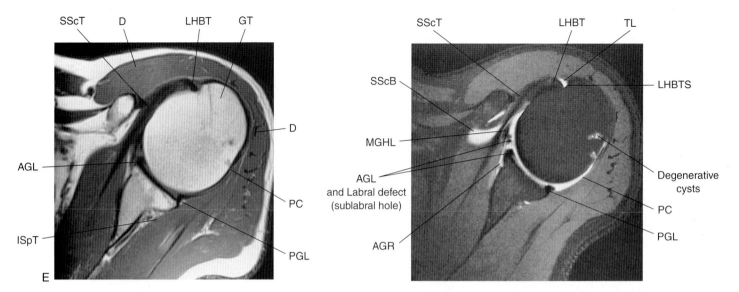

FIG. 3. E: Series of nine anatomically closed matched pairs of axial MR images of a left shoulder. T1-weighted images without **(left)** and T1-weighted fat-saturated images after intraarticular application of dilute gadolinium **(right)** from the same volunteer are displayed in sequence from cranial to caudal. AGL, anterior glenoid labrum; AGR, anterior glenoid recess; D, deltoid muscle; GT, greater tuberosity; ISpT, infraspinatus tendon and/or muscle; LHBT, long head biceps tendon; LHBTS, long head biceps tendon sheath; MGHL, middle glenohumeral ligament; PC, posterior capsule; PGL, posterior glenoid labrum; SScB, subscapularis bursa; SScT, subscapularis tendon and/or muscle; TL, transverse humeral ligament.

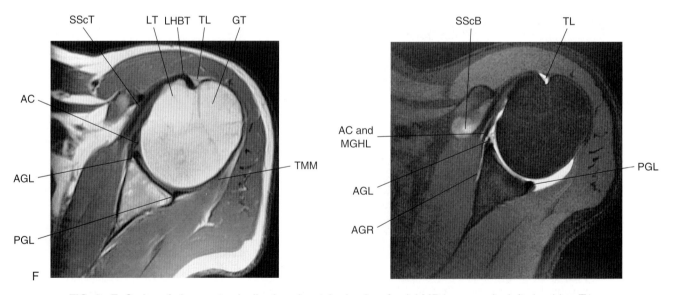

FIG. 3. F: Series of nine anatomically closed matched pairs of axial MR images of a left shoulder. T1-weighted images without **(left)** and T1-weighted fat-saturated images after intraarticular application of dilute gadolinium **(right)** from the same volunteer are displayed in sequence from cranial to caudal. AC, anterior capsule; AGL, anterior glenoid labrum; AGR, anterior glenoid recess; GT, greater tuberosity; LHBT, long head biceps tendon; LT, lesser tuberosity; MGHL, middle glenohumeral ligament; PGL, posterior glenoid labrum; SScB, subscapularis bursa; SScT, subscapularis tendon and/or muscle; TL, transverse humeral ligament; TMM, teres minor muscle.

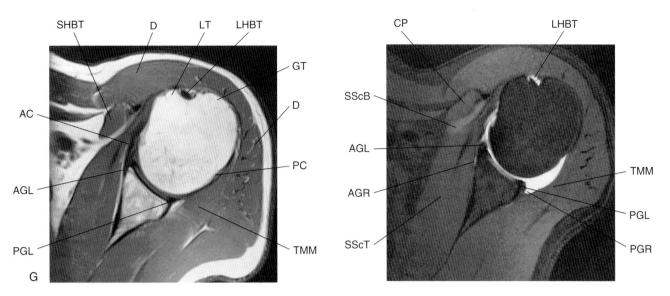

FIG. 3. G: Series of nine anatomically closed matched pairs of axial MR images of a left shoulder. T1-weighted images without **(left)** and T1-weighted fat-saturated images after intraarticular application of dilute gadolinium **(right)** from the same volunteer are displayed in sequence from cranial to caudal. AC, anterior capsule; AGL, anterior glenoid labrum; AGR, anterior glenoid recess; CP, coracoid process; D, deltoid muscle; GT, greater tuberosity; LHBT, long head biceps tendon; LT, lesser tuberosity; PC, posterior capsule; PGL, posterior glenoid labrum; PGR, posterior glenoid recess; SHBT, short head biceps tendon; SScB, subscapularis bursa; SScT, subscapularis tendon and/or muscle; TMM, teres minor muscle.

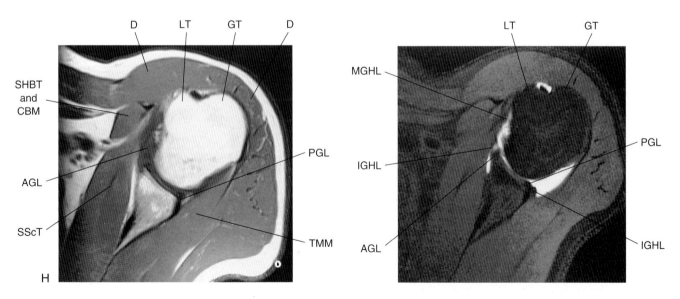

FIG. 3. H: Series of nine anatomically closed matched pairs of axial MR images of a left shoulder. T1-weighted images without **(left)** and T1-weighted fat-saturated images after intraarticular application of dilute gadolinium **(right)** from the same volunteer are displayed in sequence from cranial to caudal. AGL, anterior glenoid labrum; CBM, coracobrachialis muscle; D, deltoid muscle; GT, greater tuberosity; IGHL, inferior glenohumeral ligament; LT, lesser tuberosity; MGHL, middle glenohumeral ligament; SHBT, short head biceps tendon; SScT, subscapularis tendon and/or muscle; TMM, teres minor muscle.

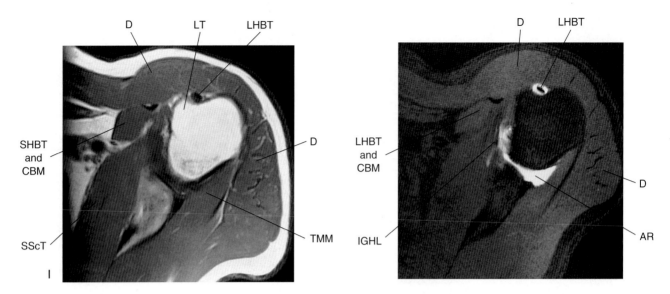

FIG. 3. I: Series of nine anatomically closed matched pairs of axial MR images of a left shoulder. T1-weighted images without **(left)** and T1-weighted fat-saturated images after intraarticular application of dilute gadolinium **(right)** from the same volunteer are displayed in sequence from cranial to caudal. AR, axillary recess; CBM, coracobrachialis muscle; D, deltoid muscle; IGHL, inferior glenohumeral ligament; LHBT, long head biceps tendon; LT, lesser tuberosity; SHBT, short head biceps tendon; SScT, sub-scapularis tendon and/or muscle; TMM, teres minor muscle.

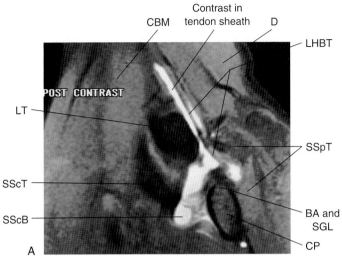

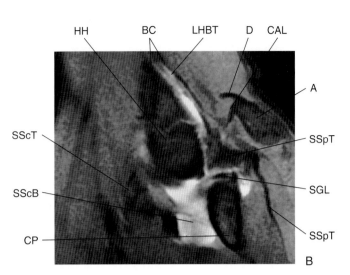

FIG. 4. A: Series of seven modified oblique axial MR images of the left shoulder with the arm in abduction and external rotation displayed in sequence from cranial to caudal. These T1-weighted short TR and short TE fat-saturated spin-echo images were obtained after intraarticular gadolinium injection. BA, biceps anchor; CBM, coracobrachialis muscle; CP, coracoid process; D, deltoid muscle; LHBT, long head biceps tendon; LT, lesser tuberosity; SGL, superior glenoid labrum; SScB, subscapularis bursa; SScT, subscapularis tendon and/or muscle; SSpT, supraspinatus tendon and/or muscle.

FIG. 4. B: Series of seven modified oblique axial MR images of the left shoulder with the arm in abduction and external rotation displayed in sequence from cranial to caudal. These T1-weighted short TR and short TE fat-saturated spin-echo images were obtained after intraarticular gadolinium injection. A, acromion; BC, bony cortex; CAL, coracoacromial ligament; CP, coracoid process; D, deltoid muscle; HH, humeral head; LHBT, long head biceps tendon; SGL, superior glenoid labrum; SScB, subscapularis bursa; SScT, subscapularis tendon and/or muscle; SSpT, supraspinatus tendon and/or muscle.

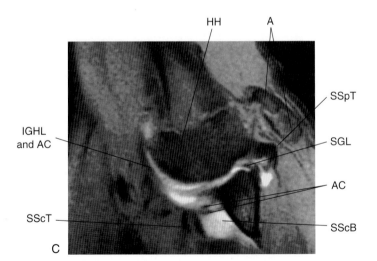

FIG. 4. C: Series of seven modified oblique axial MR images of the left shoulder with the arm in abduction and external rotation displayed in sequence from cranial to caudal. These T1-weighted short TR and short TE fat-saturated spin-echo images were obtained after intraarticular gadolinium injection. A, acromion; AC, anterior capsule; HH, humeral head; IGHL, inferior glenohumeral ligament; SGL, superior glenoid labrum; SScB, subscapularis bursa; SScT, subscapularis tendon and/or muscle; SSpT, supraspinatus tendon and/or muscle.

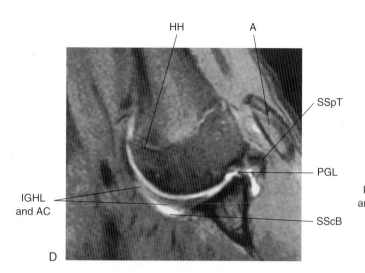

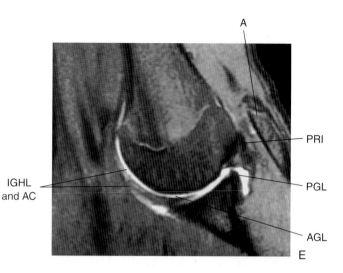

FIG. 4. D: Series of seven modified oblique axial MR images of the left shoulder with the arm in abduction and external rotation displayed in sequence from cranial to caudal. These T1-weighted short TR and short TE fat-saturated spin-echo images were obtained after intraarticular gadolinium injection. A, acromion; AC, anterior capsule; HH, humeral head; IGHL, inferior glenohumeral ligament; PGL, posterior glenoid labrum; SScB, subscapularis bursa; SSpT, supraspinatus tendon and/or muscle.

FIG. 4. E: Series of seven modified oblique axial MR images of the left shoulder with the arm in abduction and external rotation displayed in sequence from cranial to caudal. These T1-weighted short TR and short TE fat-saturated spin-echo images were obtained after intraarticular gadolinium injection. A, acromion; AC, anterior capsule; AGL, anterior glenoid labrum; HH, humeral head; IGHL, inferior glenohumeral ligament; PGL, posterior glenoid labrum; PRI, posterior rotator interval.

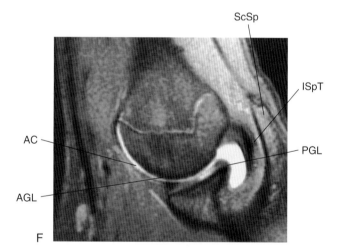

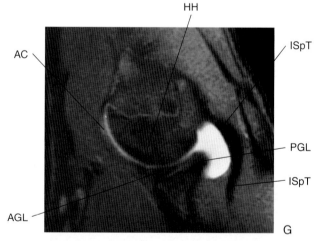

FIG. 4. F: Series of seven modified oblique axial MR images of the left shoulder with the arm in abduction and external rotation displayed in sequence from cranial to caudal. These T1-weighted short TR and short TE fat-saturated spin-echo images were obtained after intraarticular gadolinium injection. AC, anterior capsule; AGL, anterior glenoid labrum; ISpT, infraspinatus tendon and/or muscle; PGL, posterior glenoid labrum; PGR, posterior glenoid recess; ScSp, scapular spine.

FIG. 4. G: Series of seven modified oblique axial MR images of the left shoulder with the arm in abduction and external rotation displayed in sequence from cranial to caudal. These T1-weighted short TR and short TE fat-saturated spin-echo images were obtained after intraarticular gadolinium injection. AC, anterior capsule; AGL, anterior glenoid labrum; HH, humeral head; ISpT, infraspinatus tendon and/or muscle; PGL, posterior glenoid labrum.

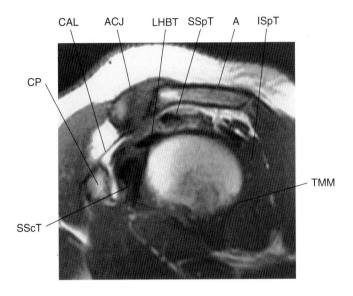

CAL   ACJ   LHBT SSpT   A   ISpT

CP

TMM

SScT

FIG. 5. T1-weighted oblique sagittal MR image displaying the normal anatomic osseous and ligamentous components of the coracoacromial arch with the tip of the coracoid process, coracoacromial ligament of 1 mm thickness, acromioclavicular joint, and acromion. Interposed between the humeral head and the coracoacromial arch are the structures of the rotator cuff including the subscapularis muscle and tendon, the long head of the biceps tendon, the supraspinatus, infraspinatus and teres minor muscles, and tendons. A, acromion; ACJ, acromioclavicular joint; CAL, coracoacromial ligament; CP, coracoid process; ISpT, infraspinatus tendon and/or muscle; LHBT, long head biceps tendon; SScT, subscapularis tendon and/or muscle; SSpT, supraspinatus tendon and/or muscle; TMM, teres minor muscle.

TABLE 1. *Prevalence of acromial types*

	Type I	Type II	Type III	Type IV
All shoulder examinations (n = 420)	196 (47%)	165 (39%)	45 (11%)	14 (3%)
Group I				
Supraspinatus tendon tear at surgery (n = 45)	17 (38%)	18 (40%)	8 (18%)	2 (4%)
Normal cuff at surgery (n = 3)	12 (39%)	15 (48%)	1 (3%)	3 (10%)
Group II				
Asymptomatic volunteers (n = 57)	25 (44%)	20 (35%)	7 (12%)	5 (9%)

Note: Group II did not have surgical examination of the rotator cuff.
From ref. 7, with permission.

Coracoacromial Arch

The coracoacromial arch is a strong bony and ligamentous structure that forms a protective roof for the humeral head, rotator cuff tendons, long head of the biceps tendon, joint capsule, and capsular ligaments. It also lies above potential fluid spaces and areolar gliding zones, the subacromial and subscapularis bursae. It serves as an attachment site for many of the muscles and tendons that affect the function of the shoulder joint. It limits the space available to the rotator cuff tendons physiologically during abduction and serves as a mechanical restraint for the humeral head.

The coracoacromial arch is composed of the acromion and the acromioclavicular joint, the distal clavicle, the coracoid process, and the coracoacromial ligament (see Figs. 1*D* and *E* and Fig. 5). The shape of the acromion is well evaluated on oblique sagittal MR images, two or three slices lateral to the acromioclavicular joint depending on slice thickness and interval applied. Acromial shapes have been emphasized and classified by Bigliani and co-workers (6). Their frequency of occurrence in symptomatic patients and asymptomatic volunteers was recently documented by Farley and colleagues (7) (Table 1). The more common type I configuration of the acromion can be found in 47% of asymptomatic shoulders (Fig. 6). It has a flat undersurface. The Type II acromion (39%) has a concave undersurface. The type III acromion (11%) is concave or flat inferiorly with an anterior "hook." Some authors differentiate between a congenital and acquired origin for this anterior hook. Differentiation between congenital type III and acquired type III acromions may be difficult (8). Farley and colleagues also reported a type IV acromion (3%), distinguished by a convex inferior surface without a discernible association with rotator cuff pathology. The relative percentage of acromial shapes varies between patient and specimen populations, including between males

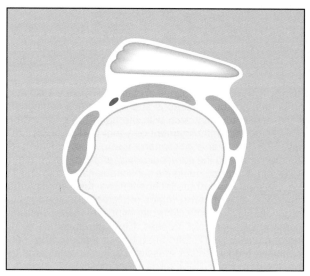

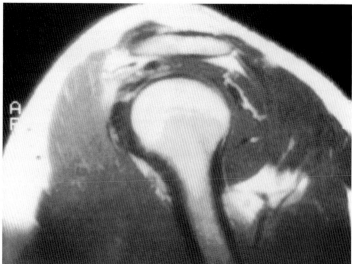

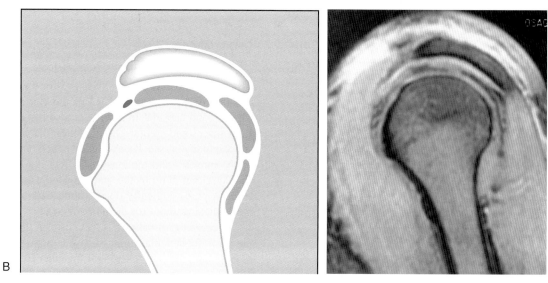

FIG. 6. Drawings and corresponding MR images of the anatomic classification of acromial shapes. **A:** Type I with a flat undersurface. Spin-echo TR 500/TE 20. **B:** Type II with a concave undersurface. Gradient echo TR 250/TE 12/flip angle 10.

and females. No relationship between acromial shape and age is known (7,8). It appears that there is an association of the type III acromial shape with an increased incidence of rotator cuff pathology (7,9).

On an oblique-coronal MR image, the acromioclavicular relationship may demonstrate a downward or upward slant or a straight horizontal alignment (Fig. 7). A lateral downward slant of the acromion is common and is found in 56% of normal and asymptomatic individuals (7). Inferior acromial enthesophytes are common in individuals and patients older than age 50 years (Fig. 8). Presence of a laterally downsloping acromion or an enthesophyte may therefore not necessarily be associated with a subacromial space problem and impingement. Age is more likely an important confounding factor in patients in whom symptoms of impingement corre-

late with the presence of an enthesophyte (7). Thus, the issue of whether the subacromial enthesophyte causes or is caused by chronic rotator cuff impingement remains a matter of opinion.

The coracoacromial ligament is a triangular or bifid structure arising from the lateral edge of the body and tip of the coracoid process and inserting on the undersurface of the acromion. This broad insertion extends laterally from the undersurface of the anterior to the posterolateral acromion (10) (see Figs. 1D–F and 5). Clinical morphologic observations describe a ligament thickness between 2 and 5.8 mm without discrimination between impingement and asymptomatic shoulders (11). Although thought to be a broad ligamentous structure, the coracoacromial ligament is not consistently identified on MR images of asymptomatic shoulders (35%).

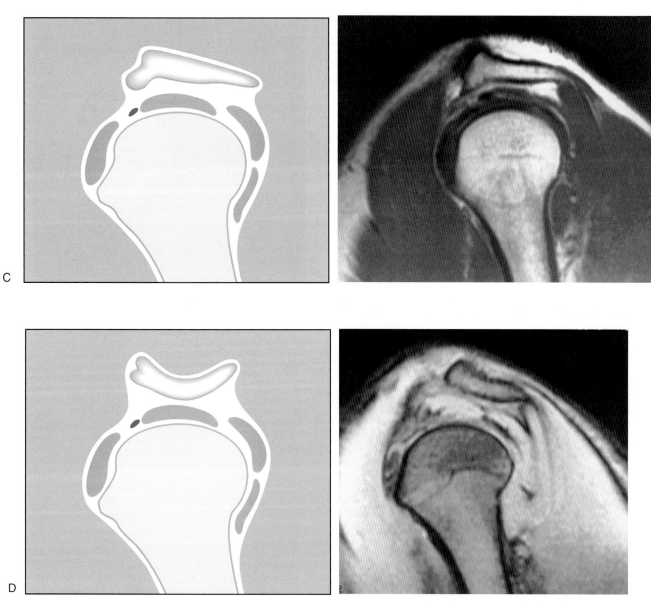

FIG. 6. *Continued.* **C:** Type III with an anterior hook or club shape. Spin-echo TR 500/TE 20. **D:** Type IV with a convex undersurface. Gradient echo TR 250/TE 12/flip angle 10. (From ref. 7, with permission.)

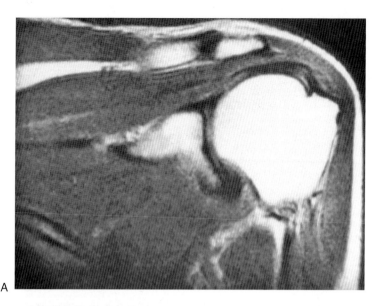

A

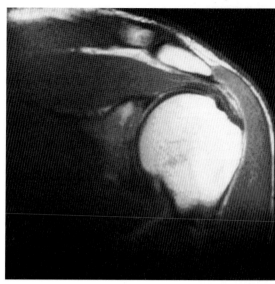

B

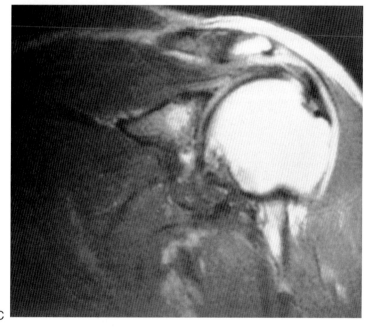

C

FIG. 7. Acromial slant. Three oblique coronal T1-weighted spin-echo images display different types of acromioclavicular alignment. **A:** Horizontal alignment. **B:** Lateral downward slant of the tip of acromion. **C:** Lateral upward slant of the tip of the acromion.

Subacromial enthesophyte

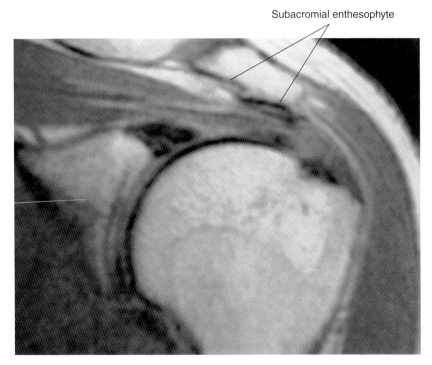

FIG. 8. The inferior acromial enthesophyte on an oblique sagittal proton density--weighted spin-echo image. This acquired change in the acromial undersurface has a statistical association with age. Its predisposing effect to the development of rotator cuff impingement remains doubtful.

This is probably because of its flat shape and oblique-helical course. On MR image, a thickness of 2 mm or less has been considered normal by some investigators based on their clinical experience, although no data supporting this definition have been published. On the other hand, a ligament thicker than 2 mm on MR image has been shown to have a statistically significant association with rotator cuff tears (7).

Subacromial/Subdeltoid Bursa

The subacromial/subdeltoid bursa is a potential space, located above the supraspinatus and superior infraspinatus tendons and below the acromion, coracoacromial ligament, acromioclavicular joint, and deltoid muscle. It is lined by fine, filmy areolar tissue. A bursa may not be seen on MR

Contiguous subacromial—subdeltoid fat stripe

Fat stripe noncontiguous under the acromion

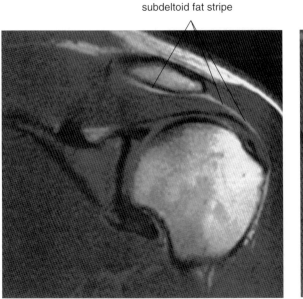
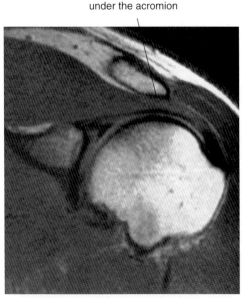

A

B

FIG. 9. The subacromial-subdeltoid fat stripe. The subacromial fat stripe can be contiguous or interrupted or even near completely absent in asymptomatic shoulders. This indirect sign previously used with plain film diagnosis of shoulder impingement is an unreliable sign with MRI and has been proven to be of poor positive predictive value for rotator cuff disease. **A:** Proton density spin-echo images of asymptomatic volunteers in oblique coronal projection showing a continuous subacromial fat stripe. **B:** A fat stripe interrupted underneath the distal clavicle.

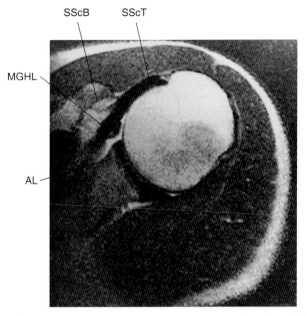

FIG. 10. Prominent subscapularis bursa under the middle glenohumeral ligament on T2-weighted axial spin-echo image. AL, anterior labrum; MGHL, middle glenohumeral ligament; SScB, subscapularis bursa; SScT, subscapularis tendon and/or muscle.

images in many asymptomatic shoulders. The bursa facilitates gliding between the deltoid and teres major muscle and the rotator cuff muscles. The subacromial bursa may connect to the subcoracoid bursa (10). A peribursal subacromial subdeltoid fat plane partially invests this bursa and can be visualized as a thin band of high signal intensity on T1-weighted images (see Fig. 2C and Fig. 9.) It may be absent or obscured in patients with rotator cuff tears, although this finding by itself on MR image is of poor predictive value because inter-

ruption of this fat plane is commonly observed in asymptomatic shoulders and normal individuals (12). Communication with the joint occurs when a full-thickness tear of the musculotendinous rotator cuff opens into the floor of the bursa. Fluid in the subacromial space is not an uncommon finding in patients without rotator cuff pathology. Rarely, however, is there absence of subacromial fluid on MR images in patients with full-thickness supraspinatus tendon tears (2).

Subscapularis Bursa

The subscapularis bursa is located between the posterior surface of the subscapularis tendon and muscle, and the anterior surface of the middle glenohumeral ligament (MGHL), scapular neck, and scapula near the base of the coracoid process (see Figs. 3B–F and 4A–D). It is normally not seen with MRI, unless an effusion is present or it is distended during intraarticular contrast injection. It can then be identified as a fluid-filled pouch underlying the coracoid process. The subscapsularis bursa communicates with the glenohumeral joint between the superior and middle glenohumeral ligaments and labrum (see Figs. 3C and D and 4D). At times, this access is facilitated by a developmental variation of the labrum in the form of a labral gap, or intralabral or sublabral hole or Buford complex. This variable defect in the labrum is clearly discernible on arthroscopy and may not be mistaken for a labral tear or capsular stripping on MR images (13) (see Figs. 3C and D). The Buford complex is discussed further in this chapter in relation to the variations of the anterior labrum, capsule, and long head of the biceps tendon. The subcoracoid bursa does not communicate with the glenohumeral joint; it lies beneath the coracoid process and coracobrachialis muscle along the anterior surface of the subscapularis muscle (Fig. 11). It can communicate with the subacromial/subdeltoid bursa.

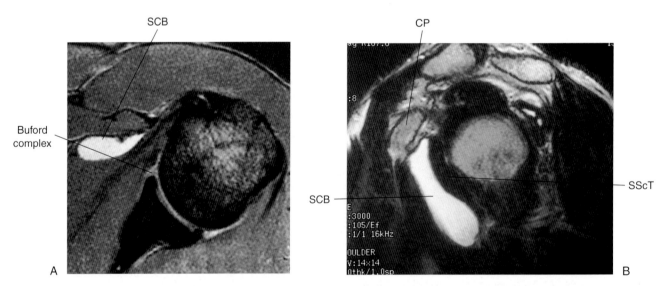

FIG. 11. The subcoracoid bursa. Its typical location is ventral to the subscapularis muscle and dorsal to the coracoid process. **A:** T2*AJR-weighted axial gradient echo image. Incidental Buford complex. SCB, subcoracoid bursa. **B:** T2-weighted fast spin-echo image in oblique sagittal plane. CP, coracoid process; SCB, subcoracoid bursa; SScT, subscapularis muscle and/or tendon.

Rotator Cuff

The rotator cuff is composed of four muscles and their tendons (see Figs. 1 and 2). The supraspinatus, infraspinatus, and teres minor muscles all originate from the dorsal aspect of the scapula and insert on the greater tuberosity of the proximal humerus. The supraspinatus tendon inserts on the promontory or highest point of the greater tuberosity, the infraspinatus tendon on the posterior aspect, and the teres minor tendon on the posterior-inferior portion. They function in abduction and external rotation. The supraspinatus assists the deltoid muscle in abduction. The infraspinatus muscle assists as a dynamic stabilizer, keeping the humeral head in the glenoid fossa. The fourth muscle of the rotator cuff is the subscapularis, which functions primarily in adduction and internal medial rotation. It originates from the costal surface of the scapula and subscapular fossa and inserts on the lesser tuberosity. Some of its distal fibers blend with the transverse ligament over the bicipital groove and joint capsule and extend to the medial anterior surface of the greater tuberosity.

The supraspinatus and infraspinatus muscles are innervated by the suprascapular nerve and brachial plexus out of the C4, C5, and C6 spinal segments; the teres minor is innervated by the axillary nerve, which originates from the brachial plexus at C4 and C5. The subscapularis muscle is innervated by the subscapular nerve, which originates from the brachial plexus at C5, C6, and C7. The suprascapular artery and circumflex scapular branches of the subscapular artery supply the supraspinatus and infraspinatus muscles. The teres minor is supplied by the posterior humeral circumflex artery and circumflex scapular branches. The subscapularis muscle is supplied by the subscapularis artery.

The tendinous portion of the teres minor, infraspinatus, and subscapularis muscles is relatively short and not well defined against muscular fascicles on MR images. The supraspinatus has a more clearly defined tendon and musculotendinous junction. Two muscle bellies may be recognized on axial MR images (Fig. 12). Their individual tendon slips join into a common musculotendinous junction and tendon. On MRI, it is defined by the most distal point at which muscle fibers can still be recognized. Recognition of the location of the musculotendinous junction can be helpful in the diagnosis of supraspinatus tendon tears. As seen on coronal MR images, the musculotendinous junction of the supraspinatus muscle usually coincides with the highest point (12-o'clock position) of the humeral head (12) (Fig. 13).

Typically, normal rotator cuff tendons are of relatively low signal intensity on all sequences. However, intermediate signal intensity on T1-weighted images is being observed in many asymptomatic patients (12) (Fig. 14) and has been reported on proton density–weighted images in up to 95% of asymptomatic shoulders (14). This may be explained by a prominent superior and inferior tendon slip attaching to separate muscle bellies of the supraspinatus muscle and allowing a layer of connective tissue in between. Some asymptomatic and, more commonly, older individuals may exhibit varying degrees of intrasubstance tendinous degeneration as

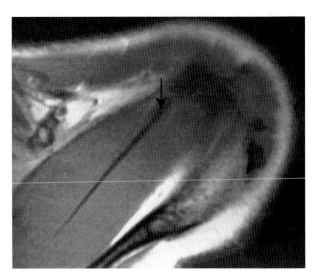

FIG. 12. Axial T1-weighted MR image through the supraspinatus tendon and muscle showing two muscle bellies around a central tendon slip (*arrow*). Partial volume averaging of the muscles with the tendon accounts for the varying signal pattern within the tendon on oblique coronal T1-, T2-, and proton density–weighted MR images.

part of the natural aging process or resulting from past trauma that is not symptomatic. The "magic angle" phenomenon is responsible for a band of intermediate signal traversing the mid and curved portion of the tendon. This is caused by the orientation of the tendon fibers at 55 degrees to the static magnetic field, with increased signal occurring at this "magic angle" of 55 degrees on short TE images (15). These variable areas of elevated signal on T1-weighted images are of low signal intensity on T2-weighted images, which should help differentiate them from significant pathology (Table 2). This is further discussed in the Chapter 6.

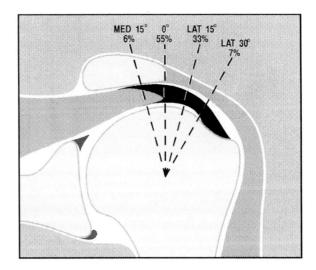

FIG. 13. Artist's rendering of the variable locations of the supraspinatus musculotendinous junction in relation to the humeral head surface by percentage as found in asymptomatic shoulders. (From ref. 12, with permission.)

TABLE 2. *Signal patterns of the supraspinatus tendon in 55 asymptomatic shoulders*

	Appearance on magnetic resonance image		No. of shoulders (%)	Clinical interpretation[a]
Type	Proton density–weighted images	T2-weighted images		
0	Signal void	Signal void	5 (9)	Normal
1	Focal, linear, diffuse intermediate signal[b]	Signal void, faint signal less than signal of fat and water	49 (89)	Normal, degeneration, "magic angle" artifact
2	Focal, linear, diffuse intermediate signal	Focal, linear, diffuse increased signal equivalent to that of water, less than full thickness	1 (2)	Partial tear
3	Focal, linear, diffuse intermediate signal	Focal, linear, increased signal equivalent to that of water extending through full thickness of tendon	0	Full tear

[a]Secondary corroborating findings such as musculotendinous retraction and atrophy of the muscle and tendon may suggest more severe disease.
[b]With or without low-signal tendon margin (types 1A–1C).
Classification adapted from ref. 2.

One of the more common pitfalls in the evaluation of the rotator cuff on shoulder MRI involves mistaking the relatively high signal intensity of the articular cartilage of the humeral head for signal within the cuff tendons (16). The anterior "rotator interval pitfall" occurs as a result of there being space between the superior border of the subscapularis and the inferior-anterior border of the supraspinatus tendons (16). This "interval" is seen at the level where the supraspinatus, subscapularis, and biceps tendons are all visualized together (see Fig. 1C). Because the anterior aspect of the distal supraspinatus tendon can curve anteriorly here, oblique coronal images may demonstrate some suspicious intermediate signal on T1- or proton density–weighted sequences just proximal to it because membranous tissue is within the rotator interval. A similar posterior rotator interval pitfall may be observed between the supraspinatus and infraspinatus muscles and tendons.

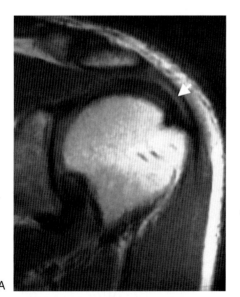
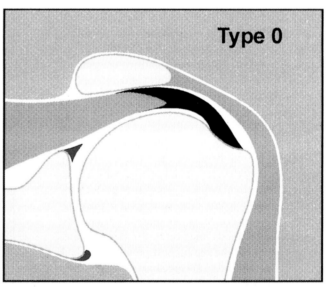

A

FIG. 14. Signal patterns of supraspinatus tendons found in asymptomatic shoulders. Artist's rendering and corresponding spin-echo MR images. Type 0 is defined as low signal on T1-, T2-, and proton density–weighted images. Type 1A is with focal increased or intermediate signal intensity on T1- or proton density–weighted images without extension to a tendon surface and no increased signal resulting from T2 prolongation on T2-weighted spin-echo images. This includes focal, linear, and diffuse distribution of this pattern within the tendon. Type 1B includes similar patterns, but with extension to one tendon surface. Type 1C is defined as a similar pattern but with the signal extending to both tendon surfaces on T1- or proton density–weighted images. Only if this increased signal intensity is confirmed and increased because of T2 prolongation on T2-weighted spin-echo images (type 2, not shown) should tendon pathology be diagnosed. **A:** Type 0 with diffuse low signal intensity *(arrow)* on T1-, T2-, and proton density–-weighted images. Artist's rendering and only T1-weighted oblique coronal spin-echo image shown. *(Continued on next page.)*

B

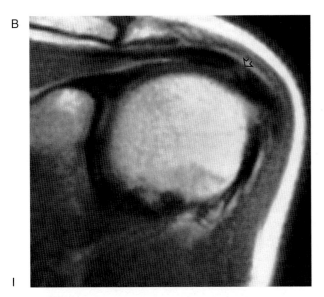

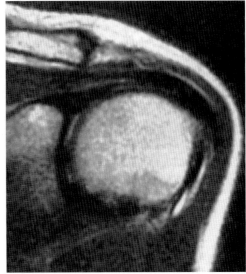

I

II

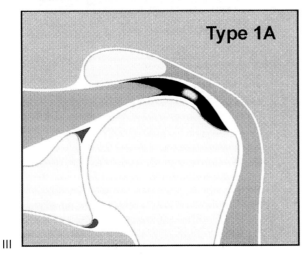

III

FIG. 14. *Continued.* **B:** Type 1A with focal central intermediate or increased signal on proton density image *(arrow)*. Artist's rendering, proton density– and T2-weighted images shown. *(Continued on next page.)*

The "muscle in place of tendon" pitfall occurs in patients whose supraspinatus tendon inserts more anteriorly than usual and in whom there is a more posterior insertion of the infraspinatus tendon (16). Mid oblique coronal sections may demonstrate intermediate signal intensity from muscle in these patients in the expected location of signal void from cuff tendons. This situation can be distinguished from a tear by the subsequent low signal seen on T2-weighted images.

Glenohumeral Joint Capsule

On MR images, the capsule presents as a low signal intensity envelope (see Figs. 3C–F). Superiorly, it encroaches on the base of the coracoid process and inserts in the supraglenoid region, thus including the long head of the biceps tendon and its insertion within the joint. Distally, the capsule inserts into the anatomic neck of the humerus and lines the bicipital groove. Anteromedially, the insertion is variable. It can attach directly into the labrum or more medially along

the scapular neck. According to the classification described by Moseley and Overgaard (17), the anterior capsule may attach on the tip or outer surface of the anterior labrum (type I), on the adjacent glenoid rim (type II), or more medially along the scapular neck (type III) (see Fig. 15). All three types can be identified on MR images of asymptomatic individuals. In general, these insertions are considered variations of attachment of the middle glenohumeral ligament or interligamentous recesses. Posteriorly, the capsular attachments are similarly defined, although only the type I attachment is considered normal (18).

Anteriorly, the capsule thickens to form the superior, middle, and inferior glenohumeral ligaments. These ligaments are variable in their morphologic makeup. Commonly they arise from the anterior aspect of the glenoid and labrum and insert with the reminder of the capsular fibers on the surface of the humeral neck and, in part, on or adjacent to the lesser tuberosity. They are best visualized with MRI in the presence of joint fluid (see Figs. 1E–H, 2B–D, 3B–I, and 4C–F). This may be achieved on T2-weighted images by the presence of a joint effusion or injection of saline. The

C

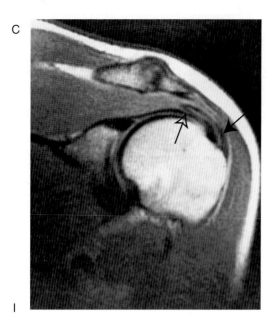

I

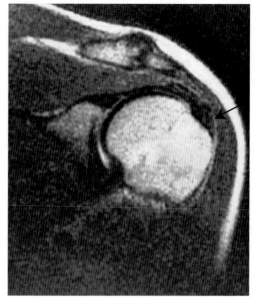

II

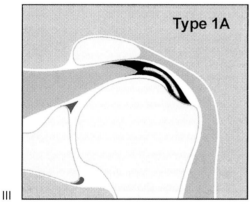

Type 1A

III

FIG. 14. *Continued.* **C:** Type 1A with linear central intrasubstance intermediate or increased signal only on proton density–-weighted image *(arrows)*. Artist rendering, proton density– and T2-weighted images shown. *(Continued on next page.)*

intraarticular injection of dilute gadolinium allows improved visualization of these ligaments on T1-weighted images. This technique is further described in Chapter 3. The superior glenohumeral ligament arises from the supraglenoid tubercle and parallels the coracoid to insert on the lesser tuberosity along with the coracohumeral ligament (see Figs. 1*F*, 3*B*, and Fig. 16*B*). The middle glenohumeral ligament is more readily recognized on MR images (see Figs. 1*E–H*, 2*B*, 3*B–F*, and 16*C*). It is variable in its attachment medial on the anterior-superior labrum or glenoid neck. It inserts along with the subscapularis tendon on the lesser tuberosity. The inferior glenohumeral ligament reinforces the capsular area between the subscapularis and the origin of the long head of the triceps muscle. It is especially well seen on MR images obtained with abduction and external rotation (see Figs. 1*G* and *H*, 2*D* and *E*, 3*H* and *I*, and 4*C–E*). On axial MR images, any of these ligaments may appear merely as a diffuse thickening of the anterior-inferior capsule and not be clearly discernible against each other. Fibers of the long head of the biceps tendon have been shown to extend into the anterior and posterior joint capsule as part of a variable insertion (13). Similarly, the aponeuro-

sis of the rotator cuff muscles and tendons, especially the subscapularis and supraspinatus, blend with the joint capsule and contribute to its fibrous matrix.

Glenoid Labrum

The glenoid labrum is a fibrous connective tissue structure that lies on the surface of the glenoid rim (see Figs. 2*B–E* and 3*B–I*). It increases the surface area for articulation with the humeral head and serves as an anchoring mechanism and distributor of stress forces for the capsular attachment rather than as a static restraint for the physiologic alignment of the humeral head with the glenoid fossa. It is usually of low signal intensity on T1- and T2-weighted images. Occasionally, the labra may be of intermediate signal on short TE MR images such as T1-weighted, proton density, and gradient echo images. This can, in part, be attributed to the magic angle phenomenon when observed in the superior and inferior portions of the anterior and posterior labrum (19). Only if high signal intensity is confirmed on T2-weighted images should a tear be diagnosed with certainty. The labra are attached to the glenoid periosteum and the glenoid articular hyaline car-

D

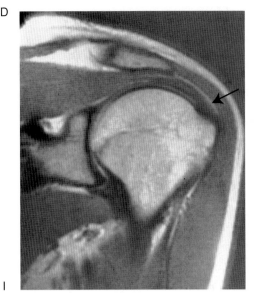

I

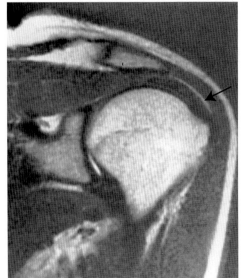

II

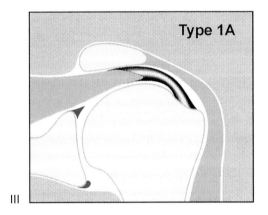

III

FIG. 14. *Continued.* D: Type 1A with diffuse increased or intermediate intratendinous signal intensity and with persistent low signal intensity tendon surface on proton density image *(arrows)*. Artist's rendering, proton density– and T2-weighted images shown. *(Continued on next page.)*

tilage, which, in contrast, is of higher signal intensity because of its greater water content. The hyaline joint cartilage in the area of the anterior glenoid rim occasionally extends partially or completely underneath the labrum, separating the labrum from the glenoid rim cortex (see Fig. 15C and Figs. 17A and 18). This has been recognized as a normal variant and should not be mistaken for a detached labrum or bucket handle tear.

The glenohumeral ligaments, joint capsule, and fibers of the long head of the biceps tendon can be understood as fibrous continuum of the anterior superior labrum. Their variable presence and thickness and point of insertion contribute to the great morphologic variabilities that the anterior labrum presents with. Normal variations in the shape of the anterior, superior, and posterior labrum have been documented on computed tomography (20) and MRI (18). The anterior labrum, although commonly having a triangular configuration (45%), may be rounded (19%), cleaved (15%), notched (8%), flat (7%), or even absent (6%) (see Fig. 17). The posterior labrum generally appears triangular (73%), although it can be rounded (12%), flat (6%), or absent (8%) (Table 3).

Cadaver studies by Petersen demonstrated further variability of the superior labral attachment to the long head of the biceps tendon, contributing to an even more variable appearance of the superior portion of the anterior labrum (21). The most common anterosuperior attachment type of the anterior labrum (55%) is into the anterior middle or inferior capsular ligament with loose areolar osseous insertion into the anterior superior glenoid. Other insertional patterns include a loose glenoid attachment (15%), a firm glenoid attachment (10%), or no glenoid attachment with a large subscapularis recess (20%) (13). On axial MR images, a distinct differentiation may sometimes be made between a labrum without a glenoid attachment, creating a sublabral foramen and Buford complex. With the sublabral foramen, a segment of the anterior-superior labrum lacks attachment to the underlying glenoid rim. With its variable fibrous continuum into the middle glenohumeral and/or long head biceps tendon, the labrum may be attached and secured to the anterior capsule instead. This variance is reported to be seen in 8% to 12% of

Text continues on page 29

E

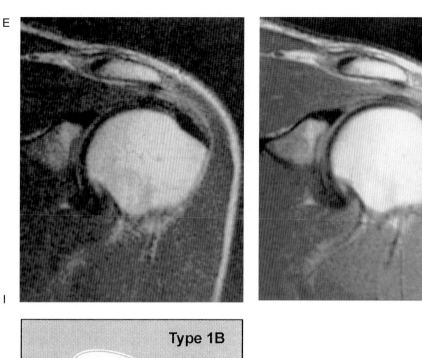

I

II

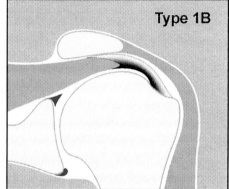

III

FIG. 14. *Continued.* **E:** Type 1B with diffuse increased intrasubstance signal extending to a tendon surface on a proton density–weighted image. Artist's rendering, proton density– and T2-weighted images shown.

F

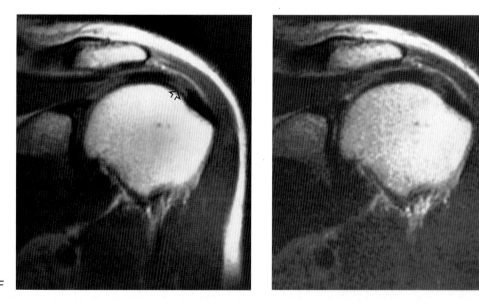

FIG. 14. *Continued* . **F:** Type 1C with central focal intermediate signal with extension to both tendon surfaces on proton density–weighted image *(arrow).* (From ref. 12, with permission.)

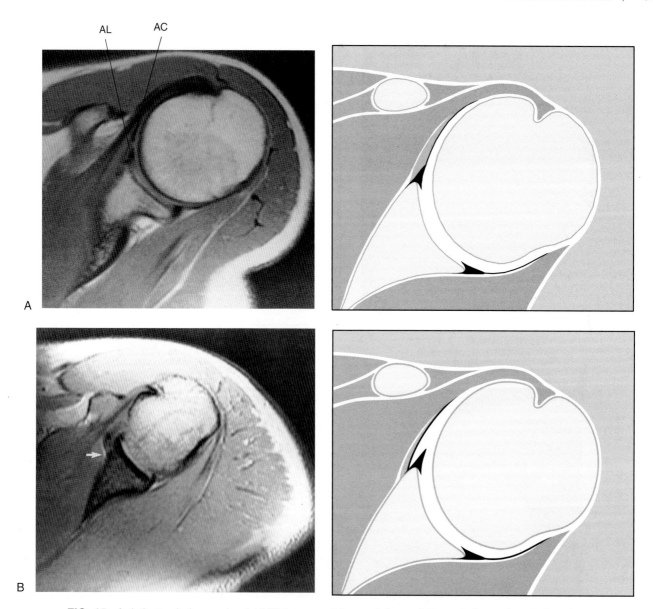

FIG. 15. Artist's rendering and axial MR images of the variations of the anterior and posterior gleno-humeral joint capsule found in asymptomatic individuals using the Moseley-Overgard classification (17). A type I capsular insertion is defined as an attachment to the tip and/or outer surface of the glenoid labrum. A type II capsule inserts on the anterior glenoid periosteum within 1 cm to the tip of the glenoid labrum. A type III attachment is more than 1 cm medial to the tip of the glenoid labrum (18). **A:** Artist's rendering and T1-weighted axial spin-echo image of a left shoulder with a type I capsular insertion. The shaded area next to the capsule demonstrates the variability within this definition. Also shown is a type I insertion of the posterior capsule. **B:** Artist's rendering and axial proton density–weighted gradient echo image of a type II capsular insertion *(arrow). (Continued on next page.)*

examined shoulders (22,23) (see Fig. 11*A*) and has been reported in 73% of cadaveric shoulders (24). With a Buford complex, a portion of the anterior-superior labrum is markedly attenuated or absent in the presence of a thick middle glenohumeral ligament. This can be found in 1.5% to 5% of shoulders studied (22,23) (see Figs. 11*B* and *C* and 16). The sublabral foramen and Buford complex provide a variation to the access into the subscapularis bursa, which, in the more common case, can be found within the labral capsular recess as an opening between capsular fibers (24a).

Tendon of the Long Head of the Biceps

The tendon of the long head of the biceps brachii muscle is surrounded by a synovial sheath and lies anteriorly in the intertubercular or bicipital groove, between the greater and lesser tuberosities. Distally it is held in place along the anterior surface of the humerus by the pectoralis major tendon. More proximally it remains confined to the intertubercular bicipital groove by the transverse humeral ligament, which lies on top of the synovial sheath of the tendon attaching to

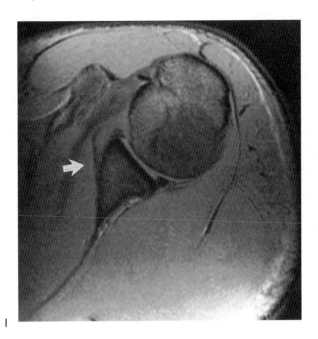

I

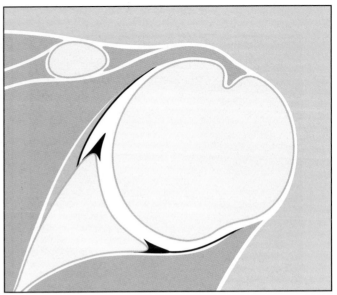

II

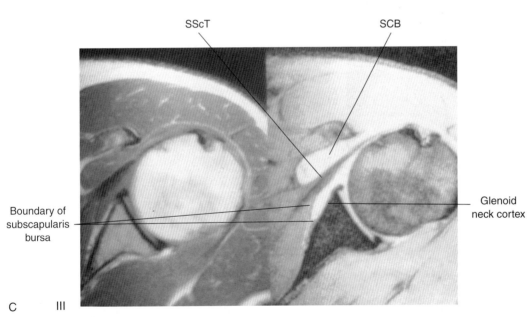

SScT   SCB

Boundary of
subscapularis
bursa

Glenoid
neck cortex

C   III

FIG. 15. *Continued.*
C: I. Type III insertion
and one that mimics a
type III capsular inser-
tion *(arrow)*. This insertion most likely repre-
sents visualization of an
interligamentous recess.
II. Gradient echo axial
image demonstrates the
medial boundary of the
subscapularis recess of-
ten confused for stripped
capsule after trauma or
a type III insertion. **III.**
Artist's rendering of a
type III capsular inser-
tion. Studies have shown
no correlation between
this type of capsular in-
sertion and instability.
(From refs. 24b, 24c.)

the periosteum of the lesser and greater tuberosity (see Figs. 1A–G, 2B and C, 3B–I, and 4A and B). This ligament also serves as part of the attachment for the tendon of the sub-scapularis muscle, which contributes to its strength and re-straining function for the long head biceps tendon. Above the transverse humeral ligament, the long head of the biceps tendon is an intraarticular structure. At this level, it is cov-ered anteriorly by the coracohumeral ligament, superior glenohumeral ligament, and margins of the supraspinatus and subscapularis tendons. Further cranially, it passes over the anterior aspect of the humeral head. Therefore, it can be impinged upon similar to the superior portion of the sub-scapularis and the anterior portion of the supraspinatus ten-dons. This commonly affected segment of the tendon is poorly visualized by MRI unless thin section multiangle

oblique views are obtained. The proximal attachment of this tendon is complex and variable, with fibrous bands extend-ing to the supraglenoid tubercle and superior labrum, as well as to the superior aspect of the anterior and posterior labrum and joint capsule (Fig. 19). Fibers may extend from the superior glenoid rim or tubercle to the posterior surface of the coracoid process. Cadaver studies have documented that insertion of this tendon into the supraglenoid region av-erages 3.5 mm medial to the glenoid rim with a range from 1 to 6 mm. Tendon fibers extend into the anterior and pos-terior labrum. Thus, both labra appear to arise from the bi-ceps tendon just before it inserts into the glenoid. In 75% of the population, a thin triangular ligament serves as a con-nection between the anterior and posterior labrum (13). Through the superior labrum, the biceps tendon may have a

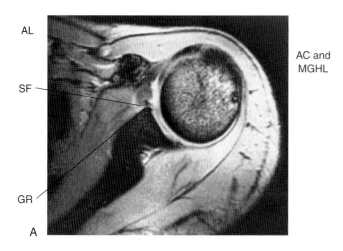

AL

SF

GR

A

AC and
MGHL

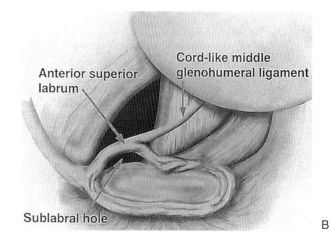

Anterior superior
labrum

Cord-like middle
glenohumeral ligament

Sublabral hole

B

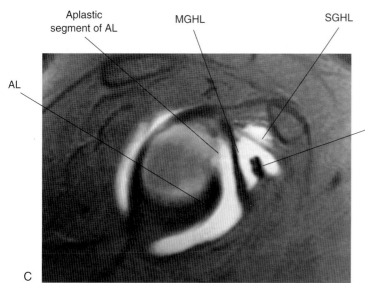

Aplastic
segment of AL

MGHL

SGHL

AL

SScT

C

FIG. 16. The sublabral foramen and Buford complex. **A:** Axial gradient echo T2-weighted MR image of the sublabral foramen. The anterior labrum being separated from the anterior glenoid attached to the middle glenohumeral ligament and anterior capsule. **B:** Artist's rendering of the sublabral hole. **C:** Oblique sagittal fat-saturated T1-weighted MR image with intraarticular gadolinium of a Buford complex showing absence of the superior anterior labrum and cord-like middle glenohumeral ligament. See also small superior glenohumeral ligament and cross section of the subscapularis tendon. (From ref. 23, with permission.) **D** and **E:** Adjacent axial fat-saturated T1-weighted images with intraarticular gadolinium showing the typical components of a Buford complex with a hypoplastic anterior labrum and thickened anterior glenohumeral ligament providing an access to the subscapularis recess or bursa. AC, anterior capsule; AL, anterior labrum; GR, glenoid rim; MGHL, middle glenohumeral ligament; SF, sublabral foramen; SGHL, superior glenohumeral ligament; SScT, subscapularis tendon and/or muscle.

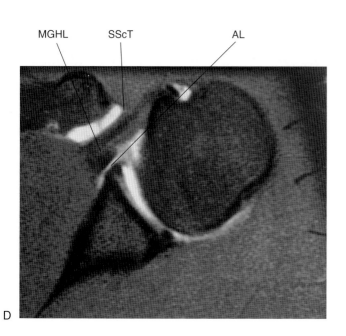

MGHL   SScT   AL

D

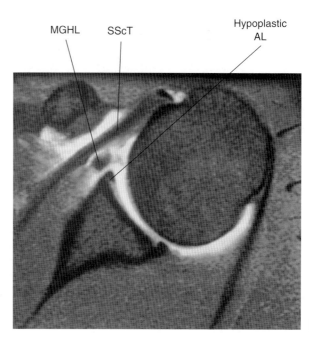

MGHL   SScT   Hypoplastic
AL

E

A

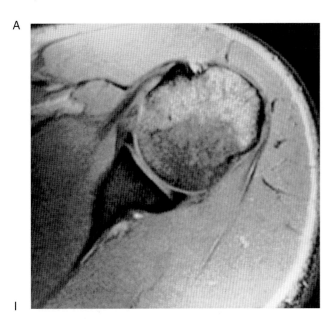

I

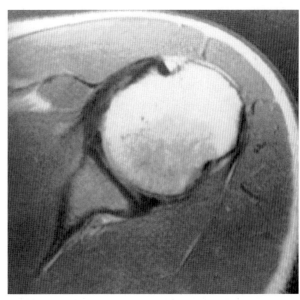

II

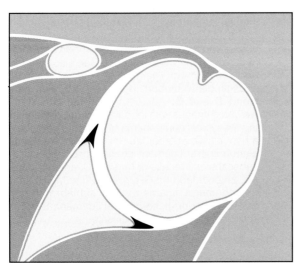

III

FIG. 17. Artist's rendering and corresponding axial MR images displaying the variations of anterior and posterior labral shapes among asymptomatic individuals. **A:** Anterior and posterior triangular shaped labrum. Artist's rendering and proton density–weighted gradient echo image. **B:** Artist's rendering of an anterior and posterior round labrum. Axial proton density–weighted gradient echo image showing a posterior round *(curved arrow)* and anterior triangular labrum *(straight arrow)*. **C:** Artist's rendering and proton density–weighted gradient echo MR images demonstrating an anterior cleaved labrum *(arrow)*. **D:** Artist's rendering and axial proton density–weighted gradient echo MR images demonstrating a notched anterior labrum *(arrow)*. **E:** Artist's rendering and proton density–weighted gradient echo MR images showing flat labra *(arrow)*. **F:** Absent labrum anterior and posterior on artist rendering and posterior on proton density–weighted gradient echo MR image *(arrow).* (From ref. 18, with permission.) *(Continued on next page.)*

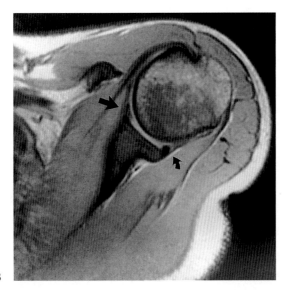

B

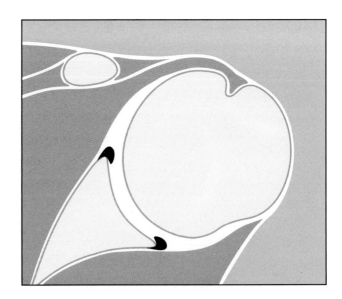

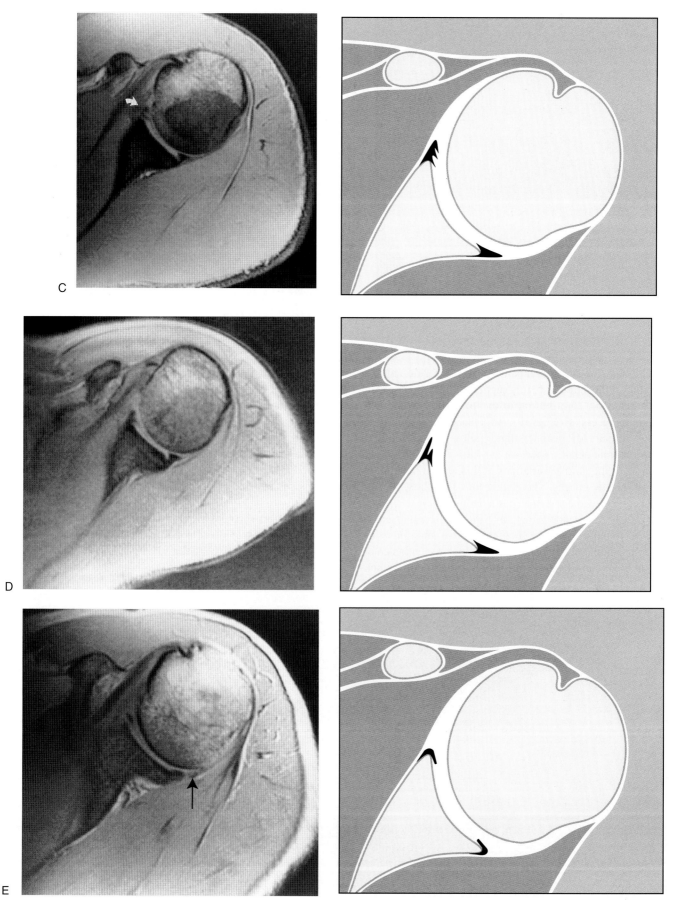

FIG. 17. *Continued.*

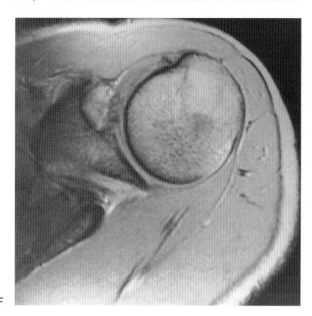
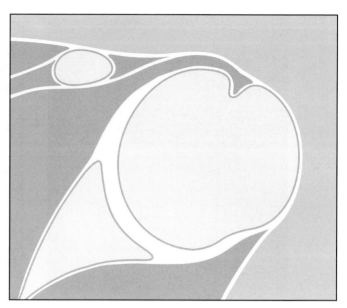

F

FIG. 17. *Continued.*

firm, loose, or no attachment to the superior anterior glenoid. In the latter case, it is supported by a direct capsular attachment, contributing to the formation of the subscapularis recess (see Fig. 19). At present, the resolution of state-of-the-art MR scanners rarely allows visualization of such anatomic detail.

Some of the normal variations of this tendon may be observed on MR images. The tendon may be split within the groove. One segment of the split tendon may lie anterior to the subscapularis tendon (Fig. 20). Similarly, a single tendon may be found outside the bicipital groove anterior to the transverse humeral ligament and subscapularis tendon entering the joint capsule above the superior margin of the sub-

scapularis tendon. These anatomic variants are important to distinguish from traumatic dislocation of the tendon out of the bicipital groove caused by tendon disruption and retraction or tearing of the transverse ligament associated with varying degrees of subscapularis tendon, coracohumeral ligament, and capsular tearing. An acute traumatic tendon dislocation can, in most cases, easily be recognized by its clinical signs and increased signal intensity, edema, swelling, and hemorrhage in adjacent connective tissue, involved tendons, ligaments, and osseous structures. In the chronic case, detectable subscapularis tendon retraction and muscular or tendinous atrophy may be the sole indicators on MRI to explain the cause of an abnormal location of the biceps tendon

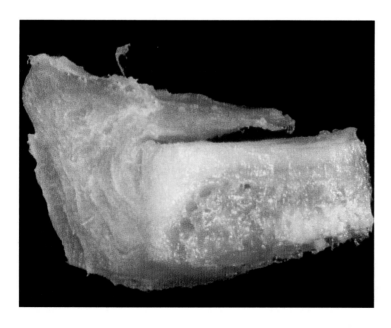

FIG. 18. Cadaveric section of the anterior glenoid labrum and rim showing hyaline joint cartilage extending around the surface of the osseous glenoid rim. This may result in the appearance of a floating or detached labrum on MR images. (Courtesy of Steve Petersen, M.D.)

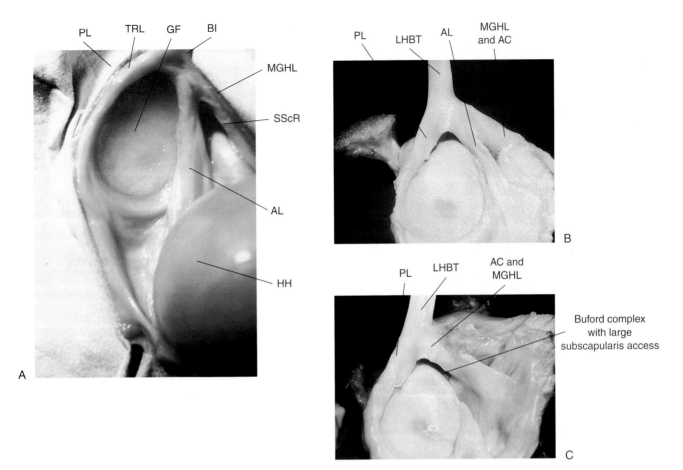

FIG. 19. Variations of the superior labrum and associated attachment of the long head of the biceps tendon on the superior glenoid demonstrated on three cadaveric specimen. **A:** Dissected partially disarticulated shoulder showing the common insertion type (75%) of the biceps tendon into the supraglenoid region just medial to the glenoid rim. The anterior and posterior superior labrum arise from the biceps tendon immediately prior to its insertion. A thin triangular ligament serves as an attachment between anterior and posterior labrum contributing to firm superior labral attachment to the glenoid. **B:** Isolated disarticulated shoulder exhibiting a loose glenoid attachment with direct capsular attachment of the long head of the biceps tendon. **C:** Isolated disarticulated shoulder showing a direct capsular rather than anterior glenoid attachment of the long head of the biceps tendon with a large subscapularis recess. AC, anterior capsule; AL, anterior labrum; BI, biceps insertion; GF, glenoid fossa; HH, humeral head; LHBT, long head biceps tendon; MGHL, middle glenohumeral ligament; PL, posterior labrum; SScR, subscapularis recess; TRL, triangular ligament. (Courtesy of Steve Petersen, M.D.)

(25). Absence of a well-developed bicipital groove favors the possibility of an ectopic variant of the tendon.

The normal biceps tendon is of low signal intensity on all MRI sequences. A small amount of central intermediate signal intensity may sometimes be observed on T1- or proton density–weighted images, probably of similar origin because of the normal variations of signal in the supraspinatus tendon. The biceps tendon sheath communicating with the

TABLE 3. *Variability in anterior and posterior labral shapes in 52 asymptomatic shoulders at inferior, mid, and superior glenoid levels*

Shape	Anterior part of labrum (%)			Posterior part of labrum (%)		
	Inferior	Mid	Superior	Inferior	Mid	Superior
Triangular	24 (46)	21 (40)	25 (49)	42 (81)	42 (81)	30 (58)
Rounded	8 (15)	4 (8)	17 (32)	7 (13)	7 (13)	5 (10)
Cleaved	9 (17)	13 (25)	2 (4)	0	0	0
Notched	7 (13)	6 (11)	0	0	0	0
Flat	2 (4)	6 (11)	3 (6)	3 (6)	3 (6)	4 (8)
Absent	2 (4)	2 (4)	5 (9)	0	0	13 (25)

From ref. 18.

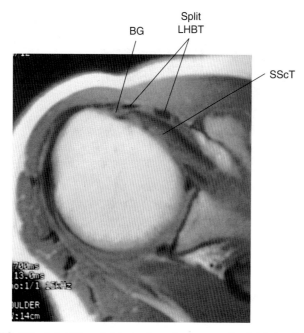

FIG. 20. Axial T1-weighted spin-echo image of a right shoulder demonstrating the normal variant of a split long head biceps tendon. One segment of the tendon is seen anterior to the subscapularis tendon. The other segment is within the bicipital groove. Both portions of the tendon have low signal intensity. BG, bicipital groove; LHBT, long head biceps tendon; SScT, subscapularis tendon and/or muscle.

shoulder joint extends at varying degrees caudally into the bicipital groove. A small amount of fluid within this synovial sheath is physiologic, correlates with the amount of synovial fluid within the shoulder joint, and does not necessarily indicate long head biceps tendon pathology.

CONCLUSION

This chapter is meant to provide anatomic insight into those morphologic structures most commonly affected in dysfunctional shoulder joints. Some of the variations are well known and generally accepted; others, such as the morphology of the biceps labral complex and classification of the anterior capsular attachment, are still the subject of investigation and controversy.

Nevertheless the morphologic-anatomic concepts in this chapter serve as a basis not only for the understanding of the subsequent clinical chapters of this book but also for the critical evaluation of new or revised anatomic concepts.

REFERENCES

1. Zlatkin MB, Iannotti JP, Roberts MC, et al. Rotator cuff tears: diagnostic performance of MR imaging. *Radiology* 1989;172:223–229.
2. Farley TE, Neumann CH, Steinbach LS, Jahnke AH, Petersen SA, Morgan FW. Full thickness tearing of the rotator cuff of the shoulder: diagnosis with MR imaging. *Am J Roentgenol* 1992;158:347–351.
3. Burk DL, Karasick D, Kurtz AB, et al. Rotator cuff tears: prospective comparison of MR imaging with arthrography, sonography, and surgery. *Am J Roentgenol* 1989;153:87–92.
4. Evancho AM, Stiles RG, Fajman WA, et al. MR imaging diagnosis of rotator cuff tears. *Am J Roentgenol* 1988;151:751–754.
5. Hodler J, Kursunoglu-Brahme S, Snyder SJ, et al. Rotator cuff disease: assessment with MR arthrography versus standard MR imaging in 36 patients with arthroscopic confirmation. *Radiology* 1992;182:431–436.
6. Bigliani LU, Morrison D, April EW. The morphology of the acromion and its relationship to rotator cuff tears. *Orthop Trans* 1986;1:228.
7. Farley TE, Neumann CH, Steinbach LS, Petersen SA. The coracoacromial arch: MR evaluation and correlation with rotator cuff pathology. *Skeletal Radiol* 1994;23:641–645.
8. Jonathan DG, Recht MP, Piraino DW, et al. Acromial morphology: relation to sex, age, symmetrie, and subacromial enthesophytes. *Radiology* 1966;199:737–742.
9. Gagey N, Ravaud E, Lassau JP. Anatomy of the acromial arch: correlation of anatomy and magnetic resonance imaging. *Surg Radiol Anat* 1993;15:63–70.
10. Detrisac DA, Johnson LL: Subacromial bursa. In: *Arthroscopic shoulder anatomy.* Thorofare, NJ: SLACK Inc, 1986:116–129.
11. Gallino M, Battiston B, Annaratone G, Terragnoli F. Coracoacromial ligament: a comparative arthroscopic and anatomic study. *Arthroscopy* 1995;11:564–567.
12. Neumann CH, Holt RG, Steinbach LS, Jahnke AH, Petersen SA. MR imaging of the shoulder: appearance of the supraspinatus tendon in asymptomatic volunteers. *Am J Roentgenol* 1992;158:1281–1287.
13. Petersen SA, Jahnke AH Jr, Noble JS, Hawkins RJ. Anatomy of the biceps-labral complex: a critical analysis. *J Shoulder Elbow Surg* 1996;5:S63.
14. Liou JT, Wilson AJ, Totty WC, Brown JJ. The normal shoulder: common variations that simulate pathologic conditions at MR imaging. *Radiology* 1993;186:435–441.
15. Erickson SJ, Cox IH, Hyde JS, Carrera GF, Strandt JA, Estkowski LD. Effect of tendon orientation on MR imaging signal intensity: a manifestation of the "magic angle" phenomenon. *Radiology* 1991; 181:389–392.
16. Zlatkin MB. Anatomy of the shoulder. In: Zlatkin MB, ed. *MRI of the shoulder.* New York: Raven Press, 1991:21–39.
17. Mosely HF, Oevergaard B. The anterior capsular mechanism and recurrent anterior dislocation of the shoulder. *J Bone Joint Surg* 1962;44B:913–927.
18. Neumann CH, Petersen SA, Jahnke AH. MR imaging of the labral-capsular complex: normal variations. *Am J Roentgenol* 1991;157: 1015–1021.
19. Suh KJ, Peterfy CG, Tirman PF, Steinbach LS, Genant HK. *Magic-angle phenomenon*: a cause of increased signal intensity in the superior glenoid labrum of the shoulder on short TE MR images. Paper and Abstract No. 165 at 80th Scientific Assembly and Annual Meeting, RSNA, Nov 27–Dec 2, 1994, Chicago, IL.
20. McNiesh LM, Callaghan JJ. CT arthrography of the shoulder: variations of the glenoid labrum. *Am J Roentgenol* 1987;149:963–966.
21. Petersen SA, Jahnke AH, Noble JS, Hawkins RJ. Anatomy of the biceps-labral complex. A critical analysis. *J Shoulder Elbow Surg* 1996;5[Suppl]:63.
22. Tuite MJ, Orwin JF. Anterosuperior labral variants of the shoulder: appearance on gradient-recalled-echo and fast spin-echo MR images. *Radiology* 1996;199:537–540.
23. Williams MW, Snyder SJ, Buford D. The Buford complex: the cord like middle glenohumeral ligament and absent antero-superior labrum complex—a normal anatomic capsulolabral variant. *Arthroscopy* 1994;10:241–247.
24. Smith DK, Chopp TM, Aufdemorte EG, Jones RC. The sublabral recess of the superior glenoid labrum: a study of cadavers with conventional nonenhanced MR imaging, MR arthrography, anatomic dissection and limited histologic examination. *Radiology* 1996;201:251–256.
24a. Tirman PFJ, Feller JF, Palmer WE, et al. The buford complex—a avariation of normal shoulder anatomy: MR arthrographic imaging features. *Am J Roentgenol* 1996;166.
24b. Tirman PFJ, Stauffer AE, Crups JV III, et al. Saline MR arthrography in the evaluation of glenohumeral instability. *Arthroscopy* 1993; 9:550–569.
24c. Palmer WE, Brown JH, Rosenthal DI. Labral–ligamentous complex of the shoulder: evaluation with MR arthrography. *Radiology* 1994; 190:645–651.
25. Erickson SJ, Fitzgerald SW, Quinn SF, et al. Long bicipital tendon of the shoulder: normal anatomy and pathologic findings on MR imaging. *Am J Roentgenol* 1992;158:1091–1096.

Shoulder Magnetic Resonance Imaging,
edited by Lynne S. Steinbach, et al.
Lippincott–Raven Publishers, Philadelphia © 1998.

CHAPTER 2

Technical Considerations

Charles G. Peterfy

After the knee, the shoulder is the most common joint referred for magnetic resonance imaging (MRI). By comparison, however, MRI of the shoulder joint poses considerably greater technical challenges and is more often the focus of debate and controversy. Some of the challenges of shoulder MRI have to do with the unique anatomy of this joint, such as its oblique orientation and extreme lateral positioning on the body, the curved course of some of its rotator cuff tendons, the noncylindrical shape of this region of the body, and the highly complex and variable morphology of labrocapsular structures. Moreover, the growing diversity of hardware and software alternatives for MRI of the shoulder make it increasingly difficult to generalize about technique and to establish standard imaging protocols. The rapid rate with which technical developments come to clinical use compound the problem by placing greater stress on radiologists to keep abreast of new techniques and to rapidly assimilate them into their practice. At the same time, there is a growing demand to contain costs and adapt to a rapidly changing health care structure. One expression of this conflict is the recent push toward tailored imaging protocols and screening examinations in place of the more comprehensive but time-consuming clinical protocols that are currently used. Focused imaging is more cost effective; however, eliminating sequences from a protocol without inadvertently discarding important diagnostic information requires a thorough understanding of the relative strengths and weaknesses of the different techniques and a sense of where any redundancy of diagnostic information might be. Otherwise, diagnostic inaccuracy can reverse the potential cost savings in monetary as well as human terms.

Accordingly, the following discussion is not only an update on current practice methods for imaging the shoulder but also as a rationale for making the sometimes difficult technical decisions necessary to adapt to the changing needs of the evolving health care system. For a comprehensive review of basic MRI physics, refer to references 1 through 6.

HARDWARE CONSIDERATIONS

MRI has benefited considerably over the years from improvements in magnet hardware. Improved gradient performance, the introduction of autoshimming, and the development of more powerful coil designs have contributed greatly to image quality in the shoulder as well as throughout the body. The following discussion addresses the practical and theoretic implications of these changes as they pertain to MRI of the shoulder.

C. G. Peterfy: Department of Radiology, University of California, San Francisco; and Arthritis and MRI Research, Osteoporosis & Arthritis Research Group, San Francisco, California 94143-0628

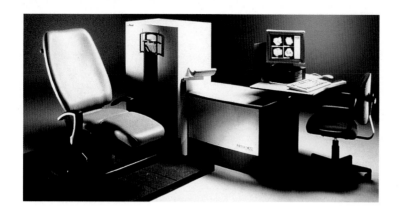

FIG. 1. Low field strength dedicated extremity MRI magnet. Artoscan MRI system with 0.2 Tesla permanent magnet can image the distal two-thirds of the arm or leg, but not the shoulder (Esaote, Genoa, Italy; US distributor is Lunar, Madison, WI).

Magnet Configuration

The demand for low-cost MRI coupled with advances in metal alloy technology and MRI engineering have spawned a greater diversity of magnet types to choose from than ever before. One of the most radical developments in this regard has been the emergence of dedicated extremity scanners, or E-MRI (7) (e.g., Artoscan, Esaote, Genoa, Italy; U.S. distributor: Lunar, Madison, WI) (Fig. 1). E-MRI offers a number of practical and economic advantages over conventional whole-body MRI for a variety of musculoskeletal applications (7). While the model shown in Fig. 1 does not accommodate shoulders, future models will have this capability.

Whole-body magnets are available in two basic configurations: closed and open. Closed, circumferential magnets (Fig. 2) are most common and have been used predominately for MRI. Most superconducting magnets are closed; accordingly, this design is used for high field strength imaging. Problems associated with the closed-bore design include occasional claustrophobia. Typically, only approximately 5% of patients cannot complete the examination because of claustrophobia, but a much larger percentage dislike the experience and often require sedation. Young children are particularly intolerant of closed whole-body MRI and in many

cases require anesthesia, which adds to the invasiveness and cost of MRI.

Open MRI systems are usually composed of two parallel permanent magnet plates, thus enabling the sides (or potentially the top) of the bore to remain open (Fig. 3). This design reduces the risk of claustrophobia, and, because permanent magnets operate at room temperature and at lower field strength than superconducting magnets, they generally cost less as well. However, lower field strength necessitates longer imaging time to achieve comparable signal-to-noise (S/N) ratio and spatial resolution (8,9), and it is generally believed to offer lower image quality than high field superconducting systems (Table 1). Exactly which field strength is most appropriate for clinical imaging continues to be a highly controversial and occasionally divisive issue among radiologists. The following discussion addresses some of the tradeoffs associated with magnetic field strength and image quality.

Magnetic Field Strength and Image Quality

There are two ways of describing the performance of any imaging modality: (a) in terms of technical parameters, such

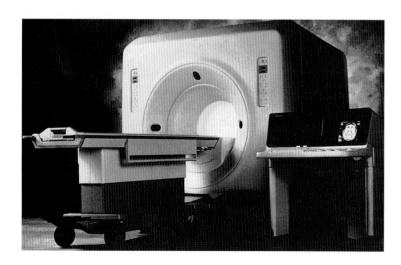

FIG. 2. Circumferential high-field, whole body MRI magnet. Signa Horizon MRI system with 1.5 Tesla superconducting magnet (General Electric, Milwaukee, WI).

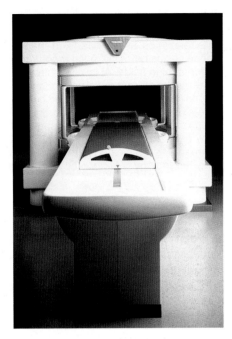

FIG. 3. Open, low-field, whole body MRI magnet. Signa Profile MRI system with 0.2 Tesla permanent magnet (General Electric, Milwaukee, WI).

TABLE 1. *Magnetic resonance imaging tradeoffs related to field strength*

	High Field	Low Field
Signal-to-noise ratio[a]	++	+
Contrast-to-noise ratio	?	?
Spatial resolution[a]	++	+
Imaging time	+	++ [b]
Contrast:		
T1 relaxation	+	+++
T2 relaxation	+++	++
Magnetic susceptibility	++	+
Fat suppression		
Chemical shift	Yes	No
STIR	Yes	Yes
Cost	++	+

[a] Improved by increasing imaging time, reducing spatial resolution, or using superconducting coils.

[b] Depends on tradeoff between faster T1 allowing shorter TR and weaker longitudinal magnetization necessitating greater signal averaging to maintain signal-to-noise ratio and spatial resolution.

as S/N ratio, contrast-to-noise (C/N) ratio, spectral separation, and so on, or (b) in terms of diagnostic parameters, such as sensitivity, specificity, and area under the receiver operator characteristic (ROC) curve. Much of the debate over field strength in MRI has focused on technical aspects of image quality. However, it is clearly diagnostic accuracy that holds the greatest clinical importance.

The most widely recognized technical limitation of low field strength MRI is decreased S/N ratio. As discussed previously, low S/N ratio usually translates into longer acquisition time or lower spatial resolution. However, C/N ratio is a more relevant parameter from the clinical standpoint because it determines the extent to which adjacent structures can be discriminated from each other and it determines the general conspicuity of lesions on MRI. Unlike S/N ratio, C/N ratio does not necessarily increase significantly with field strength (depending on the sequence used and whether receiver bandwidth is varied) (10).

Recently developed superconducting coils may offer a unique solution to the S/N ratio problem at low field strength (11). These specialized coils can offer gains in S/N ratio of twofold or more when used at low field strengths. At high field strength, most of the noise comes from the patient. Improving coil performance thus offers little gain in terms of the cumulative noise in the system. However, at low field strength, coil noise dominates over sample noise, so that improving coil conductance, for example through supercooling the conductor, can have a substantial effect on image noise. A twofold increase in S/N ratio can, in turn, be traded for a fourfold decrease in imaging time[1] or substantially improved spatial resolution.

Spectral separation (chemical shift) also scales with magnetic field strength, leading to greater fat-water separation at high field (~200 Hz at 1.5 T) than at low field (~25 Hz at 0.2 T) (Fig. 4). On the other hand, spectral resonance line widths also tend to increase with increasing field, reflecting increased local field variation. This leads to relatively decreased spectral resolution. Decreased chemical shift at low

[1] Imaging time scales as the inverse square of the improvement in S/N.

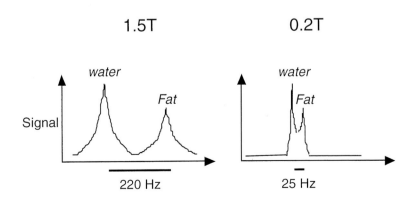

FIG. 4. Effects of field strength on spectral separation of fat and water. Spectral separation of fat and water (the chemical shift phenomenon) is decreased at low field strength. This reduces morphologic distortion but makes frequency-selective fat suppression difficult if not impossible at low fields. (From Peterfy CG, Roberts T, Genant HK. Dedicated extremity MRI: an emerging technology. *Radiol Clin North Am* 1997;35:1–20.)

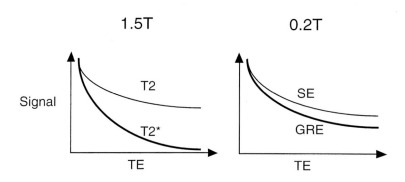

FIG. 5. Effects of field strength on T2*. T2* relaxation, which includes proton dephasing caused by T2 relaxation as well as fixed magnetic heterogeneities, is normally much greater than T2 relaxation at high fields. At low field strength, however, the effects of magnetic heterogeneities are less significant and T2* is dominated by T2. Therefore, long TE gradient echo (GRE) images show similar contrast to T2-weighted spin-echo (SE) images at low field strength. (From Peterfy CG, Roberts T, Genant HK. Dedicated extremity MRI: an emerging technology. *Radiol Clin North Am* 1997;35: 1–20.)

field strength reduces morphologic distortion and allows a smaller acquisition bandwidth but restricts the ability to perform spectral fat suppression.

Additionally, at low field strengths, where magnetic heterogeneities are less significant, T2* is dominated by T2; whereas at high field strengths, T2* is typically much shorter than T2 (Fig. 5). This is particularly significant with gradient echo imaging sequences, which are more vulnerable to magnetic susceptibility effects. The most obvious implication of this is reduced metallic artifacts and improved sensitivity for marrow pathology at low field strength.

Finally, T1 values are shorter at lower field strengths. This leads to more rapid recovery of equilibrium after excitation and hence accommodates shorter TR and more rapid imaging. The potential gain in acquisition time, however, is generally offset by the increased number of signal averagings required to maintain S/N ratio. More rapid T1 relaxation also allows short TR gradient echo sequences to tolerate larger flip angles.

Another consequence of low field strength is that gadolinium diethylenetriamine pentaacetic acid (Gd-DTPA) is more potent. This may allow smaller doses of this contrast material to be used to achieve an equivalent level of enhancement. However, adequate T1 weighting at low field strength requires shorter TR. Also, longer TEs necessitated by the use of shorter receiver bandwidths to improve S/N ratio at lower field strength introduce T2 effects, which can decrease the observed enhancement with Gd-DTPA. Moreover, if the magnitude of the effect of field strength on the T1 of a Gd-enhancing lesion is less than the effect on the T1 of surrounding normal tissue, as has been shown to be the case with certain brain tumors, lesion conspicuity may actually be lower than at high field strength (12). This is not necessarily the case for musculoskeletal tissues, but final judgment on the relative effectiveness of Gd-DTPA at low field strength must await further investigation.

Coil Selection

Numerous different coil designs are available for MRI of the shoulder. Although quadrature and phased-array coils offer the highest S/N ratio, image quality with conventional surface coils is generally sufficient for most clinical applications. Recently developed flex coils are particularly versatile and can accommodate a wide range of shoulder sizes and shapes. In most situations, a single surface coil is used. However, for imaging the shoulder in abduction and external rotation (ABER), two passively coupled coils are usually preferred.

PATIENT POSITIONING

Whole-body MRI offers only a few alternatives for patient positioning for imaging the shoulder (13). Because of the small bore size of most closed, circumferential magnets, shoulder imaging with one of these systems can only be performed when the arm is at the side or over the head. Open low field strength permanent magnets also allow the shoulder to be imaged in various degrees of abduction. However, even with these systems, the shoulder is most commonly imaged in adduction with the patient supine and the arm at the side (Fig. 6). When imaging in this position, care should be

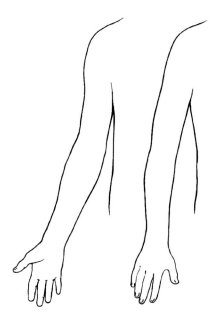

FIG. 6. Normal patient positioning. With the patient lying supine and the arm at the side, turning the thumb out rotates the shoulder externally, whereas turning the thumb in rotates the shoulder internally.

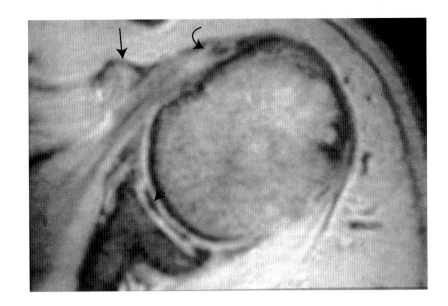

FIG. 7. Imaging in external rotation. Axial image of the shoulder shows the biceps tendon *(curved arrow)* in the intertubercular groove rotated far away from the coracoid process *(straight arrow)* indicative of external rotation of the shoulder. Note linear signal void *(arrowhead)* of gas created by vacuum phenomenon in the joint space.

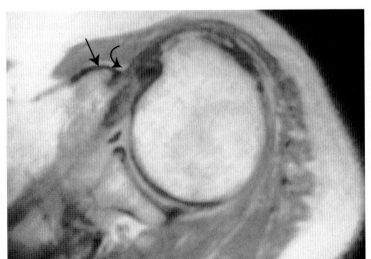

A

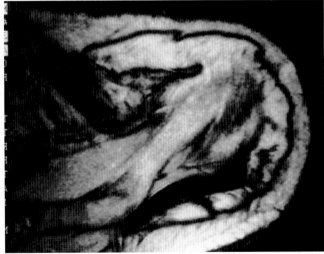

B

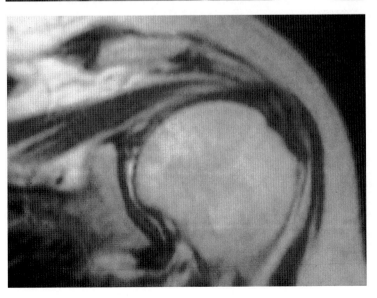

C

FIG. 8. Imaging in internal rotation. **A:** Axial image of the shoulder shows the biceps tendon *(curved arrow)* very near to the coracoid process *(straight arrow)* indicative of marked internal rotation of the shoulder. **B:** High axial section of an internally rotated shoulder shows the infraspinatus tendon overlapping the more anterior supraspinatus tendon. **C:** Oblique coronal image of the same shoulder shows a tram-track appearance of the rotator cuff caused by the overlapping tendons. Some may confuse this appearance with that of intratendonous rotator cuff tear.

taken not to place the hand on the abdomen, because this may transmit respiratory motion to the shoulder and degrade the images.

Positioning of the hand determines whether the shoulder is imaged in internal or external rotation. Exactly which position is best is controversial, and there are tradeoffs associated with each. External rotation with the thumb positioned away from the patient can be uncomfortable and tends to tighten the anterior capsule of the shoulder and obscure the anterior labrum (Fig. 7). Also, external rotation has been shown to occasionally cause gas to form in the joint because of the "vacuum phenomenon" (14). The resulting signal void and magnetic susceptibility artifact may obscure the articular surface or mimic chondrocalcinosis but usually does not pose major problems in terms of image interpretation. External rotation does, however, align the tendons of the rotator cuff well for oblique coronal imaging, and placing the patient's palm under the buttock aids immobilization of the shoulder during imaging. Internal rotation of the shoulder—with the thumb turned in—slackens the anterior capsule and thus allows joint fluid to pool around the anterior labrum and better define the local morphology. This, however, is often at the expense of the visibility of the posterior labrum. Moreover, positioning the shoulder in internal rotation causes the infraspinatus tendon to overlap the supraspinatus tendon and create an appearance that may mimic rotator cuff tear (Fig. 8). Neutral positioning, with the thumb pointed up, is usually the most comfortable for the patient and, therefore, minimizes motion artifacts.

One intriguing alternative to imaging with the arm at the side is to place the patient's hand behind his head to position the arm in ABER position (15,16) (Fig. 9). This position provides superior visualization of the undersurface of the rotator cuff, delineates the important inferior glenohumeral ligament, and reorients the glenoid labrum so that the anteroinferior segment can be visualized free of "magic angle" effects.

IMAGING PLANES

Routine MRI of the shoulder is usually performed in three different planes. The axial plane is relatively straightforward but, because of the orientation of the glenohumeral joint, both the coronal and sagittal images must be obliqued. In certain circumstances, oblique axial images may also be obtained with the shoulder in ABER positioning. Although there is considerable redundancy in the anatomic information provided by each of these imaging planes, certain anatomic features are optimally evaluated in one or another of these planes (Table 2). The importance of each plane, therefore, varies with the specific clinical question posed in each case.

The following discussion describes the proper technique for acquiring each of these planes, contrasts their strengths and weakness for imaging shoulder anatomy, and identifies which anatomic structures are best delineated with each plane.

Axial

Axial images of the shoulder are used not only to evaluate the articular anatomy but also to serve as a localizer for subsequent oblique coronal and oblique sagittal images. Imaging of the shoulder thus usually begins in the axial plane. Regardless of the specific sequence chosen, it is important to ensure that the axial coverage is high enough to include the acromion (Fig. 10). The reason for this is to identify abnormalities, such as os acromiale, and to assist in proper localization of the oblique coronal sections.

Os acromiale is a failure of the distal ossification center of the acromion to fuse to the remainder of the bone during the third decade of life. Because a portion of the deltoid muscle inserts along this segment of the acromion, mobility at this site during abduction may result in depression of the distal acromion and impingement of the rotator cuff. Os acromiale

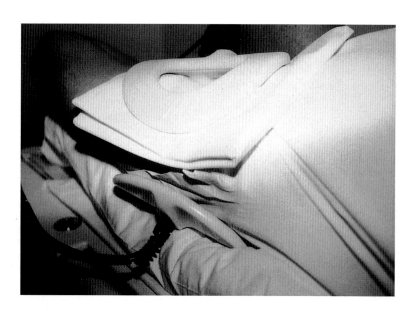

FIG. 9. Abduction and external rotation positioning. Placing the hand behind the head of a supine patient positions the ipsilateral shoulder in abduction and external rotation (ABER). A 3 coil in front of the shoulder coupled to a 5 coil behind the shoulder is the preferred configuration.

TABLE 2. *Structures best delineated in each imaging plane*

Imaging plane	Anatomical structures
Axial	Acromion (os acromiale)
	Labrum (anterior, posterior)[a]
	Middle and superior glenohumeral ligaments
	Glenohumeral articular surfaces
	Biceps tendon (intertubercular portion)
	Subscapularis tendon
	Spinoglenoid notch (suprascapular n.)
	Supraspinatus and infraspinatus tendons
Oblique coronal	Labrum (superior, inferior[b])
	Biceps tendon (labral insertion)
	Glenohumeral articular surfaces
	Acromioclavicular joint
	Suprascapular notch (suprascapular n.)
	Rotator cuff muscles
Oblique sagittal	Coracoacromial arch
	Subacromial-subdeltoid bursa
	Acromioclavicular joint
	Biceps tendon (intra-articular portion)
	Rotator cuff interval
Abducted and externally rotated Oblique axial	Spinatus tendons (undersurface)
	Inferior glenohumeral ligament
	Labrum (anteroinferior)

[a]With gadolinium (Gd)-contrast or effusion in the joint, the anterosuperior, anteroinferior, posteroinferior, and posterosuperior labra are also well delineated in this plane.
[b]Visualization of inferior labrum usually requires Gd-contrast or effusion in the joint.

may not be visible during routine shoulder arthroscopy, and thus may become a cause of failed shoulder surgery. Even though it is possible to diagnose this anomaly on images acquired in other planes, it is best shown on axial images (see Fig. 10).

Other structures well imaged in the axial plane include the following:

- Portions of the articular surfaces of the glenohumeral joint. Partial volume averaging limits evaluation of the superior and inferior surfaces of the humeral head.
- Anterior and posterior labrum. Intraarticular Gd contrast is usually necessary to delineate the anterosuperior, anteroinferior, posterosuperior, and posteroinferior segments of the labrum on short TE images, whereas the superior and inferior labral segments are obscured by partial volume averaging.
- Superior and middle glenohumeral ligaments. The important inferior glenohumeral ligament is lax and folded over on itself when the arm is in an adducted position, and, although portions of the ligament can be seen when Gd contrast fills and distends the joint, abnormalities are difficult to delineate.
- Subscapularis tendon.
- Quadrilateral space, which conveys the axillary nerve.
- Intertubercular portion of the tendon of the long head of the biceps. Partial volume averaging and magic angle effects on short TE images limit visualization of the superior portion and the tendon as it curves over the humeral head.
- Spinoglenoid notch of the scapula, where the suprascapular nerve can be found.

Oblique Coronal

The oblique coronal plane is best selected off a relatively cephalad section of an axial localizer, where the course of the supraspinatus can be followed directly (Figs. 11 and 12). Although the muscle bellies of the supraspinatus and infraspinatus follow the spine of the scapula, their tendons curve anteriorly beneath the acromion toward their insertion on the greater tuberosity of the humerus. Therefore, the usual

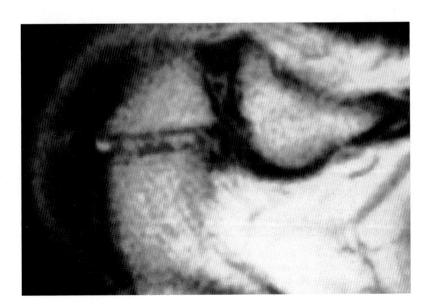

FIG. 10. Os acromiale on high axial localizer. The acromion of this 40-year-old patient with symptoms of rotator cuff impingement shows a non-united ossification center anterolaterally known as the os acromiale. Contraction of the deltoid muscle, which inserts along the acromion, during abduction can close the os acromiale on the retracting supraspinatus tendon and cause impingement syndrome.

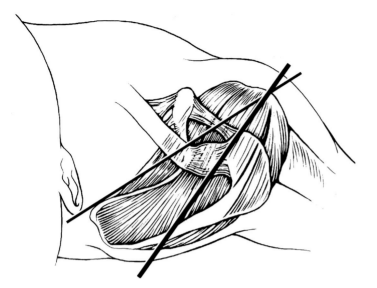

FIG. 11. Oblique coronal plane for imaging the spinatus tendons. Bird's-eye view shows the relationship between the muscles and tendons of the rotator cuff and the bones of the shoulder. The thick line marks the optimal plane for sectioning the supraspinatus tendon along its long axis. The thin line marks a less desirable plane parallel to the spine of the scapula but oblique to the spinatus tendons.

practice of aligning the oblique coronal plane with the spine of the scapula on a mid glenoid slice of the axial localizer tends to section the anterior portion of the supraspinatus tendon—where most tears of the rotator cuff arise—obliquely and anterior to the supraspinatus muscle (Fig. 13). Without the supraspinatus muscle to landmark the tendon, anterior tears may be mistaken for partial-volume averaging of the rotator cuff interval. The more familiar appearance of the supraspinatus muscle and tendon can be seen on more dorsal sections. However, once again because of the curvature of the spinatus tendons, what appears to be the supraspinatus musculotendinous unit may in fact be the supraspinatus muscle aligned with the infraspinatus tendon. Because it is the spinatus tendons and not their respective muscles that are of primary clinical interest in most cases, oblique coronal images should ideally be aligned with the tendons themselves,

and these are visible only on the superior sections of the axial images (see Fig. 12).

In some cases, it may not be possible to acquire sufficiently obliqued coronal images. With some MRI systems, for example, fast spin-echo images cannot be obliqued as much as the conventional spin-echo images because of insufficient gradient strength (see Fig. 13). Understanding of the effects of inadequate obliquity of the coronal images, however, is usually sufficient to allow one to sort out the anatomy and avoid serious diagnostic misinterpretations.

Anatomic structures best shown with oblique coronal images include the following:

- Spinatus tendons of the rotator cuff. The subscapularis and teres minor are better seen in axial and oblique sagittal planes.
- Superior labrum and biceps tendon insertion. The inferior

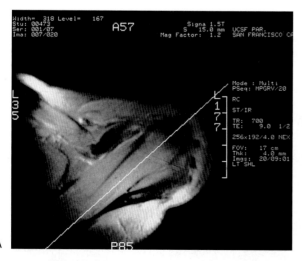

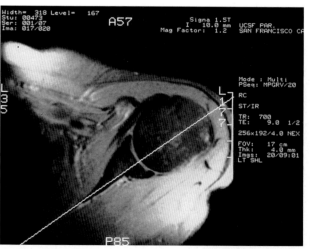

FIG. 12. High versus mid axial localizer for the oblique coronal plane. **A:** High axial section at the level of the supraspinatus tendon allows alignment of oblique coronal sections directly with the tendon. **B:** Aligning oblique coronal sections with the spine of the scapula using a mid glenoid localizer underestimates the degree of obliquity necessary to section the supraspinatus tendon longitudinally.

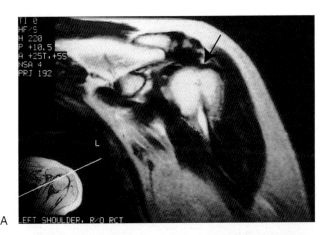

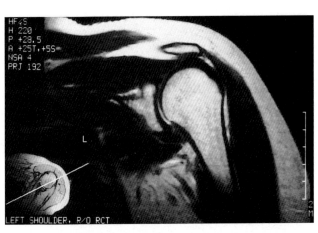

A

B

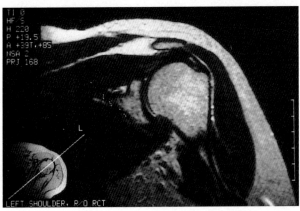

C

FIG. 13. Consequences of inadequate obliquity of coronal imaging of the supraspinatus tendon. **A:** Inadequately angled 0.5 Tesla T2-weighted fast spin-echo oblique coronal image depicts the anterior portion of the supraspinatus tendon, where most tears *(arrow)* arise, without its corresponding muscle belly to serve as anatomic reference. **B:** A more posterior section through the supraspinatus muscle also passes through the infraspinatus tendon, and thus artificially combines these two structures on a single image. **C:** A more angulated T2-weighted conventional spin-echo image properly aligns the supraspinatus tendon and muscle.

labrum is usually obscured by redundant synovial tissue in the axillary pouch unless the joint is distended with effusion or intraarticular Gd contrast.

- Articular surfaces of the glenohumeral joint.
- Undersurface of the acromion.
- Acromioclavicular joint.
- Suprascapular notch of the scapula.

Oblique Sagittal

The oblique sagittal plane is also obtained from an axial localizer, but is parallel to the articular surface of the glenoid fossa and perpendicular to the spine of the scapula (Fig. 14). The oblique sagittal plane is useful for evaluating the muscles of the rotator cuff, particularly the subscapularis and

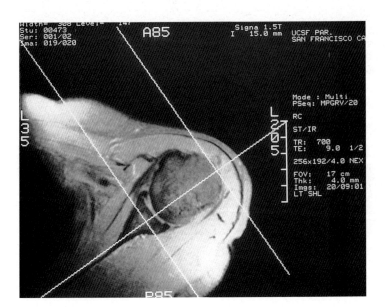

FIG. 14. Axial localizer for the oblique sagittal plane. Oblique sagittal sections are acquired with a mid scapular localizer, parallel to the articular surface of the glenoid but perpendicular to the spine of the scapula.

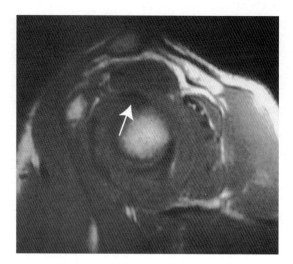

FIG. 15. Oblique sagittal plane for evaluating the muscles of the rotator cuff. Oblique sagittal image shows all the muscles of the rotator cuff and the intraarticular component of biceps tendon *(arrow)*.

teres minor, which are more difficult to evaluate in other planes (Fig. 15). The quadrilateral space, which conveys the axillary nerve, is also well seen on these images. The oblique sagittal plane is optimal for evaluating the coracoacromial arch, which is composed of the coracoid process anteriorly, the acromion posteriorly, and the coracoacromial ligament that stretches between them. It is based on the oblique sagittal images that the acromion is classified as type 1, 2, or 3 (see Chapter 6). Although an os acromiale is most easily identified on axial images, it can also be diagnosed in the oblique sagittal plane by the presence of a second synarthrosis distal to the acromioclavicular joint (Fig. 16). Sometimes the coracoacromial ligament (Fig. 17) can be delineated throughout its course on a single oblique sagittal image, although this usually requires a less oblique plane than the one described here. At present, the value of delineating the coracoacromial ligament on MR images remains controversial, and thus changing the standard orientation of the oblique sagittal plane simply to provide better visualization of this structure is probably not warranted. The subacromial-subdeltoid bursa, which curves over the anterior portion of the

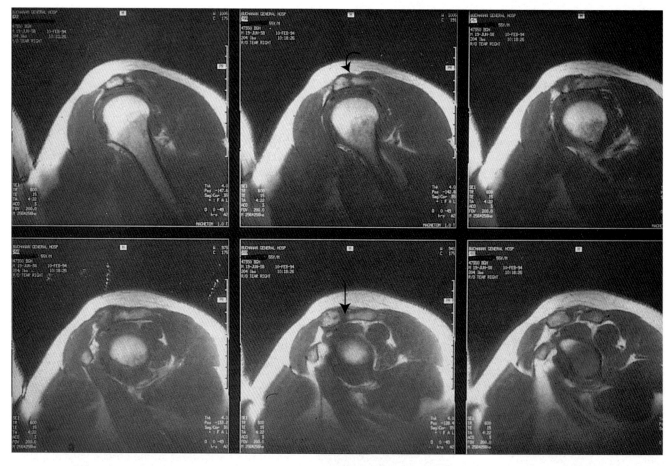

FIG. 16. Appearance of os acromiale on oblique sagittal images. Os acromiale is disclosed on the oblique sagittal images by a double acromioclavicular joint appearance produced by the additional vertically oriented articulation of the nonfused synchondrosis of the os acromiale *(curved arrow)*. Acromioclavicular joint *(straight arrow)*.

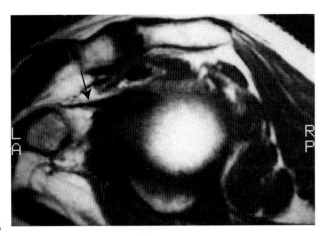 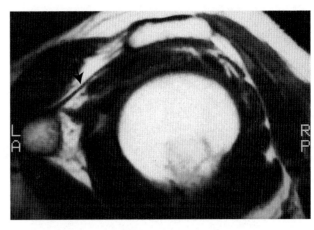

A   B

FIG. 17. Coracoacromial and coracohumeral ligaments on oblique sagittal images. **A:** The coraco-humeral ligament *(arrow)* is well seen on oblique sagittal images as a low low signal intensity band extend-ing through the rotator cuff interval from the coracoid process to the intertubercular groove of the humerus and silhouetted by fat on either side. **B:** The coracoacromial ligament *(arrow)* can be seen more laterally, but typically appears discontinuous on conventionally oriented oblique sagittal images.

joint and lies just beneath the coracoacromial arch, is also optimally visualized in the oblique sagittal plane (Fig. 18). Between the supraspinatus and subscapularis tendons lies the rotator cuff interval. One important structure in this space that is best seen on oblique sagittal images is the coraco-humeral ligament (see Fig. 17). This ligament supports the humerus in abduction and stabilizes the intertubercular por-tion of the tendon of the long head of the biceps.

Oblique Axial (ABER Positioning)

As discussed previously, ABER positioning is achieved in the supine patient by placing the patient's hand behind his or her head. Oblique axial images of the shoulder are then ob-tained by aligning sections with the long axis of the humerus using a direct coronal localizer (Fig. 19). This plane is par-ticularly useful for evaluating the spinatus tendons (16) (Fig.

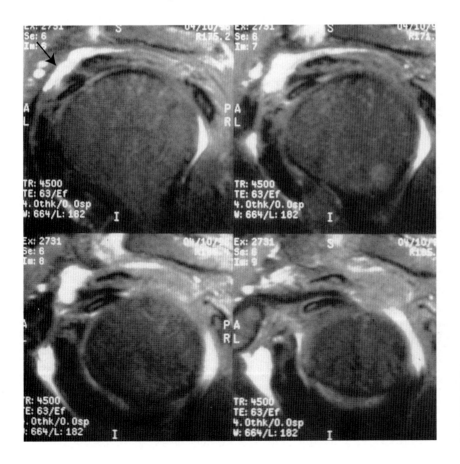

FIG. 18. Subacromial bursa on oblique sagittal images. Oblique sagittal T2-weighted fat-suppressed images show fluid in the subacromial bursa *(arrow)* draping over the coracoid process anteri-orly on oblique sagittal images.

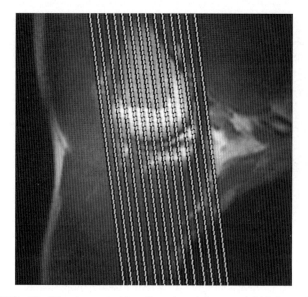

FIG. 19. Direct coronal localizer for oblique axial abducted and externally rotated (ABER) images. Oblique axial sections are aligned with the long axis of the humerus on a coronal localizer acquired with the patient in the ABER position.

20). Sections anterior to the scapular spine show primarily the supraspinatus tendon, whereas sections posterior to the spine show the infraspinatus tendon. ABER images are unique in their depiction of the inferior glenohumeral ligament under tension. ABER images are also useful for show-

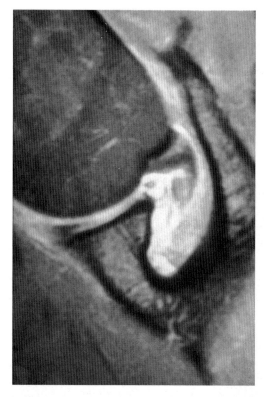

FIG. 20. Oblique axial plane in the abducted and externally rotated position. Image shows section through the spine of the scapula.

ing the anteroinferior segment of the labrum free of magic angle effects (see Fig. 20).

PULSE SEQUENCES

Sequence options for imaging the shoulder include conventional spin-echo and gradient echo techniques, fast spin-echo, short tau inversion recovery (STIR), and fast STIR. Each of these have strengths and weaknesses that must be considered in the design of any imaging protocol (Table 3).

Spin-Echo

As with most of musculoskeletal MRI, conventional T1-weighted and T2-weighted spin-echo have been the workhorse sequences for imaging the shoulder. T1-weighted spin-echo is a relatively rapid technique, easy to use, and consistently offers high contrast between fat and water (Fig. 21). It can be used with both high-field and low-field magnets, although shorter TRs are necessary at low magnetic field strengths to achieve comparable T1 weighting because of more rapid T1 relaxation.

T1-weighted images provide high sensitivity for conditions that elevate the water content of fatty marrow (e.g., hematopoietic reconversion, bone contusion and fracture, osteomyelitis, ischemia, and infiltrating neoplasm). Certain fat planes of interest, such as those lining the subacromial bursa, separating individual muscle groups, and surrounding neurovascular structures, are also well seen on T1-weighted images. T1-weighted spin-echo is also used to identify areas enhanced by Gd-contrast administered either intravenously or by direct intraarticular injection. In such cases, frequency-selective fat suppression is often included to provide contrast between fat and Gd-enhanced tissues, which may otherwise show similar signal intensities. Fat suppression can also be used to augment contrast between nonfatty structures of in-

TABLE 3. *Visibility of pathology with different pulse sequence*

Pulse sequence	Pathology			
	Marrow	Rotator cuff	Labral tear	Bursa/cysts
T1 SE[a]	+++	+	++	+
T2 SE	++	+++	+[b]	+++
PD SE[a]		+	++	+
T2* GRE[a]	+	+	++	+++
T2 FSE	+	+++	+[b]	+++
T2 FSE fat sat	+++	+++	+[b]	++++
STIR/FSTIR	++++	+++	+[b]	++++

PD, proton-density–weighted; GRE, gradient echo; SE, spin-echo; FSE, fast spin-echo; FSTIR, fast STIR.
[a]Magic angle effects limit specificity of signal changes in nondisplaced tears of tendons, ligaments and labrum.
[b]Only displaced tears are visible.

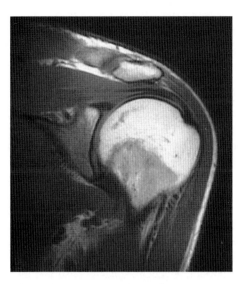

FIG. 21. T1-weighted spin-echo. Oblique coronal T1-weighted spin-echo image of the shoulder offers high contrast between fat and water but limited contrast between free and bound water.

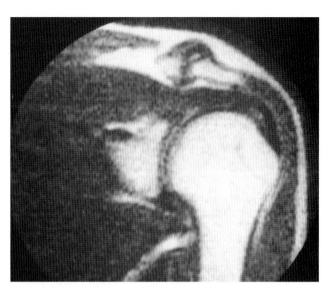

FIG. 23. Limited signal-to-noise (S/N) ratio on T2-weighted spin-echo. Oblique coronal T2-weighted spin-echo image shows poor S/N ratio.

termediate and long T1 (e.g., articular cartilage and joint fluid) by rescaling their respective pixel intensities (Fig. 22). Limitations of T1-weighted spin-echo include vulnerability to magic angle effects, which can both mimic and obscure important findings in certain tissues, and relatively poor discrimination between free and bound water, which limits the ability to detect most inflammatory, infectious, traumatic, and neoplastic conditions in nonfatty tissues.

T2-weighted spin-echo, on the other hand, generates contrast primarily on the basis of tissue differences in free and bound water, and is therefore more sensitive for inflammation, infection, trauma, and neoplasia. Also, because of the long TE, T2-weighted images are relatively unaffected by the magic angle phenomenon. The problem with T2-weighted imaging relates principally to long imaging time and limited S/N ratio (Fig. 23). This restricts the maximum spatial resolution that can be attained within a reasonable clinical protocol, although this is not a significant limitation for most clinical indications when using modern MRI hardware and software. Increasing the number of excitations in order to

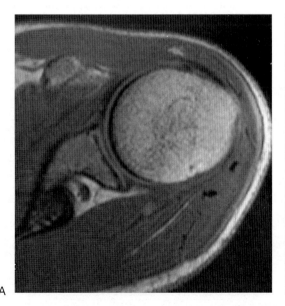

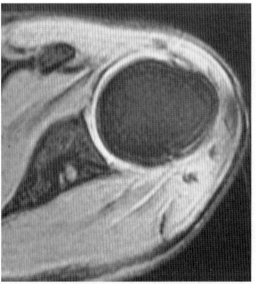

A

B

FIG. 22. Augmenting T1 contrast with fat suppression. Oblique coronal T1-weighted spin-echo image of the shoulder before **(A)** and following **(B)** fat-suppression T1-weighted three-dimensional gradient echo image shows high contrast between articular cartilage and adjacent synovial fluid based on differences in T1 that are normally overshadowed by fat.

boost S/N ratio is usually not an option because of the already lengthy acquisition times involved. S/N ratio can be improved by increasing the field strength, but this also increases imaging time by prolonging T1 and therefore necessitating longer TRs. Accordingly, the most viable approach to increasing S/N on T2-weighted images is the use of quadrature or phased-array coils. Recently developed superconducting coils may prove useful for this purpose on low field strength systems.

Gradient Echo

One alternative to lengthy T2-weighted spin-echo imaging is partial flip angle gradient echo imaging. Gradient echo sequences are substantially faster and, because they use short TEs (<30 msec), they show greater sensitivity for nondisplaced labral tears, which, like meniscal tears, are poorly depicted on long TE images. Moreover, the high speed of gradient echo sequences makes three-dimensional imaging feasible. Three-dimensional technique permits thinner sections and offers higher S/N ratios than two-dimensional images with comparable voxel size. Three-dimensional imaging also facilitates multiplanar reformatting by providing well-shaped, contiguous sections, potentially with isotropic voxels. Balanced against these advantages are a number of limitations. First, the restriction to short TE imaging makes gradient echo vulnerable to magic angle effects, which limit specificity for tendinitis and ligamentous injuries in certain locations. Short TE imaging also limits sensitivity for chondromalacia, which can be seen as foci of T2 prolongation within the normally short T2 articular cartilage (see Chapter 10). Another important limitation of gradient echo, particularly for musculoskeletal imaging, is its vulnerability to fixed magnetic heterogeneities. This manifests as signal loss

and morphologic distortion near metallic implants (Fig. 24) and collections of gas (see Fig. 7), and limits the utility of gradient echo imaging following surgery or air contrast arthrography. T2* effects are also prominent in the marrow cavity where differences in magnetic susceptibility between trabecular bone and adjacent marrow tissue produce field heterogeneities that dephase protons near these interfaces. Because of this, fat generally appears lower in signal intensity in the marrow cavity than it does in adipose tissue on gradient echo images (see Fig. 24). More importantly, water protons in the marrow also show more rapid T2* relaxation and this reduces the sensitivity of gradient echo images for trauma, infection, or infiltrating neoplasms, as long as the trabecular network remains intact. Once these processes begin to destroy trabeculae, their conspicuity on gradient echo images increases accordingly (Fig. 25).

It is important to recognize that these susceptibility effects scale with the magnetic field strength. Accordingly, metallic artifacts are less severe and early marrow disease is more conspicuous on images acquired at low field strength.

Fast Spin-Echo

The development of fast spin-echo, or RARE as Henning (17) originally called it, was a breakthrough in modern MRI that provided heavily T2-weighted images in only a fraction of the time and with greater resolution than was possible with conventional spin-echo techniques (Fig. 26). Accordingly, fast spin-echo was rapidly incorporated in clinical MRI protocols. The key to fast spin-echo was incorporating multiple 180-degree refocusing pulses and phase-encoding steps into each TR (18) (Fig. 27). The higher amplitude phase encodings carry most of the high-frequency spatial information, but they are inherently dephasing and therefore

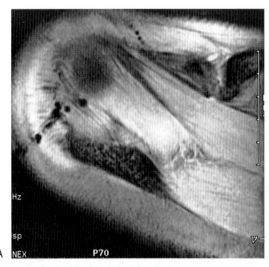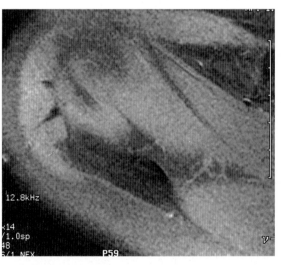

FIG. 24. Limitations of gradient echo imaging. **A:** Axial T2*-weighted three-dimensional gradient echo image of a shoulder after subacromial decompression surgery shows numerous metallic artifacts in the surgical bed. **B:** T1-weighted fat-suppressed spin-echo image at the same level fails to reveal the metallic artifacts.

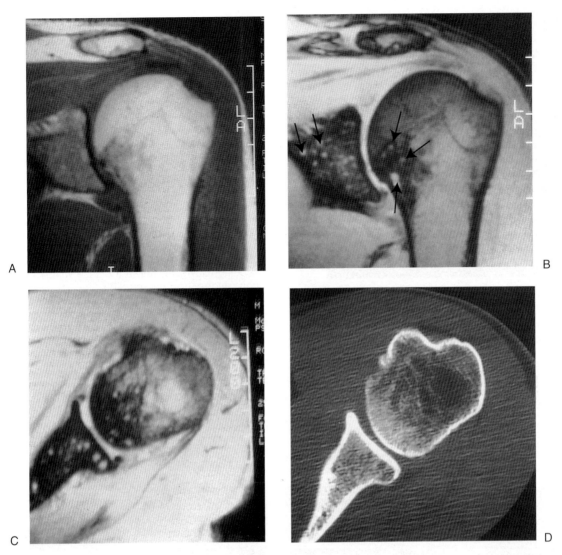

FIG. 25. Effect of trabecular destruction on lesion conspicuity on gradient echo images. **A:** Mild heterogeneity of the marrow in the proximal humerus of a patient with multiple myeloma is difficult to distinguish on T1-weighted spin-echo images from residual hematopoietic tissue commonly present in this location. **B:** T2*-weighted gradient echo images of the same shoulder reveal foci of trabecular destruction *(arrows)* that are typical of multiple myeloma but not seen in normal hematopoietic marrow. Foci of trabecular destruction are more apparant on axial T2*-weighted gradient echo images **(C)** than on computed tomography images **(D).**

generate relatively small echoes. Low-amplitude phase-encoding steps, on the other hand, provide less spatial information but generate large echoes and therefore dominate in terms of image signal. The TE of the lowest amplitude phase-encoding step (TE$_{eff}$) thus determines the degree of T2 contrast in the final image. One implication of this approach is that by ordering the signal-poor high-amplitude phase-encoding steps early in the sequence (i.e., during the signal-rich portion of the T2 decay curve), high-frequency spatial information is emphasized in the final image. T2-weighted fast spin-echo images accordingly show higher resolution than do conventional spin-echo images. Additionally, fast spin-echo is less vulnerable to magnetic susceptibility effects than is any other commercially available pulse sequence.

For these reasons, many institutions have turned to fast spin-echo for their T2-weighted imaging sequence in the shoulder. However, a few technical caveats are important to bear in mind. First, unlike conventional spin-echo imaging, in which an additional short TE (proton density weighted) image could be acquired in a dual-echo sequence without any additional imaging time, because multiple echoes are used to generate each set of fast spin-echo images, dual-echo fast spin-echo imaging requires two separate acquisitions and therefore considerably increased imaging time (Fig. 27) excluding the prescan. Moreover, short TE fast spin-echo images tend to show "blurring" and may thus obscure fine anatomic detail (Fig. 28). Blurring can be reduced by decreasing the echo spacing; however, not all MRI systems

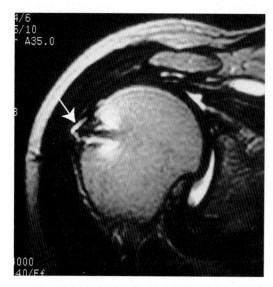

FIG. 26. Fast spin-echo imaging. Oblique coronal T2-weighted fast spin-echo image of the same shoulder depicted in Fig. 24 shows pronounced T2 contrast, high spatial resolution, and considerably diminished metallic artifact *(arrow)*.

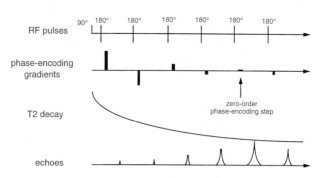

FIG. 27. The fast spin-echo pulse sequence. Long TE fast spin-echo sequences offer the optimal trade-off between signal loss resulting from T2 decay and that resulting from phase encoding. However, unlike the case with conventional spin-echo, dual-echo imaging with fast spin-echo requires re-ordering the echoes and therefore increased imaging time. (From Peterfy C, Linares R, Steinbach L. Recent advances in magnetic resonance imaging of the musculoskeletal system. *Radiol Clin North Am* 1994;32:291–311.)

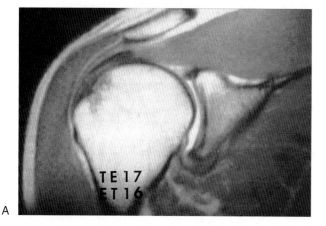

A

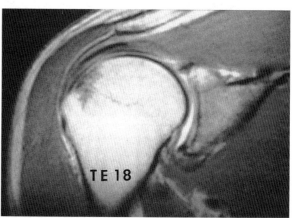

B

FIG. 28. Blurring on short TE fast spin-echo. Proton-density–weighted fast spin-echo image (TR = 2000 msec, TE = 17 msec, 16 echoes) **(A)** is blurred compared to a conventional spin-echo image acquired with the same imaging parameters **(B)**.

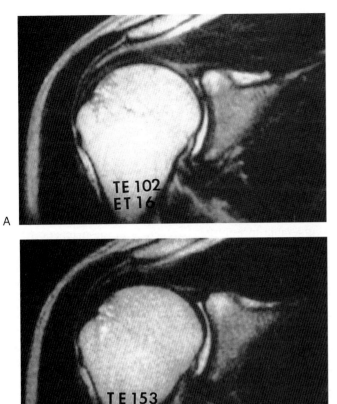

A

TE 102
ET 16

B

TE 80

C

TE 153
ET 16

FIG. 29. Poor fat-water contrast on T2-weighted fast spin-echo. T2-weighted fast spin-echo (TR = 2500 msec, TE = 120 msec) **(A)** shows higher signal intensity in fat, and therefore lower fat-water contrast, than does conventional T2-weighted fast spin-echo with a shorter TE (80 msec) **(B)**. Lengthening TE (140 msec) improves fat-water contrast, but at the expense of overall S/N ratio **(C)**.

have sufficient gradient strength to do this adequately. Also, the utility of the proton-density–weighted image in shoulder MRI is probably only marginal anyway. Even though fast spin-echo does provide greater sensitivity than long TE images for nondisplaced labral tears, blurring often makes fast spin-echo less reliable than conventional spin-echo. Moreover, the original motive of using proton-density–weighted images to provide anatomic reference to long TE images, which show inferior S/N ratio and spatial resolution, is not justified with fast spin-echo, because its long TE images already show high resolution, in fact, higher resolution than the short TE images, in those circumstances in which there is blurring. Accordingly, the tradition of dual-echo imaging should be reconsidered when using fast spin-echo.

Another caveat associated with fast spin-echo is that fat remains high in signal intensity on T2-weighted images (19,20) (Fig. 29). This lowers contrast between fat and fluid in the subacromial bursa as well as the bone marrow. Use of extremely long TEs (>140 msec) improves the contrast between fat and free water, but at the expense of overall S/N ratio. Frequency-selective fat presaturation can be added to T2-weighted fast spin-echo sequences to suppress the high signal intensity of fat (Figs. 30 and 31), but field heterogeneities about the shoulder often produce uneven fat suppression (21) that may mimic fluid in the subacromial bursa or bone marrow (Fig. 32). Typically, these heterogeneities are most severe near the greater tuberosity where the spinatus tendons insert. If the frequency shift is large enough, inadvertent water saturation may also occur and ironically suppress signal from a torn rotator cuff.

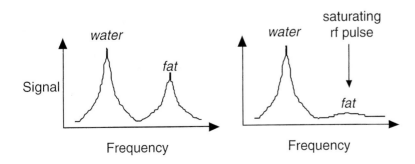

FIG. 30. Frequency-selective fat presaturation. In spectral fat suppression, a saturating RF pulse tuned specifically to the resonant frequency of fat is administered at the beginning of the pulse sequence. Effectiveness of this technique depends on homogeneity of the magnetic field and sufficient magnetic field strength to adequately separate the two resonant frequencies.

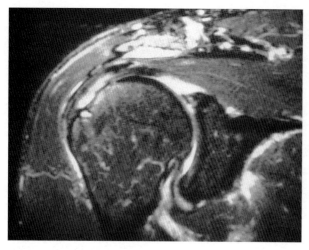

FIG. 31. Fat-suppressed T2-weighted fast spin-echo imaging. Homogeneous fat suppression on T2-weighted fast spin-echo images increases the sensitivity for marrow edema and most soft-tissue abnormalities, with the exception of certain calcified and fibrotic processes.

One approach to correcting this problem is to place fluid-filled pouches around the shoulder in an effort to correct the inherent anatomic irregularities. Even though commercially available devices specially designed for this purpose show promise, the approach does not always work. Shimming the magnet before imaging can improve the homogeneity of the field and therefore of fat suppression. In the past, this was too tedious and time consuming to be feasible for clinical use, but recently introduced autoshimming methods available on many state-of-the-art MRI systems allows this correction to be made in only a few seconds. Some patients' shoulders, however, are positioned very laterally and therefore are situated in a very heterogeneous portion of the magnetic field that is more difficult to shim. In such cases, or when autoshimming or special pouches are not available, an alternative method of fat suppression, such as STIR, may be necessary.

STIR

STIR imaging provides robust fat suppression that is less vulnerable to mild heterogeneities in the magnetic field (22,23) (Fig. 33). Additionally, the technique is extremely sensitive to the presence of free water protons and depicts both long T1 and long T2 substances with high signal intensity. However, conventional STIR is a lengthy imaging technique and offers relatively poor spatial resolution and anatomic coverage. The reduced number of slices available with STIR is particularly problematic in the axial plane. Fast STIR provides similar contrast more rapidly (24), but because it is a fast spin-echo technique, images acquired with a short TE can appear blurred (see Fig. 33). Blurring can be reduced by decreasing echo spacing and lengthening the TE, but this increases imaging time and magnetization transfer (MT) in the muscles associated with multislice fast spin-echo imaging, excessive signal loss in the soft tissues about the shoulder can actually reduce the overall interpretability of the image by obscuring anatomic landmarks (25).

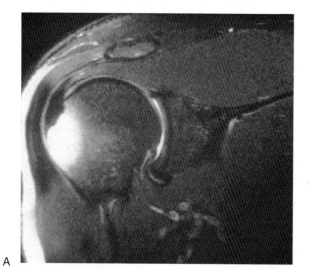

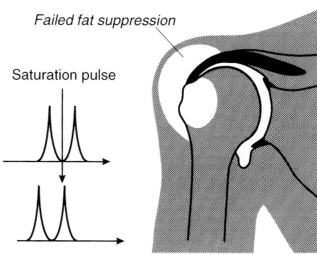

Failed fat suppression

Saturation pulse

A

B

FIG. 32. A and **B:** Failed frequency-selective fat suppression of the shoulder. The curved shape of the shoulder perturbs the static magnetic field and interferes with spectral fat suppression. Failure of fat suppression over the greater tuberosity on T2-weighted images results in local unmasking of high signal intensity marrow fat and may thus mimic traumatic, infectious, ischemic, or neoplastic disorders. Note the loss of signal from the deltoid muscle indicating inadvertent water suppression resulting from the extreme frequency shift in this region of the shoulder. Water suppression may extend over the insertion of the supraspinatus tendon and may thus obscure rotator cuff tendonitis or tear.

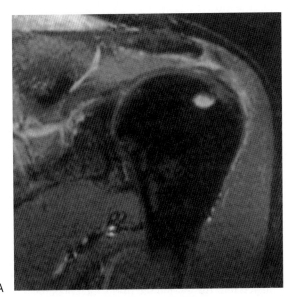 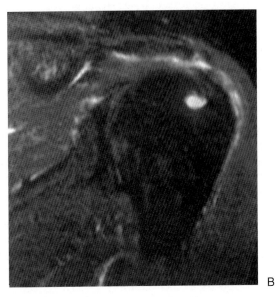

A   B

FIG. 33. STIR imaging of the shoulder. **A:** Conventional STIR images of the shoulder offer more homogeneous fat suppression and high sensitivity for free water, but they take longer to acquire and often suffer poor resolution. **B:** Fast STIR images require only a fraction of the imaging time required for conventional STIR, but also show even fat suppression and similar contrast. Fast STIR may, however, show blurring when short TEs are used, as in this case. Long TE fast STIR images show less blurring but exhibit signal loss because of T2 decay and magnetization transfer effects in skeletal muscle and other soft-tissues that may obscure anatomic landmarks and thus lower the interpretability of fast STIR images. Note the lower signal intensity in muscle on the fast STIR images relative to that on the conventional STIR images despite similar TE. This difference can be attributed to magnetization-transfer effects in fast STIR.

COLLAGEN-RELATED EFFECTS ON CONTRAST

Magnetization Transfer Contrast

Magnetization transfer, or saturation transfer as it is sometimes called, is a relaxation mechanism that under certain circumstances can cause signal loss in a variety of tissues, particularly those that contain collagen (26–30) (Fig. 34). Normally, all MRI signals are derived from mobile protons in water and fat. Protons in macromolecules, such as collagen, are relatively immobile and therefore show rapid T2 relaxation (<0.1 msec). Accordingly, even the shortest TE attainable with conventional MRI is too long to detect any signal from this restricted proton pool. This MRI-invisible macromolecular pool is, however, in thermodynamic equilibrium, both chemically and magnetically, with the MRI-visible pool in water. Therefore, effects on macromolecular protons can influence the status of protons in the water pool and thus affect the MR signal indirectly. Under certain conditions, macromolecular protons become selectively saturated. This evokes a transfer of longitudinal magnetization from the unsaturated water pool in order to maintain equilib-

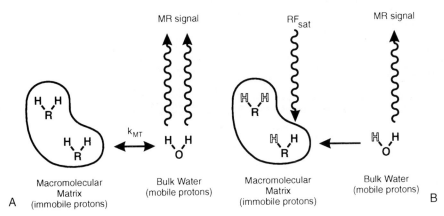

A   B

FIG. 34. Basic principles of magnetization transfer. **A:** Normal magnet equilibrium between immobile protons associated with macromolecules (MR-invisible) and mobile protons in bulk water (MR-visible). **B:** Selective saturation of immobile protons results in magnetization transfer from unsaturated water protons to the immobile protons, which manifests as a net loss of MR signal.

rium, consequently decreasing tissue signal in proportion to the relative concentrations of the two proton pools.

In a manner analogous to fat suppression, macromolecular protons can be selectively saturated with special pulse sequences that exploit differences in resonant frequency or relaxation time between the restricted and mobile pools. Accordingly, irradiation just off the resonant frequency of water produces strong MT effects in susceptible tissues. Alternatively, a series of short, intense binomial pulses timed in such a way as to selectively refocus long T2 species while dephasing the short T2 macromolecular protons (i.e., pulsed MT) can also be used (28,31). Some degree of MT effect occurs in conventional multislice spin-echo imaging as "waiting" slices are irradiated off-resonance during the selection of other slices (32). This effect is relatively small, however, because of the need for a minimal RF amplitude to saturate the restricted protons. Somewhat greater off-resonance radiation occurs with fast spin-echo sequences because several-fold more RF pulses are delivered per TR. The effect accordingly increases with the number of slices used (32).

These MT effects have a number of potential implications. First, tissue MT can be harnessed to generate contrast between structures that may otherwise appear isointense. As discussed previously, collagen is a strong substrate for MT. Therefore, MT sequences and multislice fast spin-echo suppress signal in hydrated, collagen-containing tissues, such as articular cartilage and skeletal muscle. MT may also suppress signal in granulation tissue, however, and thus lower

the diagnostic sensitivity of fast spin-echo for tendonitis. Although this has not yet been formally tested, it has been anecdotally noted in some cases of rotator cuff tendonitis (Fig. 35).

Magic Angle Phenomenon

Another important factor in determining the signal intensity of collagen-containing tissues is the orientation of the constituent collagen fibrils relative to the static magnetic field (B_0) (33–35). This phenomenon of angular anisotropy of T2 relaxation is known as the *magic angle phenomenon,* and was first described in tendons. Tendons are relatively acellular structures composed of densely arranged collagen fibers embedded in an amorphous ground substance. Much of the tensile strength of collagen derives from its highly organized microstructure: microfibrils of tropocollagen are arranged into fibrils, and the fibrils then organized into fibers. The regularity of this structure also confers an extremely short T2 relaxation time (<1 msec) to water protons constrained by collagen in tendons and other fibrous tissues (Fig. 36). Accordingly, normal tendons appear to have no signal on conventional MR images. Increased signal intensity within a tendon on T2-weighted images is always abnormal and indicative of rupture or active inflammation. Increased intratendinous signal on short TE images, such as T1-weighted and proton-density–weighted spin-echo se-

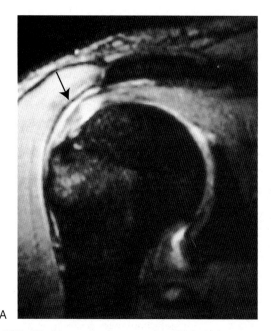
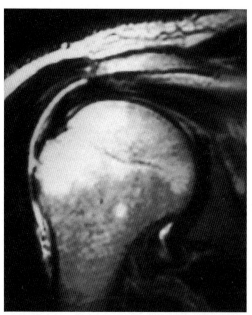

FIG. 35. Magnetization transfer effects in fast spin-echo imaging. **A:** T2*-weighted gradient echo image of the shoulder shows high signal intensity *(arrow)* indicative of tendinosis or partial tear within the otherwise intact supraspinatus tendon. **B:** On T2-weighted fast spin-echo images of the same shoulder, the elevated water signal in the supraspinatus tendon is markedly less detectable. (From Peterfy C, Linares R, Steinbach L. Recent advances in magnetic resonance imaging of the musculoskeletal system. *Radiol Clin North Am* 1994;32:291–311.)

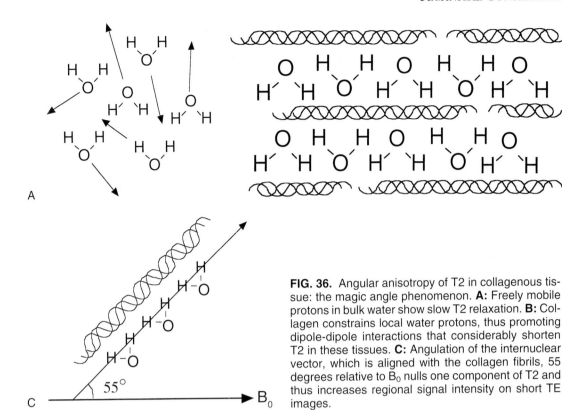

FIG. 36. Angular anisotropy of T2 in collagenous tissue: the magic angle phenomenon. **A:** Freely mobile protons in bulk water show slow T2 relaxation. **B:** Collagen constrains local water protons, thus promoting dipole-dipole interactions that considerably shorten T2 in these tissues. **C:** Angulation of the internuclear vector, which is aligned with the collagen fibrils, 55 degrees relative to B_0 nulls one component of T2 and thus increases regional signal intensity on short TE images.

quences and all gradient echo sequences, is generally considered indicative of so called "tendinosis" or myxoid degeneration. However, under certain conditions, the presence of intermediate signal within tendons on short TE sequences can be a normal finding (36) solely because of variation of tendon T2 relaxation with the orientation of the tendon relative to B_0 (i.e., angular anisotropy of T2 relaxation).

Because of structural anisotropy, T2 decay in tendons slows markedly as orientation of the tendons relative to B_0, which is aligned with the long axis of the magnet bore in most superconducting systems, approaches the magic angle of 55 degrees. Accordingly, under these conditions, signal emerges in tendons that otherwise have no signal as TE decreases below approximately 40 msec. In the shoulder, this phenomenon commonly manifests in the spinatus tendons where they pass through 55 degrees near their insertion on the greater tuberosity of the humerus (Fig. 37). The tendon of the long head of the biceps also exhibits this phenomenon as it curves over the humerus to insert on the superior glenoid rim and labrum (Fig. 38). Disappearance of intratendinous signal on long TE sequences distinguishes these magic angle effects from active tendinitis or rupture, which exhibit per-

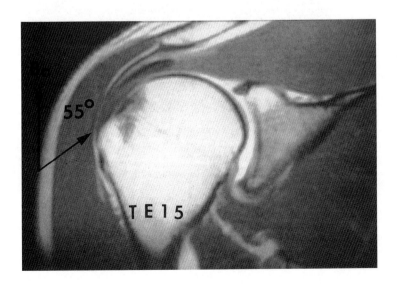

FIG. 37. Magic angle effects in the rotator cuff. T1-weighted oblique coronal image of the shoulder shows increased signal intensity due to magic angle phenomenon in the supraspinatus tendon where it curves through 55 degrees relative to B_0 to insert on the greater tuberosity.

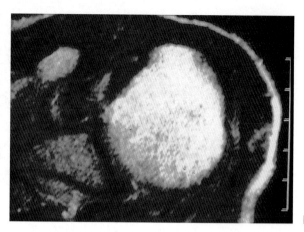

FIG. 38. Magic angle effects in the biceps tendon. **A:** T1-weighted axial image shows increased signal intensity *(arrow)* in the biceps tendon where the tendon begins to curve over the humeral head. **B:** Increased signal in the biceps tendon subsides as the TE becomes sufficiently long on the T2-weighted image.

sistently increased signal intensity on T2-weighted images. Reorientation of the tendons by abducting the arm can also reduce this potential artifact, but this is only feasible in magnets with an open-bore configuration. Magic angle effects are independent of the plane of section, and they are related entirely to the orientation of the tendon within the magnet bore.

The magic angle phenomenon is not exclusive to tendons but is a feature of most collagen-containing tissues, including ligaments (Fig. 39), menisci, labra (Fig. 40), and hyaline

articular cartilage. The implications of angle-dependent T2 relaxation must therefore be kept in mind while imaging these tissues. The magic angle phenomenon can be seen at several sites in the glenoid labrum, which contains circumferentially oriented collagen fibers. This may account for the rather poor sensitivity reported in the recent literature for MRI detection of labral tears. Options for evading these

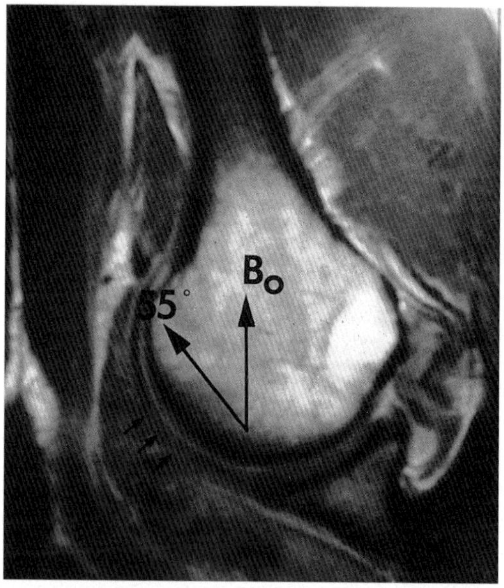

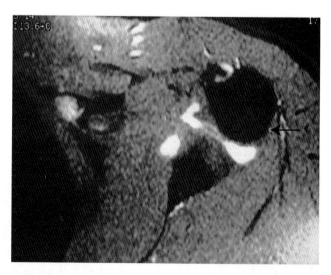

FIG. 40. Magic angle effects in the glenoid labrum. Axial T1-weighted spin-echo (TR = 500 msec, TE = 6 msec) image shows increased signal in the anteroinferior segment of the labrum *(arrow)* resulting from magic angle phenomenon. The labrum is well delineated in this case because of the presence of intraarticular gadolinium-containing contrast material from direct arthrography, but would otherwise contrast poorly against the isointense neighboring soft tissues. Increased labral signal can reduce the conspicuity of nondisplaced tears, and thus lower the sensitivity of short TE magnetic resonance imaging.

FIG. 39. Magic angle effects in the glenohumeral ligaments. T1-weighted oblique axial abducted and externally rotated image shows increased signal in a segment of the inferior glenohumeral ligament *(arrows)* where the ligament curves through 55 degrees relative to B_0.

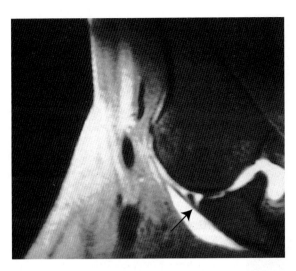

FIG. 41. Imaging the labrum in the abducted and externally rotated (ABER) position. Positioning the shoulder in ABER reorients the anteroinferior labrum *(arrow)* relative to B_0 and thus eliminates the effects of magic angle phenomenon. This increases the sensitivity of MRI for abnormalities of this important labral segment. Note the partial avulsion of the anteroinferior labrum still attached to the glenoid by its periosteal sleeve.

magic angle effects in the labrum are limited: long TE sequences are inherently insensitive for nondisplaced labral tear, rotating the body in the magnet does not reorient the labrum relative to B_0, and positioning the body transverse to B_0 is feasible only in open magnets. One option in circumferential whole-body magnets is to image the shoulder in ABER positioning (Fig. 41). Magic angle effect may still occur but at different sites in the labrum, and by comparing these images with those obtained with arm at the side, each labral segment can be thoroughly examined. Another alter-

native is to delineate the labrum with intraarticular contrast material, that is, by MR arthrography.

MAGNETIC RESONANCE ARTHROGRAPHY

There are two fundamental approaches to MR arthrography: (a) direct intraarticular injection of contrast material (15,16,37); and (b) indirect arthrography with intravenous Gd-containing agents (38). Direct MR arthrography has been the most widely used technique and is most analogous to other forms of arthrography. Typically, 15 to 20 mL of a 1/200 dilution of Gd-contrast in saline (100 μL in 20 mL) is injected directly into the glenohumeral joint under fluoroscopic guidance. This technique provides sufficient image contrast and joint distention to delineate the labrocapsular anatomy and other small structures on T1-weighted images (Fig. 42). Image contrast can be further augmented with frequency-selective fat suppression, as long as care is taken to ensure homogeneity of the field. STIR is not an appropriate method of fat suppression in this setting because T1 shortening by Gd lowers the signal intensity of the joint fluid and thus reduces image contrast. Also, because intraarticular injection of Gd-containing contrast material has not yet been formally ratified by the FDA, some researchers advocate injecting only saline into the joint and imaging with T2-weighted spin-echo or gradient echo sequences (Fig. 43).

The problem with direct MR arthrography is that the need for fluoroscopic guidance complicates the procedure and adds to its cost. One alternative is "indirect" MR arthrography (38), in which a normal dose of Gd contrast is injected intravenously and allowed to diffuse into the joint through the highly vascular synovial lining. Actively mobilizing the joint before imaging stimulates blood flow and diffusion, and speeds up the process considerably. Ten to 15 minutes of mobilization is usually sufficient to produce a substantial

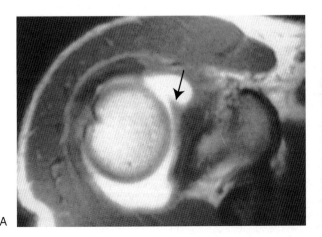

A

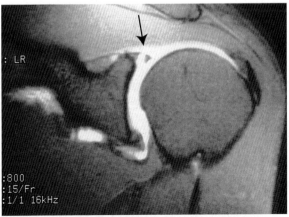

B

FIG. 42. Direct magnetic resonance arthrography with gadolinium (Gd)-containing contrast material. **A:** Axial T1-weighted spin-echo direct Gd arthrogram shows marked joint distention with high signal intensity fluid delineating small articular structures *(arrow)*. **B:** Fat suppression augments Gd contrast in oblique coronal T1-weighted spin-echo image showing a tear of the superior labrum *(arrow)*.

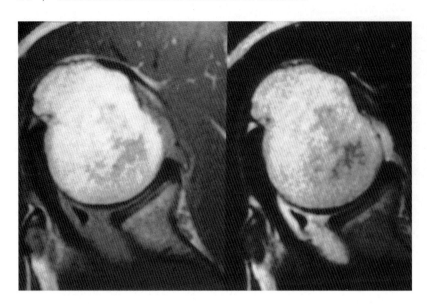

FIG. 43. Direct magnetic resonance arthrography with saline. Saline arthrography mimics a joint effusion and delineates articular structures better on T2-weighted images **(B)** than on proton-density–weighted images **(A)**.

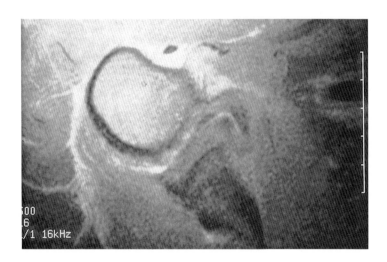

FIG. 44. Indirect magnetic resonance arthrography. Axial T1-weighted spin-echo image following intravenous injection of gadolinium-containing contrast shows contrast within the synovial fluid. Although the amount of contrast-enhanced fluid in the joint is scant and the joint is not distended, a thin film delineates the anteroinferior labrum despite local magic angle effects.[1]

---

[1] Imaging time scales as the inverse square of the improvement in S/N.

TABLE 4. *General protocol for magnetic resonance imaging of the shoulder*

Plane	Sequence	TR	TE	θ/TI	FOV	Matrix	Slice/gap	NEX	ETL
Axial	T2* GRE	500	24	20°	16	256 X 192	4/1	2	
Oblique coronal	T1 SE	500	12		14	256 X 192	4/1	2	
	T2 FSE + fat sat	3000	90		14	256 X 192	4/1	2	8
	FSTIR	2500	34	160°	14	256 X 192	5/1	2	8
Oblique sagittal	T2 FSE	3000	140		14	256 X 192	4/1	2	8
ABER	T2 FSE	3000	140		14	256 X 192	4/1	2	8

Parameters optimized for 1.5 T MRI. TR, TE and TI expressed in msec; field of view (FOV) expressed in cm; slice/gap expressed in mm.

NEX, number of excitations; ETL, echo train length; GRE, gradient echo; SE, spin-echo; FSE, fast spin-echo; STIR, short tau inversion recovery; *FSTIR,* fast STIR; ABER, abducted and externally rotated.

FSTIR is recommended if fat suppression fails on the T2 FSE sequence.

arthrographic effect and improve the delineation of labro-capsular structures (Fig. 44). However, enhancement is generally lower with this method than with direct MR arthrography, despite the larger and therefore more expensive dose of contrast material. Another limitation of the indirect technique is the lack of joint distention, which normally serves to separate adjacent labrocapsular structures. Also, intravenous administration of contrast material directly enhances a number of extraarticular structures, such as the subacromial bursa, thus eliminating extravasation of contrast as a useful diagnostic sign.

CONCLUSION

Based on the principles outlined in this chapter, one can propose the following general protocol for routine MRI of the shoulder (Table 4), accepting that a variety of different approaches may be equally valid, depending on local hardware and software constraints, the dynamics of the practice, and certain special needs of the referring physician or patient.

The protocol begins with an axial scan acquired with a T2*-weighted gradient echo sequence and high anatomic coverage. These axial images serve as localizers for the oblique-coronal scan, which is acquired with T1-weighted spin-echo and fat-suppressed T2-weighted fast spin-echo. Care must be taken to use a sufficiently high axial image to allow proper alignment of the oblique-coronal sections along the supraspinatus tendon. Autoshimming or special pouches may be necessary to ensure homogeneous fat suppression on the T2-weighted images. Alternatively, fast STIR could be used. Oblique sagittal T2-weighted fast spin-echo images are also obtained, with or without fat suppression. If fat suppression is not used, the TE should be long (e.g., 140 msec) to increase fat-water contrast. If oblique axial imaging with ABER positioning is also to be included, sequences should include T2-weighted fast spin-echo with long TE and no fat suppression, and/or MR arthrography. MR arthrography can be performed with saline and T2-weighted fast spin-echo or with Gd-contrast and T1-weighted spin-echo with fat suppression. MR arthrography is most informative in the axial and oblique coronal planes when using conventional positioning and in the oblique axial plane when ABER positioning is used.

As health care in the United States focuses increasingly on matters of cost and efficiency, there is growing pressure on radiologists to justify their practice methods. Of all the imaging tools available to them, none have the power and sophistication that MRI has for solving costly and frustrating medical problems. It is not surprising, therefore, that other physicians want to covet this technology. Proper use of MRI, however, requires considerably greater technical sophistication on the part of the physician and continuous effort to keep up with new developments in this rapidly paced field. It is

critical, therefore, that radiologists working with MRI make every effort to maintain a high level of sophistication with this modality in order to maximize their contribution to patient management as well as to ensure continued stewardship of this powerful technology by members of the radiologic community.

REFERENCES

1. Abragam A. *The principles of nuclear magnetism.* London: Oxford University Press, 1983.
2. Budinger T, Lauterbur P. Nuclear magnetic resonance technology for medical studies. *Science* 1984;226:288–298.
3. Haacke E, Tkach J. Fast MR imaging: techniques and clinical applications. *Am J Roentgenol* 1990;155:951–964.
4. Pykett I. NMR imaging in medicine. *Sci Am* 1982;246:78–88.
5. Young S. *Magnetic resonance imaging: basic principles.* New York: Raven Press, 1988.
6. König S, Brown R. Determinants of proton relaxation in tissue. *Magn Reson Imag* 1984;1:437–449.
7. Peterfy CG, Roberts T, Genant HK. Dedicated extremity MRI: an emerging technology. In: Kneeland JB, ed. *Radiol Clin North Am* 1996;24:1–20.
8. Hoult DI, Chen CN, Sank VJ. The field dependency of NMR imaging. *Magn Reson Med* 1986;3:722–746.
9. Boska MD, Hubesch B, Meyerhoff DJ, et al. Comparison of P-31 MRS and H-1 MRI at 1.5 and 2.0 T. *Magn Reson Med* 1990;13:228–238.
10. Rutt BK, Lee DE. The impact of field strength on image quality in MRI. *JMRI* 1996;6:57–62.
11. van Heteren JG, James TW, Bourne LC. Thin film high temperature superconducting RF coils for low field MRI. *Magn Reson Med* 1994;32:396–400.
12. Elister AD. Field-strength dependence of gadolinium enhancement: theory and implications. *AJNR* 1994;15:1420–1423.
13. Boorstein JM, Kneeland JB, Dalinka MK, Iannotti JP, Suh JS. Magnetic resonance imaging of the shoulder. *Curr Probl Diagn Radiol* 1992;21:7–27.
14. Davis SJ, Teresi LM, Bradley WG, Ressler JA, Eto RT. Effect of arm rotation on MR imaging of the rotator cuff. *Radiology* 1991;181:265–268.
15. Tirman PFJ, Bost FW, Garvin GJ, et al. Posterosuperior glenoid impingement: MRI and MR arthrographic findings with arthroscopic correlation. *Radiology* 1994;193:431–436.
16. Tirman PFJ, Bost FW, Steinbach LS, et al. MR arthrographic depiction of tears of the rotator cuff: benefit of abduction and external rotation of the arm. *Radiology* 1994;192:851–856.
17. Henning J, Nauerth A, Freidberg H. RARE imaging: a fast imaging method for clinical MR. *Magn Reson Med* 1986;3:823–833.
18. Listerud J, Einstein S, Outwater E, Kressel HY. First principles of fast spin echo. *Magn Reson Q* 1992;8:199–244.
19. Constable RT, Anderson AW, Zhong J, et al. Factors influencing contrast in fast spin-echo MR imaging. *Magn Reson Imag* 1992;10:497–511.
20. Henkelman R, Hardy P, Bishop J, et al. Why fat is bright on RARE and fast spin-echo imaging. *JMRI* 1992;2:533–540.
21. Anzai Y, Lufkin RB, Jabour BA, Hanafee WN. Fat-suppression failure artifacts simulating pathology on frequency-selective fat-suppression MR images of the head and neck. *AJNR* 1992;13:879–884.
22. Dwyer AJ, Frank JA, Sank VJ, et al. Short-TI inversion recovery pulse sequence: analysis and initial experience in cancer imaging. *Radiology* 1988;168:827–836.
23. Bydder GM, Young IR. MR imaging: clinical use of the inversion recovery sequence. *J Comput Assist Tomogr* 1985;9:659–675.
24. Fleckenstein JL, Archer BT, Barker BA, et al. Fast short-tau inversion-recovery MR imaging. *Radiology* 1991;197:499–504.
25. Smith R, Constable R, Reinhold C, McCauley T, Lange R, McCarthy S. Fast spin echo STIR imaging. *J Comput Assist Tomogr* 1994;18:209–213.

26. Woolf SD, Chesnick S, Frank JA, Lim KO, Balaban RS. Magnetization transfer contrast: MR imaging of the knee. *Radiology* 1991;179:623–628.
27. Yeung HN, Aisen AM. Magnetization transfer contrast with periodic pulsed saturation. *Radiology* 1992;183:209–214.
28. Hu BS, Conolly SM, Wright GA, Nishimura DG, Macovski A. Pulsed saturation transfer contrast. *Magn Res Med* 1992;26:231–240.
29. Hajnal JV, Baudouin CJ, Oatridge A, Young IR, Bydder GM. Design and implementation of magnetization transfer pulse sequences for clinical use. *J Comput Assist Tomogr* 1992;16:7–18.
30. Peterfy CG, Majumdar S, Lang P, van Dijke CF, Sack K, Genant H. MR imaging of the arthritic knee: improved discrimination of cartilage, synovium and effusion with pulsed saturation transfer and fat-suppressed T1-weighted sequences. *Radiology* 1994;191:413–419.
31. Miyazaki M, Takai H, Kojima F, Kassai Y. *Control of magnetization transfer effects in fast SE imaging.* Chicago: Radiological Society of North America, 1994:306.
32. Yao L, Gentili A, Thomas A. Incidental magnetization transfer contrast in fast spin-echo imaging of cartilage. *JMRI* 1996;6:180–184.
33. Erickson SJ, Cox IH, Hyde JS, Carrera GF, Strandt JA, Estkowski LD. Effect of tendon orientation on MR imaging signal intensity: a manifestation of the "magic angle" phenomenon. *Radiology* 1991;181:389–392.
34. Erickson SJ, Prost RW, Timins ME. The "magic angle" effect: background physics and clinical relevance. *Radiology* 1993;188:23–25.
35. Peterfy CG, Janzen DL, Tirman PFJ, van Dijke CF, Pollack M, Genant HK. Magic-angle phenomenon: a cause of increased signal in the normal lateral meniscus on short-TE MR images of the knee. *Am J Roentgenol* 1994;163:149–154.
36. Mirowitz SA. Normal rotator cuff: MR imaging with conventional and fat-suppression techniques. *Radiology* 1991;180:735–740.
37. Palmer WE, Brown JH, Rosenthal DI. Labral-ligamentous complex of the shoulder: evaluation with MR arthrography. *Radiology* 1994;190:645–651.
38. Vahlensieck M, Peterfy CG, Wischer T, et al. Indirect MR-arthrography: optimization and clinical applications. *Radiology* 1996;200:249–254.

Shoulder Magnetic Resonance Imaging,
edited by Lynne S. Steinbach, et al.
Lippincott–Raven Publishers, Philadelphia © 1998.

CHAPTER 3

MR Arthrography

Phillip F.J. Tirman

Magnetic resonance imaging (MRI) has become a popular imaging modality for investigation of the shoulder because of its inherent improved soft tissue contrast, oblique imaging plane capability, and excellent resolution using surface coils. Whereas conventional MRI allows direct visualization of major anatomic structures, smaller intraarticular structures, including the glenoid labrum, glenohumeral ligaments, and articular surface of the rotator cuff tendon, can be difficult to evaluate in the absence of a joint effusion. There is some controversy over the accuracy of MRI of the nondistended glenohumeral joint in detecting partial undersurface tears of the supraspinatus tendon and tears of the glenoid labrum and capsule (1–4). Several researchers have said that to improve the diagnostic accuracy of MRI, the glenohumeral joint should be distended with fluid before imaging (1,2,5–8). This chapter reviews the techniques used in performing MR arthrography, imaging characteristics of MR arthrography, and diagnostic utilization of the technique.

TECHNIQUE

Two standard techniques for direct MR arthrography and one indirect technique have been advocated. For direct arthrography, one technique uses dilute gadolinium diethylenetriamine pentaacetic acid (Gd-DTPA) and the other uses normal saline as the intraarticular contrast agents (1,6). Dilute gadolinium chelate is increased in signal intensity on

T1-weighted images in comparison with the decreased signal intensity of capsular structures and the tendons of the rotator cuff (Fig. 1). After the injection of intraarticular normal saline, intermediate and T2-weighted images demonstrate the glenohumeral joint surface anatomy similar to that seen in patients with a joint effusion during nonarthrographic evaluation (Fig. 2). Intravenous Gd-DTPA relies on the diffusion of gadolinium into the joint after the intravenous administration (9–12) (Fig. 3). This does not involve an injection into the joint and does not achieve joint distention, although the increase in signal intensity of joint fluid often helps delineate the labrum and capsule (10,11).

Arthrography Injection Technique

Shoulder injection techniques have been well described (5,13,14). We use the standard fluoroscopically guided anterior approach in which a 20-gauge spinal needle is placed into the joint. The injection is made between the glenoid and humerus in the lower third of the joint (5,13).

Dilute Gadolinium Chelate Technique

One milliliter of gadopentate dimeglumine (Magnevist: Berlex Laboratories, Wynne, New Jersey) in a concentration of 469.01 mg/mL is diluted into 200 mL of saline, and then approximately 12 to 20 mL of diluted gadopentate dimeglumine is injected (5,7). An easy method uses 0.1 mL of standard preparation Gd-DTPA (469.01 mg/mL) administered from a tuberculin syringe into a standard 20-mL vial of bacteriostatic saline. Gadolinium arthrography solution approximates the dilution found in the bloodstream after an intravenous injection

P. F.J. Tirman: Department of Radiology; and San Francisco Magnetic Resonance Center–St. Francis Memorial Hospital, University of California, San Francisco, San Francisco, California 94118-1944

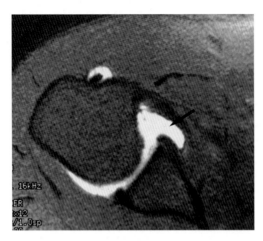

FIG. 1. Gadolinium arthrogram: Axial T1 weighted image with fat saturation after the injection of dilute gadolinium chelate demonstrates increased signal intensity fluid within the joint *(arrow)*.

and produces an increase in signal intensity on T1-weighted images. The patient's arm and shoulder are placed through a full range of motion and the patient returns to the MR unit where postinjection images are obtained. Imaging the patient within 1 hour helps ensure good joint distention with adequate gadolinium concentration. We have imaged up to 90 minutes after the injection without the use of intraarticular epinephrine and found the examination adequate.

Postinjection scan techniques are varied. Some imagers prefer the spin-echo T1-weighted images to provide crisp images with high spatial and contrast resolution. Other radiologists prefer gradient echo or volume images, allowing for thin sections and three-dimensional reconstruction. The preference depends not only on the radiologist but also on the type of MR imager, which sequences are available, and which sequences the imager performs best.

We prefer fat-saturated, T1-weighted axial, oblique coro-

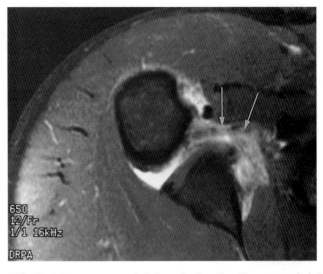

FIG. 3. Intravenous gadolinium (indirect) arthrogram: Axial T1-weighted image with fat saturation after the intravenous injection of gadolinium chelate demonstrates a torn subscapularis tendon *(arrows)* in this 35-year-old patient who suffered an anterior dislocation.

nal, and sagittal images and fast spin-echo (FSE) T2-weighted oblique coronal sequence with fat saturation. We complete the examination with abduction and external rotation (ABER) images using fat saturation.

Images obtained in the ABER position help in the detection of some undersurface tears of the rotator cuff, which may be occult in the neutral position even during arthrography (15) (Fig. 4). In the ABER position, the undersurface is free from the effacing force of the adjacent humeral head and flap tears may become displaced, allowing visualization. Additionally, imaging in the ABER position places traction on the inferior glenohumeral labral-ligamentous complex and may demonstrate an otherwise occult labral tear (5,16).

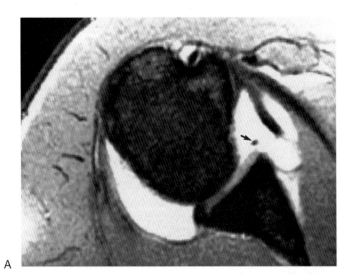

A

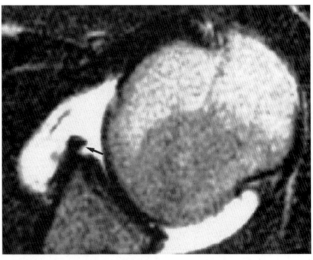

B

FIG. 2. Saline arthrogram. **A:** Gradient echo axial image through the mid portion of the joint. Fluid is of increased signal intensity on this T2*-weighted image just as in patients with a joint effusion. Note the small labral fragment *(arrow)* outlined by the fluid. **B:** Fast spin-echo T2-weighted axial image through the inferior portion of the joint. Saline acts the same as an effusion. Note the labral tear *(arrow)*.

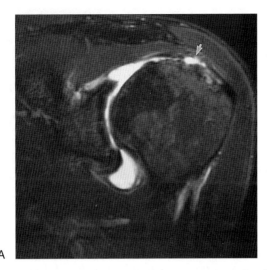
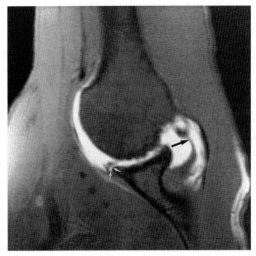

FIG. 4. Benefit of abduction and external rotation (ABER) in demonstrating and characterizing a rotator cuff tear. **A:** Fast spin-echo T2-weighted oblique coronal image with fat saturation demonstrates irregularity of the supraspinatus undersurface *(arrow)* consistent with fraying. **B:** ABER image demonstrates a large dissecting supraspinatus flap tear *(arrow)* and an unsuspected anterior labral tear *(small arrows)*.

If partial capsulolabral healing or complete healing of a tear occurs, the abnormality may go undetected (17). The joint may resynovialize the injury, making it occult at surgery (17). Placing stress on the stabilizing structures of the shoulder may bring out an otherwise undetected lesion (5,16).

This is true anteriorly and inferiorly with the use of the ABER position. ABER positioning stresses the inferior glenohumeral labral-ligamentous complex and "opens up" some partially healed or healed and incompetent labral-ligamentous attachments to the underlying glenoid (Fig. 5).

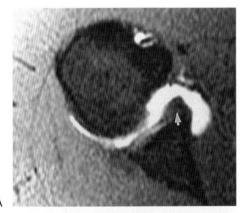
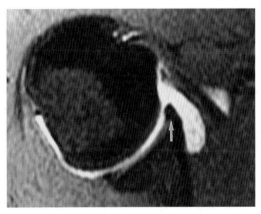

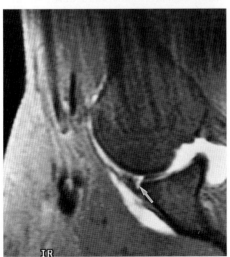

FIG. 5. A and **B:** Benefit of abduction and external rotation (ABER) in demonstrating an anterior labral tear. Axial MR arthrogram demonstrates a normal appearance to the anterior glenoid labrum *(arrows)*. **C:** Same patient as in **A** and **B** imaged in the ABER position. Note that the capsulolabral complex *(arrow)* is pulled away from the underlying glenoid. A large labral detachment was confirmed at surgery.

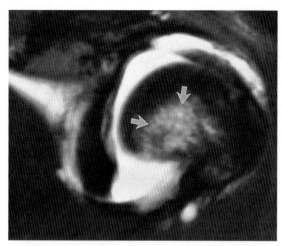
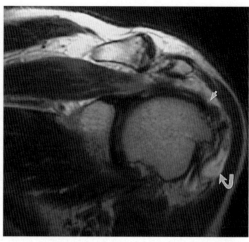

A

B

FIG. 6. A: Value of T2 weighting as a component of the arthrographic examination. Oblique coronal T2-weighted fast spin-echo (FSE) image with fat saturation demonstrates a bone trabecular injury of the anterior humerus *(arrow)* not seen on the T1-weighted images. This confirmed a suspected posterior subluxation. **B:** In another patient, oblique coronal T2-weighted FSE image demonstrates a superior surface rotator cuff tear *(arrow)* not seen on the T1-weighted arthrographic images. Note the associated bursitis *(curved arrow)*.

The T2-weighted sequence is beneficial for the evaluation of edema in structures around the joint, such as a trabecular injury of the humerus, which would be of decreased signal intensity on a T1-weighted image (Fig. 6). Also, superior surface tears of the supraspinatus that do not communicate with the joint are demonstrated using this sequence (see Fig. 6). Finally, labral cysts that have lost their communication with the joint are shown on the T2-weighted sequence.

Frequency-selective, fat-saturation techniques are beneficial when using T1-weighted sequences during dilute gadolinium arthrography (18,19). An important sign of a full-thickness tear of the supraspinatus is the observation of contrast agent within the subacromial subdeltoid bursa. Fat usually occupies this bursa and is bright on T1-weighted images. Because dilute gadolinium chelate is also increased in signal intensity on T1-weighted images, it is often difficult to diagnose with confidence a tear of the rotator cuff because contrast and fat are of similar signal intensity. Fat saturation makes signal intensity from fat decrease and removes potential confusion (18,19).

Saline Technique

In patients undergoing saline arthrography, 12 to 20 ml of sterile saline is injected until resistance is felt. The actual amount depends on the capacity of the shoulder capsule. One variation involves four to five cc of 60% iodinated contrast agent injected, followed by 8 to 15 cc of saline, allowing postexercise spot films to be obtained. The patient is then put through a simple range of motion exercise while on the way to the MRI suite.

FSE T2 images are then prescribed in three orthogonal planes: the oblique coronal, sagittal, and axial planes. We then routinely obtain FSE T2-weighted images using the ABER technique.

One potential problem with the use of the saline technique is that communication of an extraarticular fluid collection may be established with the joint. Addition of dilute gadolinium into the joint, resulting in an increase in signal intensity on T1-weighted images of an extraarticular fluid collection, confirms the communication. We therefore routinely use dilute gadolinium chelate as the contrast of choice.

Intravenous Gadolinium Technique

After the intravenous administration of 15 cc of gadopentate dimeglumine, the shoulder is exercised for 10 minutes. Exercise following the intravenous administration of gadolinium chelate encourages the development of a joint effusion and allows the diffusion of gadolinium chelate into the joint (9–12,20,21). This, in turn, allows the joint fluid to be imaged as increased signal intensity on T1-weighted MR images in contrast to the decreased signal intensity of the labrum, capsule, and rotator cuff. We then use the same imaging protocol as we did for dilute gadolinium chelate intraarticular arthrography.

PITFALLS

The most common problem with arthrography is extravasation of contrast material outside of the joint (Fig. 7). This commonly occurs through the subscapularis recess and through the thin posterior capsule. Extravasation can usually be avoided if 12 cc or less is injected into the joint. Radiologists must be careful not to underdistend the joint. Extravasation is commonly mistaken for pathologic capsular disruption, and radiologists should be careful to accurately identify the capsulolabral structures to avoid this problem.

The addition of air into the joint may also mimic intraar-

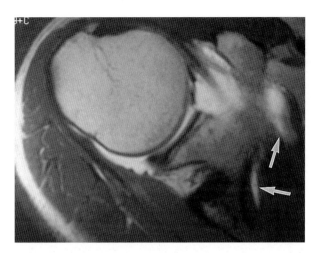

FIG. 7. Extravasation. T1-weighted arthrographic axial image demonstrates extravasation of contrast *(arrows)* medial to the coracoid process in this patient who underwent MR arthrography.

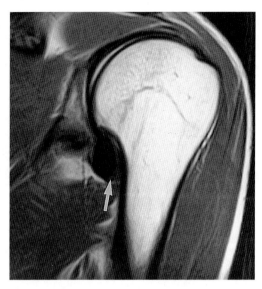

FIG. 9. Effect of too high a concentration of gadolinium. T1-weighted coronal arthrographic image demonstrates decreased signal intensity fluid within the axillary pouch *(arrow)*. The diffuse decrease in signal resulted from a mixture 1.5 cc of gadolinium to 20 cc normal saline, which caused marked T1 shortening.

ticular loose bodies (Fig. 8). Air gravitates to nondependent areas of the joint, whereas loose bodies are often located within the dependent portions and/or are surrounded by contrast elsewhere.

Use of full-strength gadolinium results in marked T1 and T2 shortening, which, in turn, leads to a marked decrease in signal intensity. In such a case, fluid is dark and of similar signal intensity to the decreased signal intensity of labrum, capsule, and rotator cuff (Fig. 9).

Although no difficulties have been reported with the use of fat saturation T1 sequences of the shoulder (18,19), we have encountered, especially on oblique coronal images, incomplete fat saturation can be caused by bulk susceptibility artifact. This artifact is caused by the curved external surface of the shoulder. This usually does not result in diagnostic difficulty except when the heterogeneous local magnetic field leads to a change in the frequency of water and fat within the

imaged volume and paradoxical partial water saturation occurs. This leads to loss of some detail of the supraspinatus insertion (22). In this setting, heterogeneous fat saturation could lead to the erroneous diagnosis of bony injury resulting from the persistence of increased fat signal from bone marrow of the humerus on fat-saturated T2-weighted images (Fig. 10). (See Chapter 2 for a more in-depth discussion on this artifact.)

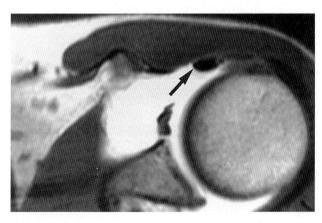

FIG. 8. Air bubble artifact. T1-weighted axial image with fat saturation demonstrates a rounded decreased signal intensity region *(arrow)*, which represented an air bubble artifact. Care must be taken to avoid the misdiagnosis of a loose body in this type of situation.

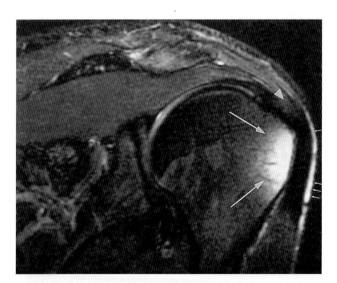

FIG. 10. Heterogeneous fat saturation. Fast spin-echo T2-weighted oblique coronal image with fat saturation demonstrates increased signal intensity within the greater tuberosity *(long thin arrows)*. This represented failure of fat saturation in this location rather than a bone trabecular injury. Note the paradoxical water saturation within the deltoid muscle, resulting in loss of signal intensity *(arrowhead)*. The subcutaneous fatty tissue *(small arrow)* has not saturated.

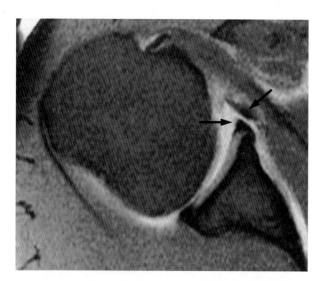

FIG. 11. Normal axial anatomy. T1-weighted arthrographic axial image demonstrates a normal anterior labrum *(arrow)* and middle glenohumeral ligament *(long arrow)*.

ARTHROGRAPHIC ANATOMY

Distending the glenohumeral joint with fluid allows diagnostic observations from a different perspective than from the nondistended joint, especially regarding the capsular structures and labrum.

Axial arthrographic images depict capsular and labral structures, the subscapularis insertion, and the biceps tendon within the intertubercular groove to the best advantage (Fig. 11).

In the neutral (conventional MRI) position, the inferior glenohumeral ligament complex (IGHLC) forms the axillary

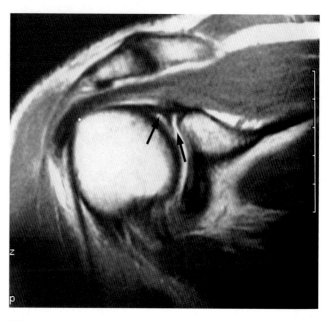

FIG. 13. Normal coronal image. T1-weighted arthrographic coronal image through the anterior portion of the joint demonstrates a normal biceps tendon insertion *(arrow)*. Note the small, normal sublabral recess *(small arrow)*.

pouch inferiorly, which is seen best in the distended state on oblique coronal images. The subscapularis bursa is present in 90% of individuals (23) and distends with the addition of intraarticular fluid. The usual communication with the joint occurs at an opening between the superior and middle glenohumeral ligaments (24,25), although an alternate or additional communication can exist at the level between the middle and inferior glenohumeral ligaments (26). The sub-

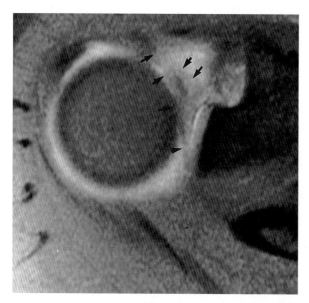

FIG. 12. Normal axial image. T1-weighted arthrographic axial image through the superior portion of the joint demonstrates a normal delta shaped biceps tendon insertion *(arrows)*.

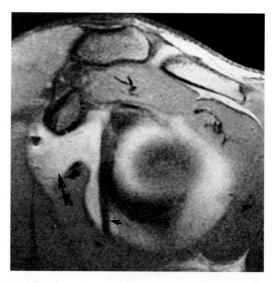

FIG. 14.. Normal sagittal image. T1-weighted arthrographic sagittal image demonstrates subcapsularis bursa saddle-bagged over the subscapularis tendon *(large arrow)*. Note the anterior band of the inferior glenohumeral ligament in this patient *(small arrow)*.

scapularis bursa commonly disrupts during the joint distention (see Fig. 7). This should not cause alarm and is not considered abnormal. The subscapularis tendon inserts into the lesser tuberosity and may be slightly lifted from its normal close approximation to the joint and lesser tuberosity by the fluid. The long head of the biceps tendon originates as a delta-shaped structure from the supraglenoid tubercle of the superior bony glenoid and courses through its intraarticular portion within the rotator cuff interval seen best on the superiormost axial images (Fig. 12). The tendon sheath communicates with the joint and usually fills with fluid during the arthrogram.

Oblique coronal images allow excellent visualization of the supraspinatus tendon, the intraarticular portion of the biceps tendon (also well seen on the oblique sagittal images), the biceps anchor, and the superior labrum (Fig. 13). A small layer of fluid can normally insinuate between the rotational cuff tendons and the hyaline articular cartilage of the humeral head.

Oblique sagittal images are useful to confirm rotator cuff

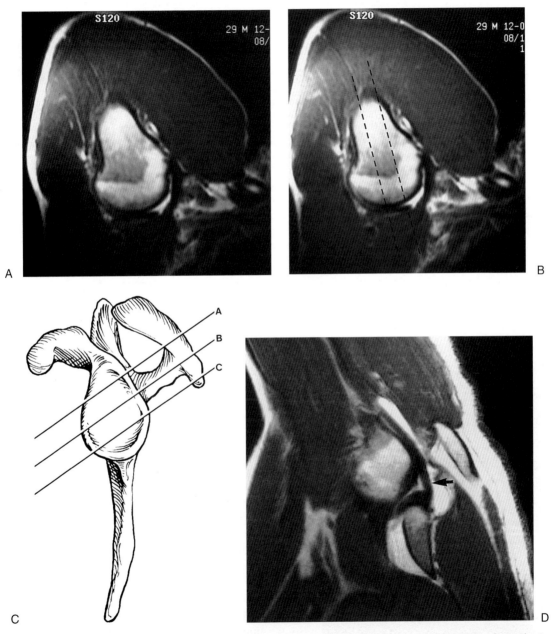

FIG. 15. Abduction and external rotation (ABER) anatomy. **A:** T1-weighted coronal localizer of a patient in the ABER position. **B:** Same image with prescription marks demonstrating the images to be obtained. The prescription marks should be oriented along the long axis of the humerus. **C:** Diagram showing the orientation of the resulting oblique axial images with respect to the scapula. **D:** ABER image of the superior joint. This image corresponds to *line A* on the diagram. Note the biceps insertion on this patient *(arrow). (Continued on next page.)*

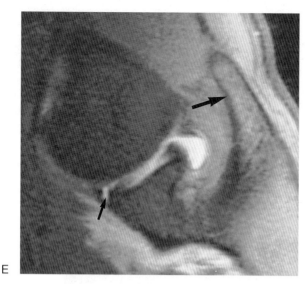

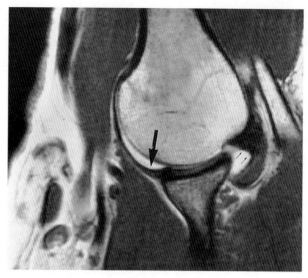

E   F

FIG. 15. *Continued.* **E:** ABER image through the mid joint. This image corresponds to *line B* on the diagram. Note the scapular spine *(large arrow)* for orientation purposes. The patient had a small labral tear *(small arrow).* **F:** ABER image through the inferior joint. This image corresponds to *line C* on the diagram. Note the normal inferior glenohumeral labral ligamentous complex insertion onto the glenoid *(arrow).* Note the normal appearing rotator cuff undersurface. (Compare to Fig. 4.)

tears and disease involving the intraarticular portion of the long head of the biceps tendon. Sagittal images are helpful in evaluating the joint cavity and bursa when searching for loose bodies. The subscapularis bursa may normally extend anteriorly over the subscapularis tendon, creating a "saddle-bag" of fluid lying underneath the coracoid process (Fig. 14).

ABER images are actually oblique axial images through the joint and oblique sagittal images with respect to the body.

The anatomy is best and most easily understood when considering the images as oblique axial to the joint (Fig. 15). For orientation purposes, it is easiest to locate the image that is oriented along the plane of the scapular spine (see Fig. 15*C*). The most useful images are then located inferior to this plane where the anterior inferior labral-ligamentous complex is shown in a position of stress and the infraspinatus undersurface is shown (Fig. 15*F*). ABER imaging may also improve detection of SLAP lesions (superior quadrant labral tear with anterior and posterior components of the tear) (Fig. 16).

ROTATOR CUFF ABNORMALITIES

Probably the most common reason to perform imaging of the shoulder is to define the status of the rotator cuff. Defining the anatomy related to impingement in order to help assess the cause and plan the treatment of disability caused by rotator cuff disease is an important reason for imaging. The spectrum of degeneration, partial tears, and full-thickness tears of the tendons of the rotator cuff can be evaluated with MRI with a relatively high degree of accuracy (27–30). Differentiating partial tears of the undersurface of the supraspinatus tendon from tendinitis/tendinosis or differentiating small partial tears of the undersurface from small full-thickness tears can be difficult. Unenhanced MRI does not perform as well in detecting partial tears as in detecting full-thickness tears (1,19,31). It was demonstrated that MR arthrography had greater diagnostic accuracy than standard MRI for partial tears involving the articular surface of the rotator cuff tendon (1,32) (Fig. 17). The sensitivity of T1-weighted MR arthrography alone was 71%, specificity 84%, and accuracy 78% when partial and full-thickness tears were

FIG. 16. SLAP lesion (superior quadrant labral tear with anterior and posterior components of the tear) on abduction and external rotation image. Note the contrast located within the posterosuperior labrum *(arrow).* The patient had a confirmed SLAP lesion at arthroscopy.

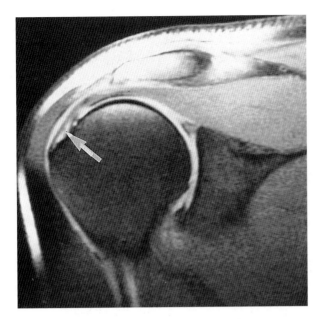

FIG. 17. Magnetic resonance arthrogram demonstrates a small undersurface partial tear of the rotator cuff *(arrow)*.

considered together versus 41%, 79%, and 61%, respectively, when intermediate and T2-weighted images were used alone. Palmer et al. (19) achieved a sensitivity and specificity of 100% in detecting full-thickness and partial tears of the rotator cuff using fat-suppressed T1-weighted arthrographic images. They also found that imbibition of contrast material into the undersurface of the cuff was representative of inflammation and degeneration, which may have implications on the surgical treatment. Tendons demonstrating imbibition are not treated as normal and are often debrided (19).

Evaluation of complete tears can also be enhanced with MR arthrography (Fig. 18). This is particularly useful if the

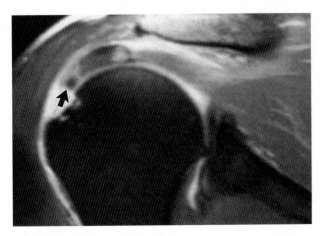

FIG. 18. Full-thickness tear. Magnetic resonance arthrogram coronal T1-weighted image with fat saturation demonstrates a full-thickness rotator cuff tear with retraction of the tendon edge medially *(arrow)*. The tendon edge is degenerated.

surgeon is interested in identifying not only the tendon tear but also the size of the tear and the condition of the tendon ends (i.e., the amount of retraction, fraying, or degeneration). As stated, extension of contrast material into the subacromial subdeltoid space confirms a full-thickness tear of the rotator cuff tendon.

In patients who have undergone prior rotator cuff surgery, MR arthrography allows more accurate evaluation for recurrent rotator cuff tear, because the rotator cuff tendon can have significant nonspecific signal alteration following rotator cuff surgery (32) (Fig. 19).

Glenohumeral Instability

The shoulder joint is considered to be the most unstable joint in the body (27,30,33). Conventional MRI has yielded mixed results in the detection of labral tears with sensitivities ranging from 44% to 90% and specificity in the range of 66% to 90% (3,4,27,34,35). MRI evaluation of capsular structures has been disappointing with respect to diagnosing instability based on capsular morphology and insertion (6,8).

Sometimes, on nonarthrographic examinations, the interface between the decreased signal intensity labrum and anterior capsule is indistinct and difficult to evaluate. This is often true in the absence of a joint effusion and is especially true in well-developed individuals such as athletes in whom muscular hypertrophy can lead to close adherence of the anterior capsule to the anterior labrum. Visualization of intraarticular surface anatomy is improved by the addition of contrast (saline or gadolinium-saline) when a paucity of joint fluid leads to difficulty in evaluating surface contours (6,36). Computed tomography (CT) arthrography is an accurate procedure in the evaluation of glenohumeral instability in which accurate delineation of anatomic derangement is necessary for surgical planning (23,37). MRI has the advantage of multiplanar imaging capability and improved soft tissue discrimination. In addition, MRI demonstrates pathologic changes within muscles, tendons, and bone, such as intrasubstance tears and bone marrow edema not shown by CT.

MR arthrography, in our experience, is most helpful in the evaluation of glenohumeral instability. The inferior glenohumeral ligamentous complex is well seen as a distinct structure. Lesions of the capsuloligamentous structures, including the anterior inferior labrum, are well defined by MR arthrography (Fig. 20). These lesions include labroligamentous detachments in the inferiormost portions of the IGHLC.

In 68 patients who underwent MR shoulder arthrography and either operative or arthroscopic therapy for a wide variety of shoulder complaints (6), sensitivity for the detection of labral tears was 89% and specificity was 98%—findings similar to some reported results obtained with unenhanced MR images (34,38,39). MR arthrographically demonstrated capsular ballooning, medial capsular insertion site, and capsular angle of insertion on the scapula, which were not found to correlate with instability examination under anesthesia

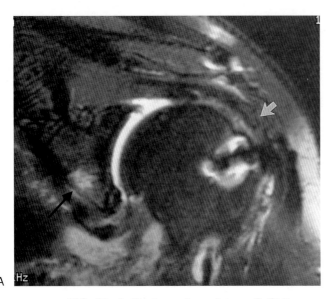
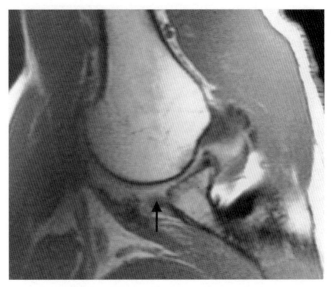

FIG. 19. A: Postoperative rotator cuff. Oblique coronal T2-weighted fast spin-echo image with fat saturation demonstrates an intact rotator cuff repair *(arrow)* after a fall. Note the bone injury of the glenoid seen only on the T2-weighted sequence *(long arrow)*. **B:** Postoperative labral tear. Note the torn detached labrum on this abduction and external rotation image *(arrow)*.

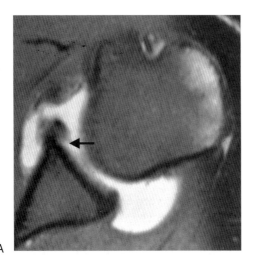
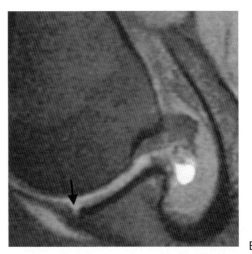

FIG. 20. Small labral tear seen at arthrography. T1 weighted arthrographic axial image demonstrates an attached but irregular anterior labrum. Abduction and external rotation image demonstrates the small labral tear *(arrow)*.

(6). Palmer (8) has also shown that capsular insertion type does not correlate with the presence of instability. Arthrographic imaging using the ABER technique further increases the sensitivity for accurate detection of labral tears to approximately 100% (5,16).

SLAP LESIONS

Snyder et al. (40) have described four types of superior labral tears anterior and posterior to the attachment of the biceps tendon. These types range from fraying and fragmentation to a bucket handle tear. MR arthrography may lift the torn labrum from the attachment to the glenoid and show insinuation of contrast material into the torn biceps anchor (see Chapter 8). In the case of the bucket handle variety of SLAP lesion, contrast may help define the fragment by lifting it from the remainder of the torn biceps anchor (Fig. 21). Care must be taken to avoid misinterpreting a sublabral hole for a SLAP lesion. This is often difficult and it may be necessary to offer a differential diagnosis.

CONCLUSION

Performing a complete MR shoulder arthrographic evaluation depends on many factors, including the following:

1. Obtaining an accurate history before the examination and being aware of the clinical suspicions. This helps determine whether to examine the patient using contrast material. Instability cases, especially in younger patients

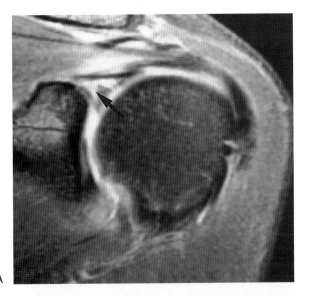
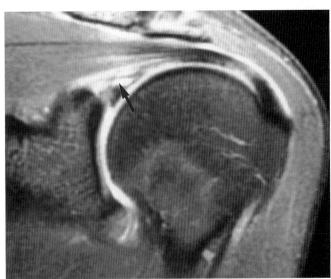
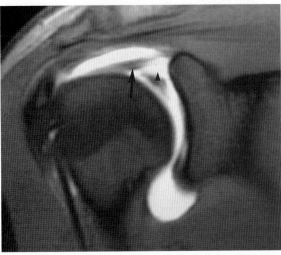
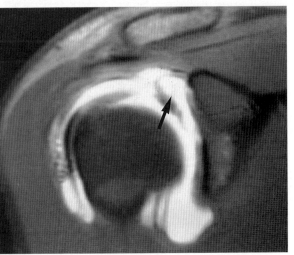

FIG. 21. SLAP lesions. **A** and **B:** Coronal T1-weighted arthrographic images with fat saturation demonstrate contrast extending into a large tear of the superior labrum *(arrows)*. **C:** Coronal T1-weighted arthrographic image with fat saturation demonstrates contrast filling a large tear of the superior labrum *(arrowhead)* at the location of the biceps tendon insertion. Note the biceps coursing through the superior joint *(arrow)*. **D:** Same patient as in **(C)**. Note the contrast extending into a large tear of the superior labrum *(arrow)*.

and in athletes of all ages, are often better served with an MR arthrogram.

2. Availability of a radiologist to perform and monitor the examination.

3. Proximity of a fluoroscopic suite. A readily available fluoroscopy room in close proximity facilitates performing shoulder injections after screening precontrast images; these examinations decrease MR scanner idle time and ensure more timely patient throughput for patients receiving precontrast examinations.

Suggested Indications

1. Instability, especially if damage to the IGHLC is suspected.

2. Partial tear versus tendinitis. Arthrography may not be necessary if change in treatment does not result from differentiation between the two.

3. Postoperative rotator cuff.

4. Further imaging evaluation of suspected abnormality on conventional MRI.

5. Evaluation of labral cysts to determine the patency of a suspected cyst–labral tear communication.

6. Labral variants—sublabral hole versus SLAP on conventional MRI.

7. Biceps anchor visualization.

8. Bursal characterization.

9. Intravenous technique can be chosen in cases of instability when intraarticular arthrography is not possible or practical.

REFERENCES

1. Flannigan B, Kursunoglu-Brahme S, Snyder S, Karzel R, Del Pizzo W, Resnick D. MR arthrography of the shoulder: comparison with conventional MR imaging. *Am J Roentgenol* 1990;155(4):829–832.

2. Hodler J, Kursunoglu-Brahme S, Flannigan B, Snyder SJ, Karzel RP, Resnick D. Injuries of the superior portion of the glenoid labrum involving the insertion of the biceps tendon: MR imaging findings in nine cases. *Am J Radiol* 1992;159:565–568.

3. Legan JM, Burkhard TK, Goff II WB, et al. Tears of the glenoid labrum: MR imaging of 88 arthroscopically confirmed cases. *Radiology* 1991;179(1):241–246.

4. Garneau RA, Renfrew DL, El MT, El-Khoury Y, Nepola JV, Lemke JH. Glenoid labrum: evaluation with MR imaging. *Radiology* 1991;179(2):519–522.

5. Tirman RM, Janecki CJ, Eubanks RG, Nelson CL. Shoulder arthrography. *Contemp Orthop* 1970;1:26.

6. Tirman PFJ, Stauffer AE, Crues JV, Turner RM, Schobert WE, Nottage WM. Saline MR arthrography in the evaluation of glenohumeral instability. *Arthroscopy* 1993;9(5):141–146.

7. Palmer WE, Caslowitz PL, Chew FS. MR arthrography on the shoulder: normal intraarticular structures and common abnormalities. *Am J Roentgenol* 1995;164(1):141–146.

8. Palmer WE, Caslowitz PL. Anterior shoulder instability: diagnostic criteria determined from prospective analysis of 121 MR arthrograms. *Radiology* 1995;197(3):819–825.

9. Drape JL, Thelen P, Gay DP, Silbermann O, Benacerraf R. Intraarticular diffusion of Gd-DOTA after intravenous injection in the knee: MR imaging evaluation. *Radiology* 1993;188(1):227–234.

10. Magre G. The use of intravenous gadolinium followed by exercise in the MRI evaluation of the shoulder. 1994, Personal communication.

11. Winalski CS, Aliabadi P, Wright RJ, Shortkroff S, Sledge CB, Weissman BN. Enhancement of joint fluid with intravenously administered gadopentetate dimeglumine: Technique, rationale, and implications. *Radiology* 1993;187(1):179–185.

12. Yamato M. Intravenous MR arthrography of the knee. *Nippon Igaku Hoshasen Gakkai Zasshi* 1995;55(7):466–469.

13. Tirman RM, Nelson CL, Tirman WS. Arthrography of the shoulder joint: state of the art. *Crit Rev Diagn Imaging* 1981;17:19–76.

14. Freiberger RH, Kaye JJ. *Arthrography*. New York: Appleton-Century-Crofts, 1979.

15. Tirman P, Bost F, Steinbach L, et al. MR arthrographic depiction of tears of the rotator cuff: benefit of abduction and external rotation of the arm. *Radiology* 1994;192(3):851–856.

16. Cvitanic O, Tirman PFJ, Feller JF, Stauffer AE, Carroll K. Can abduction and external rotation of the shoulder increase the sensitivity of MR arthrography in detecting anterior glenoid labral tears? *Am J Roentgenol* 1997;169:837–844.

17. Neviaser TJ. The anterior labroligamentous Periosteal sleeve avulsion Lesion: a Cause of anterior Instability of the Shoulder. *The Journal of Arthroscopic and Related Surgery* 1993;9(1):17–21.

18. Fritz RC, Stoller DW. Fat-suppression MR arthrography of the shoulder. *Radiology* 1992;185:614–615.

19. Palmer WE, Brown JH, Rosenthal DI. Rotator cuff: evaluation of fat-suppressed MR arthrography. *Radiology* 1993;188:683–687.

20. Daenen B, Chevrot A, Vallee C, et al. MRI of the knee. Value of delayed sequences after intravenous injection of gadolinium. *J Radiol* 1994;75(3):173–176.

21. Jerosch J, Lahm A, Castro WH, Assheuer J. Intravenous administration of gadolinium DPTA in proton spin tomography of the knee joint. *Z Orthop Ihre Grenzgeb* 1993;131(2):173–178.

22. Peterfy CG. Recent advances in magnetic resonance imaging of the musculoskeletal system. *Rad Clin* 1994;32:291–311.

23. Rafii M, Firooznia H, Golimbu C, Minkoff J, Bonamo J. CT arthrography of capsular structures of the shoulder. *Am J Roentgenol* 1986;146(2):361–367.

24. Kursunoglu-Brahme S, Resnick D. Magnetic resonance imaging of the shoulder. *Radiol Clin North Am* 1990;28(5):941–954.

25. Zlatkin MB, Bjorkengren AG, Gylys MV, Resnick D, Sartoris DJ. Cross-sectional imaging of the capsular mechanism of the glenohumeral joint. *Am J Roentgenol* 1988;150(1):151–158.

26. DePalma AF, Callery G, Bennett GA. Shoulder joint: variational anatomy and degenerative lesions of the shoulder. *Instr Course Lect* 1949.

27. Crues JV, Ryu RK. The shoulder. In: Stark D, Bradley WG, eds. *Magnetic resonance imaging*. St Louis: Mosby, 1991:2424–2458.

28. Crues JV, Fareed DO. Magnetic resonance imaging of shoulder impingement. *Top Magn Reson Imaging* 1991;3(4):39–49.

29. Tyson LL, Crues JVI. Pathogenesis of rotator cuff disease. *MRI Clin North Am* 1993;1:37–48.

30. Zlatkin MB. *MRI of the shoulder*. New York: Raven Press, 1991:174.

31. Seeger LL, Gold RH, Bassett LW, Ellman H. Shoulder impingement syndrome: MR findings in 53 shoulders. *Am J Roentgenol* 1988;150:343–347.

32. Hodler J, Kursunoglu-Brahme S, Snyder SJ, et al. Rotator cuff disease: assessment with MR arthrography versus standard MR imaging in 36 patients with arthroscopic confirmation. *Radiology* 1992;182(2):431–436.

33. O'Brien SJ, Warren RF, Schwartz E. Anterior shoulder instability. *Orthop Clin North Am* 1987;18:395–408.

34. Coumas JM, Waite RJ, Goss TP, Ferrari DA, Kanzaria PK, Pappas AM. CT and MR evaluation of the labral capsular ligamentous complex of the shoulder. *Am J Roentgenol* 1992;158:591–597.

35. Seeger LL, Gold RH, Bassett LW. Shoulder instability: evaluation with MR imaging. *Radiology* 1988;168(3):695–697.

36. Palmer WE, Brown JH, Rosenthal DI. Labral-ligamentous complex of the shoulder: evaluation with MR arthrography. *Radiology* 1994;190:645–651.

37. Rafii M, Minkoff J, Bonamo J, et al. Computed tomography (CT) arthrography of shoulder instabilities in athletes. *Am J Sports Med* 1988;16(4):352–361.

38. McCauley TR, Pope CF, Jokl P. Normal and abnormal glenoid labrum: assessment with multiplanar gradient-echo MR imaging. *Radiology* 1992;183(1):35–37.

39. Kieft GJ, Bloem JL, Rozing PM, Obermann WR. MR imaging of recurrent anterior dislocation of the shoulder: comparison with CT arthrography. *Am J Roentgenol* 1988;150(5):1083–1087.

40. Snyder SJ, Karzel RP, Del Pizzo W, Ferkel RD, Friedman MJ. SLAP lesions of the shoulder. *Arthroscopy* 1990;6(4):274–279.

Shoulder Magnetic Resonance Imaging,
edited by Lynne S. Steinbach, et al.
Lippincott–Raven Publishers, Philadelphia © 1998.

CHAPTER 4

Shoulder Biomechanics

David P. Adkison

BONY STABILITY

The bony anatomy of the glenohumeral joint contributes to overall shoulder stability (1,2). A maximum of 30% of the articular cartilage of the humeral head articulates with the articular cartilage of the normal glenoid at any time, but the concavity of the glenoid resists anterior/posterior translation. Even though Saha (3) attributed greater degrees of stability to glenohumeral articulations with greater congruity, there has only recently been biomechanical data to support such a relationship. Howell and Galinat (1) reported the average anteroposterior depth of the bony glenoid to be only 2.5 mm, whereas the average superior/inferior depth was 9.0 mm. The labrum, discussed later, deepens the glenoid articulation by 2.5 mm; providing a secure attachment site for this specialized tissue is probably the most important function of the normal glenoid.

The 30-degree retroversion of the normal humeral head, which articulates against the 7-degree retroversion of the normal glenoid, is, according to Morrey (2), necessary for proper ligament tension and does not usually contribute to posterior glenohumeral instability.

An indirect contribution to shoulder stability by the glenoid and humeral head is through maintenance of a relatively constant capsule volume and ligament tension. Patho-

logic loss of bone stock, especially of the posterior glenoid and of the humeral head, can contribute to instability. Practically, however, this is only rarely or transiently a problem because the capsule and ligaments shorten in the chronic arthritic shoulder.

MUSCULAR STABILITY

Scapulothoracic Muscles

The large muscles responsible for orientation of the scapula on the thoracic wall have an important contribution to shoulder stability. The latissimus dorsi, serratus anterior, pectoralis major, and deltoid are ideally suited to generate large torques about the shoulder joint by virtue of their cross-sectional anatomy and effective distance from the joint center of rotation. They are able to stabilize the shoulder joint against excessive retraction or protraction during vigorous activity, such as making a football tackle or performing a bench press.

An excellent study from the Kerlan-Jobe clinic demonstrated that weakness of the serratus anterior and/or the subscapularis predispose to the development of rotator cuff tendinitis symptoms in young baseball pitchers (4). Rotator cuff symptoms presumably develop because the antishear rotator cuff muscles are forced to function against a scapula that is improperly oriented with respect to the thorax, causing increased stress in the cuff musculature and underlying liga-

D. P. Adkison: Department of Orthopaedic Surgery, National Naval Medical Center, Bethesda, Maryland 20889

ments. If left unchecked, atraumatic shoulder instability can develop.

Restoration of the proper function of the large scapular rotators is the basis for modern techniques for rehabilitating the shoulder with rotator cuff tendinitis. There is little role for classic rotator cuff rehabilitation techniques in the young athlete.

Rotator Cuff Muscles

Just as the large scapulothoracic muscles are ideally suited to generate large torques and resist large forces, the rotator cuff muscles are well positioned as glenohumeral antishear muscles. They are located closer to the center of joint rotation and are intimately associated with underlying capsular ligament structures.

Large torques invariably generate shear forces across the glenohumeral joint because they are not applied through the centers of rotation of both the glenoid and humeral head. These shear forces are of much less magnitude than the torques but can still be significant. Thus, the rotator cuff can be thought of as a fine control muscle system, constantly adjusting through neuromuscular feedback systems in response to the torques required for gross motion of the shoulder.

By virtue of this fine control, the cuff muscles also act as pretensioners or cotensioners for the capsular ligaments; for example, the shoulder is in extension, external rotation, and abduction when a ball is thrown forcefully. The subscapularis, an internal rotator when concentrically contracted and a decelerator of external rotation when eccentrically contracted, cotensions the inferior glenohumeral ligament complex (IGHLC). That is, it prevents the end point of ligament function from being reached or compromised. This concept may explain why atraumatic instability develops in pitchers with subscapularis weakness as the IGHLC becomes progressively stretched.

The rotator cuff muscles also can provide some degree of compressive force across the glenohumeral articulation. By forcing the humeral head deeper into the concavity of the glenoid, rotator cuff muscles should be able to decrease shear forces and keep the head centered. This antishear function is probably facilitated by both selective contraction of cuff muscles through mechanical receptor stimuli and through the compression-concavity mechanism.

LIGAMENTOUS AND LABRAL STABILITY

Ligaments

Functionally, it is helpful to think of the glenohumeral ligaments as check reins (5). In theory, they remain essentially lax until the limit of a designated range of motion is approached, at which time they become increasingly taut and check the motion from going further. Loss of ligament competence would then be the basis for end-range instability, a concept discussed later. This is certainly a valid concept for the IGHLC in the early stages of traumatic anteroinferior glenohumeral instability, but ligamentous insufficiency in chronic instability is probably more complex and subtle.

Each of the glenohumeral ligaments primarily resists at least one humeral head motion: The superior glenohumeral ligament resists inferior translation with the adducted arm in neutral rotation; the middle glenohumeral ligament resists external rotation in the neutral adducted shoulder and resists

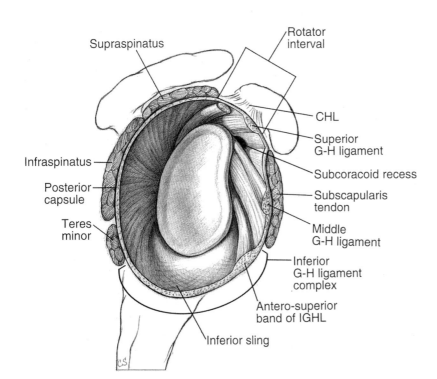

FIG. 1. Cross-sectional anatomy of the glenohumeral joint. (From Boardman, Fu. Shoulder biomechanics. In: McGinty JB, Caspari RB, Jackson RW, Poehling GG, eds. *Operative arthroscopy.* 1996;628.)

anterior translation in the shoulder abducted to 45 degrees; the inferior glenohumeral ligament complex resists anteroinferior humeral head translation, especially with the arm in external rotation, abduction, and extension. The coracohumeral ligament resists posterior and inferior translation in the suspended shoulder (Fig. 1).

More poorly understood is how these ligaments interact during complex shoulder motions that involve shifts in the centers of rotation or in translation, or how they interact during the middle ranges of motion. Sidles (5) has hypothesized a phenomenon of complementary tightening, which no longer assumes ligament function based on just a single center of rotation, but rather it conceptualizes tightening of ligaments or capsular segments in response to eccentric joint alignment. Therefore, the tension developed in the IGHLC causes a tightening of the posterior capsular structures to balance the static anterior restraint of the IGHLC. This concept is vital to current theories of shoulder instability, because ligaments that normally functional to stabilize the ligamentously well-balanced shoulder can actually participate in destabilizing the injured shoulder (Fig. 2).

Karduna et al. (6) assert that ligaments are essentially lax during the mid ranges of motion when muscle forces are the primary stabilizers. Their research focuses on the origin to insertion function ligament length (wrap length). In external rotation, long wrap lengths of the inferior glenohumeral ligament were associated with increased passive posterior glenohumeral translation.

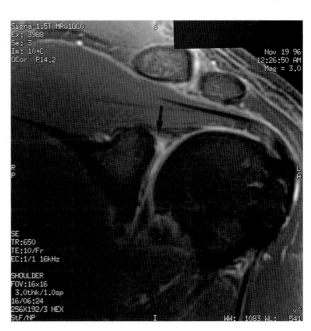

FIG. 3. Intravenous gadolinium-enhanced MR image demonstrating a type II SLAP lesion *(arrow)*, with elevation of the superior labrum.

Labrum Associated Stability

Even though the labrum does deepen the glenoid by as much as 100%, providing up to 35% of the total resistance to translation, the degree of such stability is largely dependent on joint compressive forces, labral compliance, and articular integrity. The labrum has two primary mechanical functions. First, it serves as the glenoid attachment site for the glenohumeral ligaments. Even though there are a few anatomic exceptions (such as the so-called Buford complex), the labrum is usually contiguous with the glenohumeral ligaments and is distinct from the glenoid. This histologic and gross distinction is the anatomic basis for the Bankart lesion, an end-range failure of the IGHLC resulting in avulsion of the anteroinferior labrum from the glenoid.

A second function of the labrum, probably more important in the mid ranges of shoulder motion, is that of an antishear bumper (7). The slight deepening effect and mobility of the labrum probably serve to help keep the humeral head centered in the glenoid. This may have different degrees of importance in different directions of motion. For instance, long head biceps origin instability (known as the type II SLAP lesion) may represent a loss of the superior bumper effect of the superior labrum as well as a loss of effective depressor function from the biceps tendon (Fig. 3).

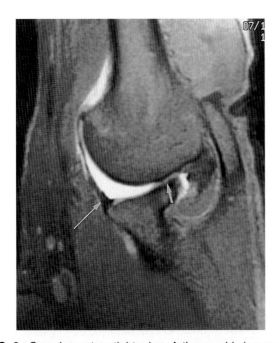

FIG. 2. Complementary tightening. Arthrographic image obtained in abduction and external rotation with anterior laxity. Notice the posterior subluxation of the joint with the contact point between the humeral head and glenoid *(short arrow)* more posteriorly located than usual. The anterior labrum/ligamentous attachment was normal *(long arrow)*.

BICEPS TENDON/ORIGIN STABILITY

Even though the role of the biceps tendon in shoulder stability has been minimized by some investigators, loss of the biceps induces increased forces in glenohumeral ligaments

(8) and is associated with a superior shift in the glenohumeral articular contact point. The biceps functions as an effective humeral head depressor, maintaining proper ligament tension in some of the glenohumeral ligaments as predicted by the complementary tightening concept of shoulder stability.

Even though most studies have examined the role of the biceps in the resting shoulder position of neutral rotation and adduction, the biceps is an effective stabilizer in other positions.

ACTIVE VERSUS PASSIVE STABILITY

Basis of Active Stability

Active stability is primarily a function of neuromuscular control. The scapulothoracic muscles orient the shoulder joint in positions that, ideally, minimize risk of instability. Rapid neural feedback in response to forces that could induce risk of ligament failure probably cause an appropriately protective reaction in most shoulders. Fu et al. (9) have recently demonstrated a loss of proprioceptive competence in unstable shoulders.

Basis of Passive Stability

In the relaxed shoulder, the humeral head is maintained centrally within the glenoid by the interaction, both actively and passively, of numerous structures. The rotator cuff, acting via capsular attachments and by direct bony insertions, provides both compressive and antishear forces. It additionally acts superiorly as a spacer when other superior constraints are lost.

Whereas active stability is primarily a function of muscle control, passive stability of the glenohumeral joint is primarily a function of the capsular, ligamentous, and labral anatomy. According to Sidles (5), the key ingredients to passive stability are a competent sealed capsule of appropriate volume, minimal joint fluid, and an intact congruent glenoid labrum (hence, normally attached ligaments).

Furthermore, the capsular ligaments must be balanced to provide passive stability during the dynamics of shoulder motion. There is increasing evidence that, for instance, in cases of inferior shoulder instability, an interplay between several variables dictates the etiology and resulting treatment options. Both rotator interval lesions, with underlying coracohumeral ligament insufficiency, and superior labral instability may contribute to inferior instability. When incompetence of either structure coincides with an increased infraglenoid capsular volume, the patient should be at increased risk for inferior instability, even in the absence of an inferior labral lesion. Indeed, Pagnani et al. (8) have shown that creation of superior labral instability causes increased tension in the inferior glenohumeral ligament complex.

END-RANGE VERSUS MID-RANGE STABILITY

The glenohumeral ligaments are usually lax when the humeral head is centered within the glenoid and when the shoulder is being moved from the resting neutral position up to end-ranges of motion. As the shoulder approaches the limits of its ranges of motion, the ligaments become progressively tighter, finally acting as check reins at the ends of motion. Therefore, forces applied to the shoulder that would increase end-range motions produce pathologic laxity as the ligaments acutely or chronically lose their ability to prevent such a motion. A force that increases the range of external rotation, extension, and abduction may produce the sudden failure of the inferior glenohumeral ligament complex known as a *Bankart lesion,* with its resulting avulsion of the glenoid labral attachments of the ligament complex.

A more subtle and repetitive forcing of end-range motion, such as in pitching a baseball, might lead to more gradual failure of ligament check-rein function; such failure could occur anywhere along the course of the ligament complex, depending on joint reaction forces, joint instant center of rotation, and associated stresses induced in other ligaments. Bankart lesions have been documented in persons who have shoulder injury from repetitive stresses and have never sustained a shoulder dislocation. However, a more likely finding in such a person would be that of increased ligament length and, subsequently, capsular volume. This increased volume is presumably the result of repetitive interstitial ligament injury with stretching and remodeling.

As capsular volume reaches some critical point, the shoulder can become unstable before reaching end ranges, that is, in the mid ranges. It is at this phase that patients may be categorized as having multidirectional shoulder instability complicating their traumatic unidirectional instability. Patients may complain of the shoulder beginning to dislocate during sleep or during routine daily activities in positions that are not normally thought to be "at-risk" positions. This characteristic may be shared with another subset of patients who have congenital joint hyperlaxity and a lifelong history of joint subluxations. Clinicians must be careful to distinguish between the subsets because the latter group almost never requires surgical stabilization whereas the former group may require a complex stabilization procedure.

Lax ligaments fail to cause the humeral head to translate as it normally should with prescribed positions. When the normal shoulder is externally rotated, extended, and abducted, the articular center of rotation experiences obligate translation of several millimeters posteriorly through the check-rein action of the inferior glenohumeral ligament complex. Patholaxity of this ligament fails to cause obligate translation, allowing the head to remain in a relative anterior position. The resulting sensation of anterior subluxation or impending dislocation is the basis for the so-called apprehension sign. The reduction or "relocation" maneuver reduces the humeral head to the proper rotation center location for a given motion.

PATHOMECHANICS

Articular Surface

Probably the most important distinction to make with regard to the articular surface is whether surface incongruities cause catching or grinding and thus simulate subluxations. Ellman (10) has noted that even partial thickness articular chondrosis may be associated with inferior glenohumeral osteophytes and that these should be noted on plain radiographs. When articular degeneration is the source of pain or catching, forcing the articular surfaces together in the grind test should elicit pain.

When severe humeral head collapse is a source of instability, the diagnosis should be obvious.

Muscular Instability

As discussed, weakness of the major scapular rotators is associated with rotator cuff tendinitis and glenohumeral instability. Dynamic scapular winging or insufficient functional scapular protraction can be a difficult diagnosis to make without the aid of electrodiagnostic studies.

Rotator cuff dysfunction does not typically cause a sensation of instability, but rotator cuff tears are secondarily associated with instability for the reasons discussed previously. Nirschl et al. (11) have demonstrated a high incidence of supraspinatus undersurface tears with anterosuperior labral lesions; Field and Savoie (12) also reported a high incidence of rotator cuff tears in association with unstable SLAP lesions. In a cadaver study, Garcia et al. (13) found no shoulders with isolated rotator cuff pathology; most specimens with cuff tears also had a labral injury.

There seems to be increasing evidence that rotator cuff tendinitis and dysfunction is initiated by glenohumeral instability in some direction and that there is little evidence for the widely held concept that acromion shape is causal in many cases of the so-called impingement syndrome. Even though acromioclavicular osteophytes can conceivably impinge on the rotator cuff, most nonarthritic acromions are concentric with the humeral head.

Burkhart (14) has demonstrated posterior rotator cuff scuffing over the posterior glenoid margin with anterior shoulder instability. Nirschl et al. found few hooked (type III) acromions in their study with 80 rotator cuff tears. A prospective, blinded study of acromion type in persons younger than age 40 years with symptomatic and asymptomatic shoulders found no difference in the incidence of acromion type between those with or without impingement syndrome (15).

Therefore, the presence of rotator cuff tendinitis or impingement syndrome, especially in young persons, should be a sign to look for labral injury, increased capsular volume, or other evidence of instability.

Ligamentous Instability

Because the ligaments, along with the labrum, serve to passively keep the humeral head centered or predictably translated with motion (16), ligamentous instability can be considered to be a loss of humeral head obligate translation. It follows that the normal complementary tightening mechanism would also be compromised with pathologic translation, perhaps even contributing to instability as the ligaments become imbalanced. The imbalance may lead to proprioceptive confusion on the patient's part about the direction of instability.

Biceps Instability

Biceps long head instability, the so-called type II SLAP lesion, is reported relatively more commonly than in the past because the arthroscope has been used with increasing frequency as an alternative to open surgery. There seems little doubt that some of the previously reported anatomic variants of the superior labrum were in fact significant labral disease. In our experience, the isolated rotator cuff tear is extremely rare; we thoroughly probe and test the labrum whenever we find a cuff tear.

We agree with Snyder (17) that superior labral detachment beyond the articular cartilage margin is significant and should be addressed. We have recently employed MRI with gadolinium intravenous contrast to preoperatively diagnose unstable SLAP lesions. This technique can be further en-

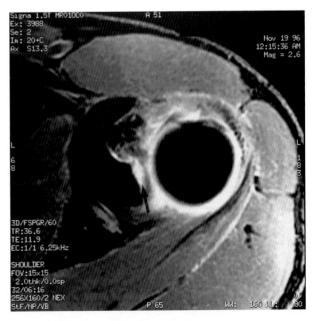

FIG. 4. Intravenous gadolinium-enhanced MR image of the superior glenoid-labral complex. Note the enhancement *(arrow)* medial to the glenoid articular surface. This represents a large superior labral detachment, which is accentuated in abduction.

hanced by having the patient abduct the shoulder 30 degrees to demonstrate superior humeral head migration with resulting elevation of the superior labrum (Fig. 4).

REFERENCES

1. Howell SM, Galinat BJ. The glenoid labral socket. A constrained articular surface. *Clin Orthop* 1989;243:122–125.
2. Morrey BF. Shoulder biomechanics. In: Rockwood CA, Matsen FA III, eds. *The Shoulder*, Philadelphia: WB Saunders, 1990:208–245.
3. Saha AK. *Theory of shoulder mechanism: descriptive and applied.* Springfield, IL: Charles C. Thomas Publisher, 1961.
4. Glousman R, Jobe F, Tibone J, et al. Dynamic electromyographic analysis of the throwing shoulder with glenohumeral instability. *J Bone Joint Surg* 1988;70A:220–226.
5. Sidles JA. *American Academy of Orthopaedic Surgeons Shoulder Course,* Waikoloa, HI, March 1993.
6. Karduna AR, Williams GR, Williams JL, Iannotti JP. Kinematics of the glenohumeral joint: Influence of muscle forces, ligamentous constraints and articular geometry. *J Orthop Res* 1996;14:986–993.
7. Lazarus MD, Sidles JA, Harryman DT, Matsen FA. Effect of a chondral-labral defect on glenoid concavity and glenohumeral stability. *J Bone Joint Surg* 1996;78-A:94–102.
8. Pagnani MJ, Deng X, Warren RF, Torzilli PA, Altchek DW. Effect of lesions of the superior portion of the glenoid labrum on glenohumeral translation. *J Bone Joint Surg* 1995;77-A:1003–1010.
9. Lephart SM, Borsa P, Fu FH, Warner JJP. *Proprioception of the shoulder joint in normal, unstable and post capsulolabral reconstructed individuals.* Presented at the tenth annual meeting of the American Shoulder and Elbow Surgeons, New Orleans, February, 1994.
10. Ellman H. *Clinical examination of the shoulder.* Presented at The Shoulder, A Comprehensive View, American Academy of Orthopaedic Surgeons, Lake Buena Vista, Florida, May, 1992.
11. Guidi EJ, Nirschl RP, Ollivierre C, Pettrone FA. *Supraspinatus labrum instability pattern lesions of the shoulder.* Presented at the 19th annual meeting of the American Orthopaedic Society for Sports Medicine, Sun Valley, Idaho, July, 1993.
12. Field LD, Savoie FH III. Arthroscopic suture repair of superior labral detachment lesions of the shoulder. *Am J Sports Med* 1993;21(6): 783–790.
13. Garcia ER, DeMaio M, Adkison DP. Rotator cuff tears are associated with significant labral pathology: a study of 100 cadaver shoulders. Presented at the annual meeting of the Society of Military Orthopaedic Surgeons, Hilton Head, SC, November, 1994.
14. Burkhart SS. Current concepts. Reconciling the paradox of rotator cuff repair versus debridement: a unified biomechanical rationale for the treatment of rotator cuff tears. *Arthroscopy* 1994;10:1–16.
15. Adkison DP, Sitler DF, DeMaio M. Acromion morphology in the asymptomatic population: a prospective controlled study. Presented at the annual meeting of the American Academy of Orthopaedic Surgeons, Atlanta, GA, February, 1996.
16. Maliky DM, Soslowsky LJ, Blasier RB, Shyr Y. Anterior glenohumeral stabilization factors: progressive effects in a biomechanical model. *J Orthop Res* 1996;14:282–288.
17. Snyder SJ. *Instructional course lecture.* Annual meeting of the Arthroscopy Association of North America, San Francisco, CA, May, 1995.

Shoulder Magnetic Resonance Imaging,
edited by Lynne S. Steinbach et al.
Lippincott–Raven Publishers, Philadelphia © 1998.

CHAPTER 5

Clinical Evaluation of the Painful Shoulder

John P. Belzer and Frederic W. Bost

<table>
<tr><td>

Documentation and Scoring
History
General Physical Examination
  Inspection
  Palpation/Crepitus/Rent
  Range of Motion—Active/Passive
  Strength Testing
  Neurologic and Vascular Examination
Specific Examinations
  Examination for Impingement, Rotator Cuff Disease,
    and Biceps Tendinitis
  Physical Examination

</td><td>

Examination for Instability
  History
  Physical Examination
    Inspection
    Palpation
    Range of Motion
    Provocative Maneuvers
    Stability Testing
  Superior Labrum–Anterior to Posterior Lesions
Examination for Miscellaneous Problems
  Adhesive Capsulitis (Frozen Shoulder)
  Specific Shoulder Disorders/Extrinsic

</td></tr>
</table>

The shoulder joint is unique in its construction, relying primarily on soft tissue restraints for stability yet maintaining the greatest mobility of any joint in the body, allowing for motion in the sagittal, coronal, and transverse planes as well as in rotation. This range of motion is necessary for the placement of the hand in position for prehension. Significant demands are placed on both the static and dynamic structures of the shoulder, which, when damaged with overuse injuries (e.g., rotator cuff disease) or (trauma such as in traumatic unidirectional instability), may lead to loss of normal shoulder function. This chapter discusses the clinical assessment of the shoulder, with special attention given to the pathologic entities best evaluated by magnetic resonance imaging (MRI).

DOCUMENTATION AND SCORING

Many scoring systems have been developed to better determine objectively preoperative symptoms and postoperative outcomes, allowing for a reproducible, controlled method of comparing treatment options from various centers. In 1978, Rowe et al. (1) published a scoring system for

the evaluation of results following surgery for glenohumeral instability. Similar scoring systems have been published in the evaluation of rotator cuff disease (2,3). A more thorough scoring system was devised by constant (4) which addressed the limitations in the aforementioned scoring systems, which were developed to quantify outcomes related to a single diagnosis. More recently, the American Shoulder and Elbow Society has adopted a standardized form that incorporates patient and physician evaluation of shoulder function, including activities of daily living, and is appropriate for the scoring of patients regardless of diagnosis (5).

HISTORY

A thorough evaluation of any orthopaedic complaint would be incomplete without a detailed history. In the examination of the shoulder, the history is even more important when physical findings are subtle and radiographs unremarkable. The mechanism of injury and the character and chronicity of the patient's symptoms help to narrow the possible causes of shoulder pain and complement the physical examination and radiographic findings in reaching a final diagnosis.

History taking commences with documentation of the patient's demographic information. The age, sex, hand dominance, vocation, and avocation are determined. Intensity of activity is recorded because it has different significance be-

J. P. Belzer and F. W. Bost: Department of Orthopaedics, University of California, San Francisco; and California Pacific Orthopaedics and Sports Medicine, San Francisco, California 94118

tween age groups; treatment of the injured shoulder in the dominant extremity of the professional athlete may be different than that necessary in the nondominant shoulder of an elderly patient. Medicolegal issues should also be determined because these may adversely affect the efficacy of treatment (6).

Information regarding the chief complaint is then obtained. Patients primarily complain of pain, but they may also complain of instability, weakness, crepitus, or stiffness or loss of motion. However, patients may complain only of loss of function if they are unable to clearly identify their symptoms. The inability to recognize symptoms is not uncommon because the deep structures of the shoulder are complex.

Each of the patient's symptoms should be addressed. If the patient complains of pain, then the location, duration, character, and timing of the pain should be determined as should factors that alter the nature of the symptoms. Often, the characteristics of the painful symptoms help focus the examiner's differential diagnosis. For instance, symptoms of night pain are classic (although not exclusive) for rotator cuff disease, whereas symptoms of the arm "going dead" acutely with overhand throwing are suggestive of anterior shoulder subluxation (7). Pain with motion of the shoulder which is associated with crepitus may indicate glenohumeral arthritis, but it may also have subacromial or scapulothoracic origins. A determination of the pain medicine requirements, including type (e.g., nonsteroidal, narcotic) and frequency of medication taken, provides an objective gauge of the patient's level of pain.

The etiology of the shoulder injury should then be determined. Shoulder injuries occur by a variety of mechanisms, including overuse injuries such as impingement (8), idiopathic processes such as adhesive capsulitis (9–11), or traumatic injuries such as glenohumeral dislocation (1,12–16) or acromioclavicular (AC) separations. Patients presenting with overuse or idiopathic shoulder problems rarely recall a specific injury, rather they see their physician because their "shoulder hurts" (17). Although patients with overuse injuries frequently do not recall the initial injury, they are usually able to articulate their symptoms and to demonstrate exacerbating motions and positions of the extremity.

Patients with idiopathic onset of shoulder pain may be experiencing the early phases of adhesive capsulitis or calcific tendinitis. The physician should note whether pain, weakness, or loss of motion represents the primary symptom. After first considering an intrinsic etiology, the physician must always be weary of extrinsic causes of shoulder pain such as brachial plexus neuropathy or cervical spine disorders (18).

In contrast, patients with traumatic shoulder injuries seek medical care because they "hurt their shoulder" (17). The mechanism of injury is recalled clearly by the patient. A fall onto an outstretched arm may result in a rotator cuff injury, labral injury, or fracture, whereas a posteriorly directed force applied to the arm with the shoulder in the position of abduction and external rotation may result in anterior glenohumeral instability. Because these patients usually present acutely, their symptoms are frequently initially global and not always specific (Table 1).

Patients who complain of shoulder instability should be questioned regarding the mechanism of the initial injury and subsequent subluxation or dislocation episodes, the frequency of instability, and the manner in which the shoulder was reduced (i.e., in the emergency department).

The physician should inquire about previous shoulder injuries or prior shoulder surgery because this information may clarify the current complaints. In addition, the type and outcome of previous interventions such as injections, physical therapy, or surgery assist in determining a diagnosis and formulating a treatment plan.

Finally, a brief medical history should be documented. Previous injuries of the cervical spine or associated neurologic problems may mimic shoulder pathology. Psoriasis may be a precursor to psoriatic spondyloarthropathy involving the shoulder, and diabetes mellitus predisposes patients to development of adhesive capsulitis. Brachial neuritis often manifests first, with shoulder pain following a viral illness or unrelated previous surgical procedure. Generalized muscular dystrophy, especially fascioscapularhumeral dystrophy, can manifest with painful shoulder dysfunction before the onset of weakness.

GENERAL PHYSICAL EXAMINATION

Physical examination of the shoulder is performed in a systemic fashion and should be carried out on both shoulders using the patient's uninvolved shoulder as a control. The examination begins with inspection of the shoulder girdle and is followed by palpation of the anatomic structures and as-

TABLE 1. *Specific injury histories*

Specific injury	Mechanism
Acromioclavicular joint dislocation	Downward blow to lateral shoulder.
Anterior glenohumeral dislocation	Forceful posterior directed blow to abducted externally rotated arm.
Posterior glenohumeral dislocation	Forceful posterior directed force to forward flexed arm.
Labrum or slap lesion	Axial force to the partially abducted or flexed arm.
Acute rotator cuff tear	Forceful abduction/flexion of arm against fixed resistance.
Acute rotator cuff tear	Suspect in anterior dislocation of shoulder in persons older than age 40.
Biceps tendon dislocation	Resistance against forceful passive external rotation or extension of arm.
Subscapularis or pectoralis major avulsion	Forceful horizontal plane extension. Posterior directed force to the 90-degrees abducted arm.

sessment of range of motion, both active and passive. The examination is completed with a series of provocative maneuvers. Each of these segments of the examination should also be performed systematically to ensure that subtle abnormalities are not overlooked. In addition, the examiner becomes increasingly comfortable with normal and abnormal findings with each examination. The examination is then documented in an organized manner so that the history and physical examination can be synthesized to arrive at a final diagnosis.

Inspection

One of the most important yet frequently unappreciated aspects of the physical examination is the visual inspection. The inspection should begin as soon as the patient interview begins. Attention to the patient's use of the shoulder when moving about the examination room before the formal examination begins may give the examiner clues into the problem. One of the more telling clues is noted when the patient protects the shoulder when removing a shirt, sling, or other protective device.

On formal inspection, the examiner looks for general asymmetry between the two shoulders. Asymmetry may be due to muscle wasting, trauma, swelling, degenerative joint disease, or extrinsic disorders such as scoliosis or hemiplegia. It is important to examine the anterior, lateral, and posterior aspects of the shoulder because each of these areas may reveal pathologic information.

Anteriorly, the clavicle and the sternoclavicular (SC) and acromioclavicular (AC) joints are the most prominent structures because their subcutaneous location makes abnormalities fairly easy to detect (Fig. 1). Asymmetry in the anterior axillary region is more difficult to detect but should not be overlooked because this area may reveal a deficiency to suggest a pectoralis major avulsion (Fig. 2) or other injury. Lat-

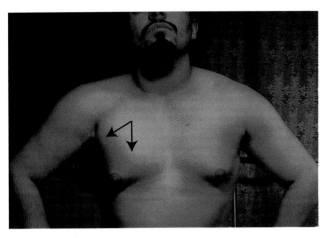

FIG. 2. Pectoralis major avulsion. The patient is contracting the pectoralis major, which reveals a defect in the anterior axillary wall and an apparent increase in the size of the pectoralis muscle (*arrows*) caused by medial retraction of the muscle.

erally, the most common asymmetry is noted in the deltoid, which may reveal wasting from axillary nerve palsy or from previous surgery, resulting in deltoid avulsion from the acromion (Fig. 3). Inferior subluxation of the glenohumeral articulation (sulcus sign) is an indicator of multidirectional instability (Fig. 4). Posteriorly, wasting of the rotator cuff muscles in the supraspinatus and infraspinatus fossa may be dramatic (Fig. 5). Wasting may be secondary to disuse atrophy, seen in glenohumeral arthritis or in chronic rotator cuff tears, or in primary neurologic causes such as suprascapular nerve palsy (Fig. 6). More isolated areas of atrophy including periscapular musculature may indicate involvement of extrinsic causes such as brachial plexus neuropathy. Patterns of muscle wasting with primary muscular dystrophy are specific, especially in fascioscapularhumeral dystrophy and it is not unusual for the orthopaedic surgeon to be the first to make this diagnosis in the patient with shoulder pain.

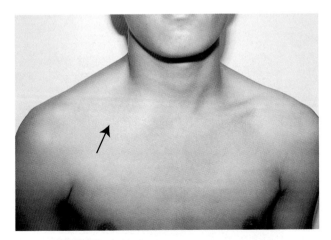

FIG. 1. Fracture of right proximal clavicle through the physeal plate with posterior displacement of the distal fragment. Note the loss of the normal prominence of the clavicle (*arrow*) compared to the normal left side.

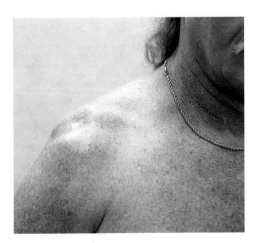

FIG. 3. Avulsed deltoid origin related to previous deltoid detachment performed during routine rotator cuff repair.

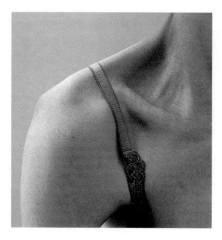

FIG. 4. Sulcus sign of the right shoulder in a patient with multidirectional instability. Note the sulcus inferior to the prominent lateral acromion.

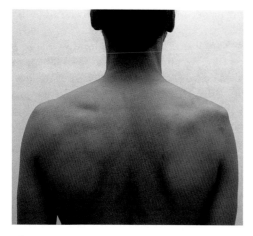

FIG. 5. Supraspinatus and infraspinatus wasting resulting from degenerative disease of the right shoulder.

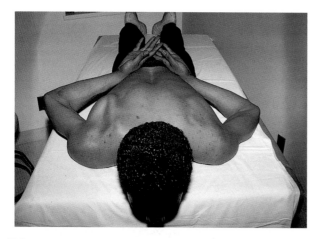

FIG. 6. Isolated infraspinatus atrophy in a professional pitcher with spinoglenoid impingement on the infraspinatus branch of suprascapular nerve.

Palpation/Crepitus/Rent

Palpation of the shoulder joint is used to identify defects, prominences, or pain in the bone and soft tissue structures of the shoulder. The examination commences with palpation of the bones and articulations, beginning with the sternoclavicular joint, where anterior or posterior dislocations and degenerative changes may occur. Palpation continues laterally along the clavicle to the AC joint. A painful AC joint may indicate an arthritic or traumatized joint. A shoulder separation is noted by the painful prominence of the distal end of the clavicle associated with hypermobility of the AC joint. Palpation is continued along the acromion and scapular spine. Finally, palpation of the proximal humerus and tuberosities is carried out, eliciting pain from fractures.

Palpation of the soft tissues is performed subsequently. This begins with palpation of the axilla to assess the pectoralis major anteriorly for ruptures. The pectoralis major may be made more prominent by having patients place their hands on their hips and press medially. The posterior boundary of the axilla is defined by the latissimus dorsi. Palpation of the deltoid is then performed, with the examiner being sure to palpate the anterior, middle, and posterior thirds of the muscle. This examination confirms findings of atrophy or injury noted on previous inspection.

Palpation of the rotator cuff is helpful in diagnosing rotator cuff disease, but it also is more difficult to perform. It is most easily executed by placing the examiner's fingers on the anterolateral aspect of the acromion with the palm of the hand resting posteriorly. The examiner's fingers then palpate in the interval between the anterior and middle thirds of the deltoid (Fig. 7). Palpation reveals tenderness in an inflamed bursa, rotator cuff, or biceps tendon. Experienced examiners may be able to palpate a defect in the rotator cuff resulting from rotator cuff rupture or biceps dislocation, or a prominence caused by calcific deposit. The examination is rendered more effective by extending the shoulder in neutral abduction to expose the tuberosities, intertubercular groove, and supraspinatus tendon anterior to the acromion.

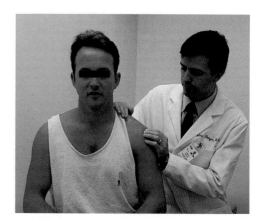

FIG. 7. Palpation of the greater tuberosity and subdeltoid bursa.

Because rotator cuff disease occurs primarily at the anterior aspect of the supraspinatus, palpation just off of the anterolateral corner of the acromion yields the most effective examination.

Anteromedial to the supraspinatus attachment to the greater tuberosity, the biceps tendon is located in the bicipital groove. It can be found most easily by palpating anteriorly on the humeral head with the arm in approximately 10 degrees of internal rotation. If in doubt about the location of the biceps tendon, the examiner can follow the easily visualized distal biceps proximally. Rotation of the humerus with the examiner's fingers over the region of the intertubercular groove assists in detecting the bicipital groove. It is important not to palpate the biceps too vigorously because a normal biceps tendon is tender when palpated forcefully, resulting in a false-positive result. An examination of the contralateral shoulder confirms the sensitivity of the biceps.

Crepitus is a nonspecific sign on physical examination because it may represent rotator cuff disease, intraarticular pathology, such as labral tears or degenerative arthritis, or scapulothoracic bursitis. With experience, the origin of crepitus may be more easily determined. Crepitus is identified when the examiner's hand rests over the region of the acromion and deltoid. Crepitus from an irregular bursa/rotator cuff articulating with a roughened undersurface of the acromion and coracoacromial ligament is best noted by bringing the patient's arm into approximately 60 to 90 degrees of forward elevation and rotating the arm internally and externally. Crepitus from an arthritic glenohumeral joint is noted by passive motion of the glenohumeral joint with the arm in neutral abduction, again rotating the arm internally and externally. Crepitus from the scapulothoracic articulation is noted posteriorly with full elevation of the upper extremity.

Range of Motion—Active/Passive

The evaluation of both active and passive range of motion is important in the complete physical examination of the shoulder. Active range of motion is tested first and identifies the functional limitations of motion. Limitations of shoulder motion may be due to true mechanical or static restrictions such as adhesive capsulitis (soft tissue contracture) or degenerative joint disease (bony obstruction), or it may be due to dynamic loss as is seen in patients with large rotator cuff tears or neurologic deficiencies. Limitations in motion may be voluntary or involuntary, depending on pain related to the underlying condition.

The Society of American Shoulder and Elbow surgeons has recommended that the evaluation of active range-of-motion tests of the shoulder should include an assessment of forward elevation, external rotation at neutral and 90 degrees of abduction, and internal rotation (19). All tests are performed preferably with the patient standing, because this position keeps the examining table from interfering with the examination. In addition, both shoulders are examined si-

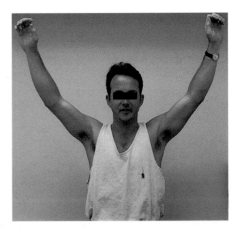

FIG. 8. Total active forward elevation is measured as maximal elevation performed with the humerus in the scapular plane located between the sagittal and coronal planes.

multaneously (except for internal rotation), allowing for the patient's contralateral shoulder to serve as a control.

Forward elevation is an examination of the patient's ability to raise his or her arm maximally in the plane of scapular motion, located between the sagittal and coronal planes (Fig. 8). Because two thirds of the overall shoulder range of motion occurs at the glenohumeral articulation and one third occurs at the scapulothoracic articulation (20), this examination evaluates the patient's true functional range of motion in overhead reaching ability. Limitations in glenohumeral range of motion can be determined by careful examination of the scapulothoracic rhythm and range. If limitations or an abnormal motion exists, the patient should be observed both anteriorly and posteriorly to determine which articulation is abnormal. A common finding in patients with a weak or painful shoulder is "hiking," which is a pathologic shoulder rhythm in which elevation or rotation of the scapula precedes glenohumeral abduction in an effort to maximize total elevation of the extremity (Fig. 9).

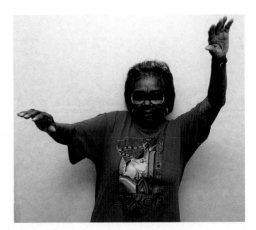

FIG. 9. This patient demonstrates the classic "hiking" of the shoulder seen in patients with massive rotator cuff tears. In an effort to increase total shoulder elevation, the patient elevates the scapula using the periscapular muscles.

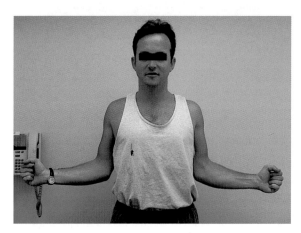

FIG. 10. Active external rotation with the elbow flexed 90 degrees and the patient standing.

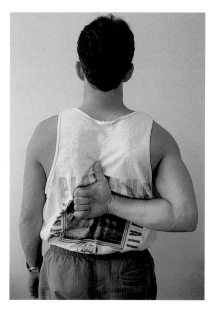

FIG. 11. Internal rotation is documented as the maximum cephalad position the patient can reach with the extended thumb.

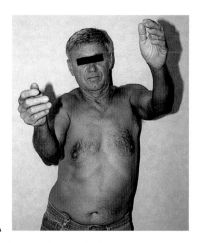

A

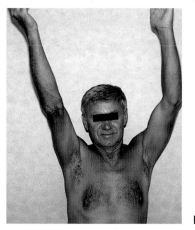

B

FIG. 12. Passive motion in all planes is measured in patients who do not have full active range of motion. **A:** In this patient, active forward elevation is limited. **B:** The examiner is able to passively position the arm in full forward elevation. Also note that the patient is able to maintain the arm in the position that it was placed.

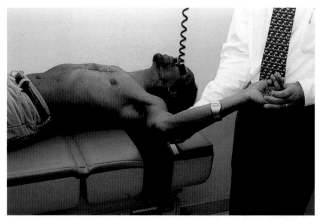

A

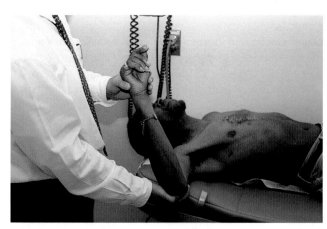

B

FIG. 13. Passive external rotation with the shoulder abducted 90 degrees is a sensitive means of determining motion abnormalities. **A:** The unaffected shoulder in a patient with adhesive capsulitis reveals normal external rotation. **B:** The affected shoulder reveals significant limitation in external rotation.

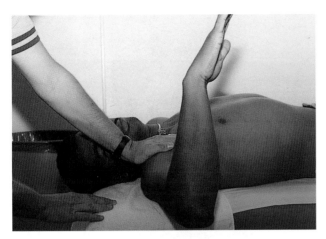

FIG. 14. Passive internal rotation with the shoulder abducted 90 degrees and the scapula stabilized reveals loss of motion. This professional baseball player exhibits a classic external rotation contracture.

External rotation is performed with the patient's elbow flexed at 90 degrees and the elbow located at the patient's side. The patient then rotates his or her forearm externally while maintaining a vertical humerus and a flexed elbow (Fig. 10). Neutral rotation is defined when the forearm is directly anterior, that is, in the sagittal plane, and 90 degrees external rotation is noted when the forearm is rotated directly laterally in the coronal plane.

Internal rotation is evaluated by instructing patients to place their hand behind their back and reach their thumb as high as possible. This examination is not performed simultaneously but rather sequentially, to minimize interference between the two extremities. The maximum height that the patient is able to reach the thumb is documented by the anatomic level, for instance, the iliac crest, lumbar spine, or thoracolumbar junction (Fig. 11).

Measurements of passive range of motion are performed when limitations in active motion are noted. An increase seen in passive range of motion over that noted in active range of motion suggests a functional cause for motion loss. The most common diagnosis resulting in this discrepancy is large and massive rotator cuff tears, although neurologic causes may result in a similar clinical picture (Fig. 12). Passive range of motion may be performed with the patient supine to increase patient comfort.

Determination of the subtle loss in range of motion is essential in the throwing athlete because contractures frequently limit internal rotation and horizontal adduction in this patient population. These alterations in the normal mechanics of the shoulder, if not addressed, may result in increased stresses on the anterior capsule and secondarily on the elbow. Subtle restrictions of passive motion again can be detected by measuring internal and external rotation of the shoulder with the humerus abducted 90 degrees and the scapula stabilized by the examiner's hand (Fig. 13). Alternatively, internal rotation loss can be quickly detected (but not quantitatively measured) by observing scapular winging on standing or prone patients with their hands clasped behind their back (Fig. 14). An external rotation contracture (limited internal rotation) is frequently noted (Fig. 15).

Strength Testing

Strength testing is an integral part of the shoulder examination. It exposes weakness that may be primarily related to mechanical damage to the soft tissues, to neurologic causes, or secondarily to pain inhibition. It is thus imperative that the strength examination evaluate all of the major structures of the shoulder to delineate the structures that are injured or dysfunctional. The supraspinatus strength is tested by resisted forward elevation with the arm maximally internally rotated and shoulder abducted 60 degrees (Fig. 16). Resisted external rotation in neutral abduction tests the infraspinatus–teres minor complex (Fig. 17). Strength of the subscapularis is tested with resisted internal rotation and the lift-off test (Fig. 18), which is described in later paragraphs.

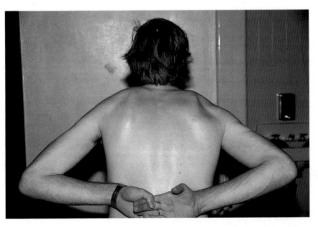
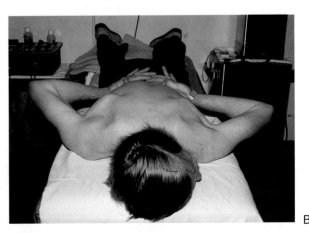

A   B

FIG. 15. External rotation contracture may be demonstrated by two methods. **A:** Abduction rotation testing. **B:** Scapular winging in the prone patient with the hands placed on the lumbar spine.

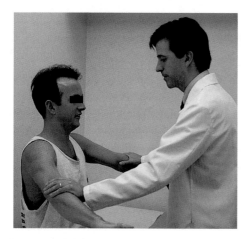

FIG. 16. Supraspinatus strength is tested with the patient's arm in a position of 60 degrees of forward elevation with the shoulder internally rotated and the elbow extended. A downward force applied by the examiner is resisted by the patient.

Neurologic and Vascular Examination

In patients with subtle complaints of shoulder pain or weakness, a thorough neurologic examination must be performed. This includes an examination of sensory, motor, and reflex functions of the upper extremity because cervical spine conditions may mimic shoulder conditions. Careful attention should be paid to the evaluation of the external rotators of the shoulder because suprascapular nerve entrapment at the level of the suprascapular notch or the spinoglenoid notch may lead to paralysis of the supraspinatus and infraspinatus or the infraspinatus alone, respectively (21). This denervation results in shoulder pain as well as weakness in shoulder elevation and external rotation. Frequently, these patients have clinical findings that are consistent with rotator cuff disease.

Finally, in patients with shoulder pain of unclear origin, a vascular examination should be performed to evaluate the patient for thoracic outlet syndrome (TOS) or axillary ve-

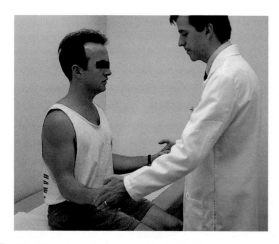

FIG. 17. External rotation is tested with the patient's arm at the side and the elbow flexed 90 degrees. The patient resists a medially directed force applied by the examiner to the dorsum of the patient's hand.

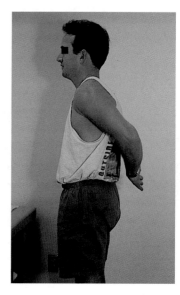

FIG. 18. The lift-off test is performed to evaluate subscapularis strength. The patient is asked to actively lift the hand off of the lumbar region.

nous occlusion. The Adson's test, which is used to determine TOS, is performed by palpating the patient's radial pulse. The patient's arm is then placed in abduction and external rotation while the pulse is maintained. Patients are then instructed to rotate their head to the involved shoulder. A diminished pulse confirms TOS. In overhead athletes, axillary venous occlusion can occur through repetitive impingement with abduction and is manifested by pain and venous engorgement of the upper extremity.

SPECIFIC EXAMINATIONS

There are many afflictions of the shoulder that may be adequately evaluated using a thorough general examination complemented by an appropriate radiographic examination. These afflictions include most fractures and acute dislocations, glenohumeral and acromioclavicular arthritis, and calcific tendinitis. The clinical evaluation of soft tissue injuries of the shoulder, which are some of the more common causes of a symptomatic shoulder, may be much more elusive. These injuries include impingement syndrome and rotator cuff disease, glenohumeral instability, and superior labral lesions. In the evaluation of these entities, many special signs and tests have been described to aid in the evaluation of these processes. MRI is also an important adjunct because of its ability to accurately evaluate soft tissue structures of the shoulder. The following is a discussion of the evaluation of those entities in which MRI is most effectively used to improve diagnostic accuracy.

Examination for Impingement, Rotator Cuff Disease, and Biceps Tendinitis

A thorough history and physical examination of the shoulder by an experienced examiner results in an examination with 84% to 90% sensitivity and 75% to 95% specificity when evaluating for rotator cuff tears (22,23). The history generally reveals chronic symptoms of pain, which may be aggravated with overhead activity of the shoulder. An acute incident such as a fall may worsen an already painful shoulder and may result in greater weakness. This may represent an acute additional tear in an already torn rotator cuff and can greatly influence the goals and success of surgical intervention. The location of pain is nonspecific, but generally is located over the lateral aspect of the deltoid. Classically, patients complain of night pain that awakens them from sleep.

Physical Examination

The visual examination of the shoulder with rotator cuff disease may reveal previous incisions or other conditions related to previous surgery (Fig. 19). Supraspinatus or infraspinatus fossa atrophy suggests disuse of the rotator cuff resulting from long-standing pain with or without tearing of cuff tissue. Inspection of the distal arm may reveal a distally migrated bulk of the biceps muscle caused by rupture of the long head of the biceps tendon (Fig. 20).

Palpation of the rotator cuff may reveal tenderness of the cuff in various positions, suggesting an impingement process. The palpation examination is facilitated by extending the shoulder. With subsequent external rotation, the anterior portion of the supraspinatus is palpated. With progressive internal rotation, the more posterior aspect of the rotator cuff is exposed. Crepitus is a common complaint in patients with rotator cuff disease. It is tested by bringing the arm into approximately 60 degrees of forward elevation and then rotating the arm internally and externally. The roughened cuff

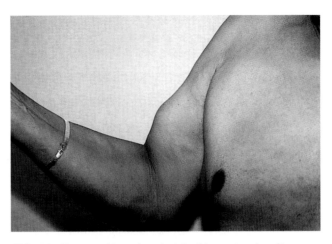

FIG. 20. Ruptured long head of the biceps tendon. Because of the tendon rupture, the muscle belly has retracted distally, resulting in the characteristic "Popeye" appearance.

and bursa rotating under the acromion and coracoacromial ligament create the crepitus, which is palpated by the examiner's fingertips.

Range of motion of the shoulder with rotator cuff deficiency is frequently not affected. A small percentage of patients with massive rotator cuff tears may be able to fully elevate the arm. These patients may have proximal migration of the humeral head such that it contacts the undersurface of the acromion. This contact point functions as a fulcrum, allowing for near normal elevation of the shoulder with deltoid contraction, despite the absence of the rotator cuff. For this reason, examination of the rhythm of shoulder motion is essential in the diagnosis of rotator cuff disease. An often subtle finding on range-of-motion examination in patients with rotator cuff disease is the characteristic hiking of the shoulder or elevation of the scapula with the trapezius muscle. An even more subtle observation, which is best appreciated when viewed posteriorly, is the abnormal rhythm accompanying excessive scapular rotation in abduction or flexion.

In patients who do exhibit limits in range of motion, an examination of passive motion is carried out. This important aspect of the examination helps distinguish impingement syndrome and rotator cuff disease from other conditions, most notably adhesive capsulitis. Whereas in adhesive capsulitis there are similar limits in both active and passive range of motion, rotator cuff disease generally does not limit passive range of motion unless secondary adhesive capsulitis has developed. Additionally, those patients with massive tears who are unable to actively elevate the arm above 90 degrees may be able to actively maintain the arm in full abduction when placed in this position by the examiner.

While testing range of motion, the examiner should look for a painful arc of motion. The painful arc is a nonspecific examination, but it is suggestive of rotator cuff disease (24). The painful arc usually occurs when the patient actively elevates the arm between approximately 60 and 100 degrees (Fig. 21). This motion arc is painful because of the passing of the greater tuberosity under the anterolateral edge of the acromion, causing increased discomfort in an irritated rota-

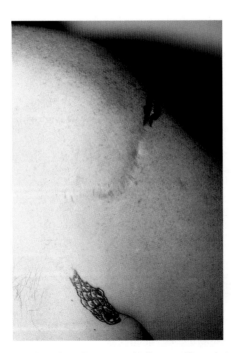

FIG. 19. Previous incisions may indicate prior related surgical procedures.

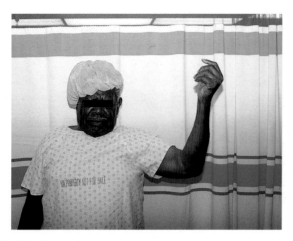

FIG. 21. The painful arc is noted when the patient elevates the shoulder through an arc between 60 and 100 degrees. This patient had impingement without a rotator cuff tear and improved with subacromial decompression.

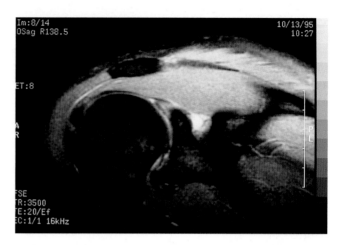

FIG. 22. An example of a ganglion cyst in the spinoglenoid notch impinging on the infraspinatus branch of the supras-capular nerve with electromyographically documented neu-ropraxia of the infraspinatus.

tor cuff or biceps tendon. A similar painful arc may also be seen when performing the passive supine abduction rotation test. Patients may experience painful symptoms when the arm is taken from neutral to 60 degrees of external rotation and from neutral rotation into approximately 45 degrees of internal rotation, which causes abrasion of the inflamed ro-tator cuff or biceps tendon against the undersurface of the acromion or coracoacromial ligament.

After range of motion has been assessed, strength testing of the supraspinatus, external (infraspinatus/teres minor), and internal (subscapularis) rotators is performed to further highlight suspected weakness. Supraspinatus function is evaluated by testing the patient's ability to resist a downward force applied to the humerus with the elbow extended and the arm in a position of internal rotation and 45 degrees of forward flexion. Pain, weakness, or both symptoms may re-sult in the patient's inability to resist.

If the patient is sufficiently weak or painful, he or she may exhibit a drop-arm test (25). The drop-arm test is positive when the patient is unable to slowly lower the maximally el-evated arm to the side because of pain or weakness. Instead, the patient drops the affected extremity to his or her side.

Strength of the infraspinatus and teres minor is evaluated by assessing the patient's ability to resist inwardly applied force to the forearm with the shoulder in a position of neutral abduction with the elbow flexed 90 degrees. Weakness in ex-ternal rotation suggests a large or massive cuff tear, although it may also represent a palsy of the infraspinatus branch of the suprascapular nerve (Fig. 22). A confirmatory indicator of a large or massive rotator cuff tear is the dropping test (24). In this test, the examiner holds the patient's involved extremity in external rotation. The patient is asked to main-tain the arm in the externally rotated position. Because the infraspinatus and teres minor are the primary external rota-tors of the shoulder, a patient's inability to maintain external rotation suggests a massive tear involving the infraspinatus and often the teres minor.

The internal rotation strength of the shoulder is evaluated by the lift-off test (26). Because internal rotation of the shoulder in neutral rotation is performed by not only the sub-scapularis but also the pectoralis major, teres major, and latissimus dorsi, it is necessary to isolate the subscapularis by placing these other external rotators at a mechanical dis-advantage. This is achieved by internally rotating the shoul-der and positioning the forearm behind the patient's back. The patient is then asked to lift his or her hand off of the lum-bar region of the spine, an action that requires further active internal rotation of the shoulder. Alternatively, the physician may hold the hand away from the patient's lumbar spine and then ask the patient to maintain the position when the hand is released. An inability to do so suggests dysfunction of the subscapularis.

Pathology of the long head of the biceps tendon often ac-companies rotator cuff conditions and occasionally can be seen in isolation (8). Because of this, it is imperative that the biceps tendon be examined in isolation. Speed's test is the most useful of the many tests that evaluate the biceps tendon

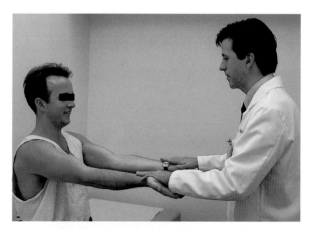

FIG. 23. Speed's test assessing tendonitis of the long head of the biceps is demonstrated.

(19). In the Speed's test, the patient resists a downward force applied to the arm in 90 degrees of forward flexion with the palms facing up and the elbows straight (Fig. 23). Pain at the shoulder suggests biceps pathology, either at its origin, at the superior labrum or within the bicipital groove; however, this test may elicit similar symptoms in patients with supraspinatus conditions. A confirmatory test is the Yergason's sign in which the patient simultaneously resists a pronation force applied to the forearm and an external rotation force applied to the shoulder by the examiner (27).

The impingement signs are provocative maneuvers that are helpful in clarifying the diagnosis of rotator cuff disease or biceps tendinitis. Two signs of impingement are routinely examined and may be performed with the patient in the upright or supine positions. The first sign, described by Neer (8), is pain elicited with maximal passive glenohumeral forward flexion with the shoulder in neutral rotation, which impinges the inflamed supraspinatus and biceps tendons and the subacromial bursa under the anterolateral edge of the acromion (Fig. 24). The second sign, described by Hawkins and colleagues (19,24,28), is pain elicited with glenohumeral forward flexion to 90 degrees, slight horizontal adduction, and internal rotation, which compresses the inflamed supraspinatus insertion at the greater tuberosity and subacromial bursa under the coracoacromial ligament (Fig. 25).

Once the entire physical examination is completed, a diagnostic subacromial impingement test may be performed to confirm the diagnosis of rotator cuff disease (8). In this test, 5 to 10 cc of 1% lidocaine is injected into the subacromial bursa to temporarily eliminate the patient's symptoms of pain. Cortisone may also be included in the injection as a therapeutic treatment (Fig. 26). Patients with true impingement or rotator cuff disease should receive greater than 50% relief of pain when the impingement signs are repeated. In addition to pain relief, the cause of weakness elicited on examination is clarified. Weakness may be secondary to pain inhibition, muscular atrophy, or tendon rupture. If weakness persists despite the relief of pain following the injection, the

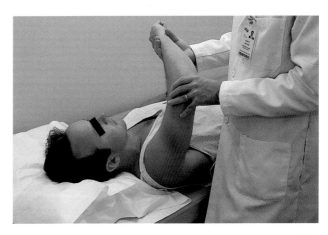

FIG. 25. Secondary or impingement II (Hawkins' sign) is noted as pain with passive internal rotation of the shoulder in a position of 90 degrees of forward flexion.

rotator cuff is usually torn. Persistent pain should lead the physician to suspect other sources of shoulder pain.

Frequently, acromioclavicular arthritis accompanies rotator cuff disease in the elderly patient. Symptoms referable to the AC joint are clarified by the "cross-body" or horizontal adduction test. In this test, the arm is brought into 90 degrees of forward flexion. The arm is then adducted maximally, creating compression of the AC joint. Pain suggests pathology of this articulation. Subsequent injection of 2 cc of 1% lidocaine into the AC joint assists in determining the contribution of an AC condition to the patient's symptoms.

Examination for Instability

Instability of the shoulder remains one of the more complex and interesting aspects of shoulder pathology. In recent years, a more thorough understanding of the variations in normal glenohumeral translation has evolved. Additionally, there continues to be advancements in the understanding of

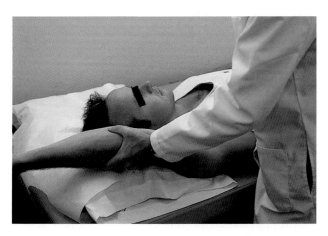

FIG. 24. Primary or impingement I (Neer's sign) is noted as pain with maximal passive elevation of the shoulder.

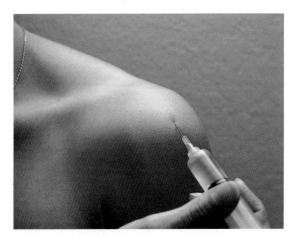

FIG. 26. The impingement test. The eradication of pain following the injection of lidocaine confirms rotator cuff disease.

the true spectrum of the pathology associated with glenohumeral instability, including its relationship to rotator cuff disease. These changing concepts of the causes of shoulder symptoms as they relate to shoulder instability is evident in the overhead throwing athlete in whom secondary impingement of the articular rotator cuff has been identified as a cause of shoulder pain related to instability (29).

The most common mechanism of shoulder instability is trauma, which may be acute or recurrent. The initial episode of instability usually is due to a major force and frequently requires manipulation by a health care worker to achieve a reduction. Subsequent dislocations may occur with less force. Patients who present with traumatic instability have been classified by the acronym TUBS (*t*raumatic, *u*nidirectional, *B*ankart, *s*urgical, which is most appropriately treated by *s*urgery) (15).

Atraumatic instability of the shoulder, which represents the more complex patient profile to evaluate and treat, has gained more attention recently. Some of these patients have an underlying collagen disorder, which results in laxity of all joints. Because of the global laxity of all structures of the shoulder, these patients present with multidirectional instability, which occurs as a result of minor trauma. The minor trauma may lead to disuse of the shoulder, which allows for weakening of the rotator cuff and further symptomatic instability of the shoulder. These patients have been classified by the acronym AMBRI (*a*traumatic, *m*ultidirectional, *b*ilateral, *r*ecurrent, *i*nstability, which is most appropriately treated by *r*ehabilitation aimed at strengthening the rotator cuff, and when indicated, surgery consists of an *i*nferior capsular shift) (15).

A third group of patients are those in whom symptoms of unidirectional or multidirectional instability develop following repetitive microtrauma. This group includes the athletic population, especially throwers and other athletes who use overhead motion, in whom secondary impingement related to either underlying traumatic instability or congenital ligamentous laxity develops (29,30). These patients may have symptoms of pain consistent with rotator cuff tendinitis instead of symptoms of instability.

History

Determining the origin of shoulder instability is essential in properly diagnosing and treating the unstable shoulder. The initial history addresses whether the patient's instability is traumatic or atraumatic. The patient with traumatic instability should be asked about the position of the shoulder when the dislocation occurred and the magnitude and direction of the force that led to the dislocation. Additionally, patients should be asked about the frequency and the magnitude of the forces required to create recurrence of instability.

The more common anterior dislocation (31) occurs when a force is applied to the abducted and externally rotated upper extremity and frequently occurs in sporting activities such as basketball, football, volleyball, and water polo. Pos-

terior shoulder dislocation is a much less common injury than anterior dislocations and for this reason these patients are frequently misdiagnosed. Traumatic posterior instability classically occurs during a seizure or from electric shock (19), but it may also be caused by a posteriorly directed force applied to the extremity when the arm is forward flexed to 90 degrees, for example, in a motor vehicle accident when the patient's hand is on the steering wheel or when a football player's arms are in a blocking position.

Patients with multidirectional instability may be anterior dominant or posterior dominant depending on the direction of greatest laxity. Their history is much less well described. Patients may complain of either pain or instability, or they may not realize that their shoulder is unstable at all but they are unable to perform certain activities. Patients with multidirectional instability often do not recognize episodes of instability because the shoulder rarely stays subluxated or dislocated. The onset of their symptoms is usually insidious. An additional crucial component of the history is whether the instability is voluntary or involuntary; patients with voluntary instability are poor surgical candidates (32).

Throwers and other athletes who use overhand motion and who have shoulder pain should always be suspected of having instability as a cause for their symptoms. The description of a dead-arm sensation may indicate a momentary instability episode during a violent overhand throw (7). Such persons may complain of night pain and other symptoms of rotator cuff disease as previously discussed (29).

Physical Examination

Inspection

The physical examination of a reduced glenohumeral joint in a patient with symptomatic instability may be unremarkable. Simple inspection of the shoulder at rest infrequently reveals findings of significance in the unstable shoulder, which, at the time of examination is reduced. The examiner should inspect the patient's shoulder girdle for evidence of a sulcus sign, which suggests inferior translation of the glenohumeral joint (Fig. 27). The examiner should evaluate the patient for findings of systemic laxity, which may contribute to multidirectional instability. These findings include the ability to hyperextend the elbows, hyperextend the metacarpophalangeal joint of the index finger, abduct the thumb so that it reaches the volar surface of the forearm, and hyperextend the elbows (Fig. 28). If the examiner suspects an underlying collagen disorder such as Marfan's disease, a brief ocular inspection and cardiac examination should be performed.

The acutely dislocated shoulder has the exaggerated sulcus noted below the acromion caused by the medial shift of the proximal humerus. In posterior dislocation, the arm is only comfortable to the patient in internal rotation while the appearance of the shoulder is near normal. These subtle findings may easily be missed by even the experienced exam-

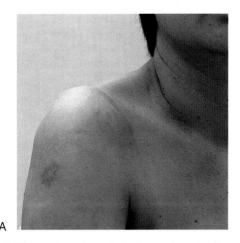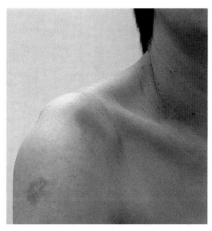

FIG. 27. The sulcus sign. **A:** In the resting position, the patient's shoulder has a relatively normal appearance. **B:** The examiner applies axial traction on the extremity, resulting in the sulcus being inferior to the lateral edge of the acromion.

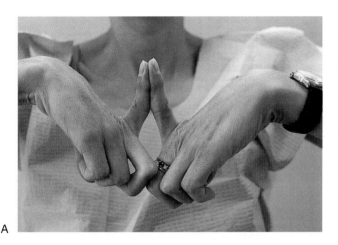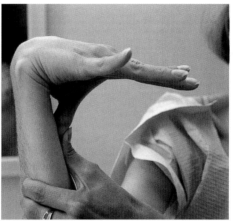

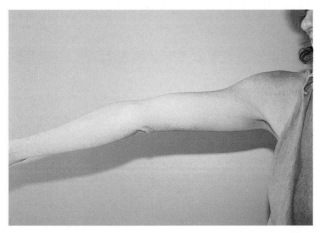

FIG. 28. In patients with suspected multidirectional instability, findings of joint laxity in other joints should be noted. **A:** Hyperflexibility of the index metacarpophalyngeal joint. **B:** The ability to touch the thumb to the volar surface of the forearm. **C:** The ability to hyperextend the elbow.

iner. The most helpful inspection aid is the examination from above and behind the seated patient. From this vantage point, the examiner can appreciate differences in the anterior and posterior shoulder contours, which may be the most notable physical finding.

Palpation

Palpation of the unstable shoulder may, on occasion, reveal an inferior sulcus sign. This may be bilateral in patients with multidirectional instability. If the examiner palpates the shoulder while moving the shoulder, crepitus may be evident. This is rare but may be present in patients with numerous dislocations or subluxations in whom traumatic degenerative changes, Hill-Sachs lesions, or labral lesions are beginning to develop.

Range of Motion

Active and passive range of motion are rarely limited in patients with instability of the shoulder. However, patients who have recently experienced dislocations may experience apprehension or pain when the shoulder is put in a position of risk, for instance, abduction and external rotation in a patient who has recently experienced an anteroinferior dislocation.

Provocative Maneuvers

Following the passive range of motion portion of the physical examination, the apprehension test can be performed. The apprehension test is a provocative maneuver to evaluate the shoulder for anterior instability (Fig. 29A). This test is best performed with the patient supine. In this posi-

tion, the patient is comfortable, thus eliminating extraneous symptoms and allowing a focused examination on anterior capsulolabral stressing. The examiner brings the arm into 90 degrees of abduction. Slowly the arm is brought into increased external rotation. As the shoulder reaches approximately 90 degrees of external rotation, the humeral head may begin to subluxate anteriorly in a patient with anterior instability, making the patient apprehensive that dislocation is imminent (25). If the patient complains of only pain with the apprehension testing, this may be a symptom related to impingement syndrome, rotator cuff disease, biceps tendinitis, or labral lesions. To confirm that symptoms are originating from the anterior subluxation of the humeral head, the examiner performs the Jobe relocation test. In this test, the examiner attempts to reduce the anterior subluxation of the glenohumeral joint by applying a gentle posteriorly directed pressure on the anterior aspect of the proximal humerus while the shoulder is maintained in the position of apprehension (Fig. 29B). If the patient's symptoms are related to anterior instability, this maneuver will relieve the patient's symptoms.

Posterior instability is tested by the posterior stress test. This test is performed on the seated or side-lying patient with the humerus forward flexed 90 degrees, adducted, and internally rotated, and with the examiner applying a posteriorly directed force on the elbow, forcing the humeral head over the posterior rim of the glenoid. Because posterior instability is more frequently a subluxation than a true dislocation, patients do not react as strongly to this maneuver, but rather confirm that this position recreates their shoulder symptoms.

Stability Testing

Stability testing, although often difficult to perform effectively because of patient guarding, represents the mainstay

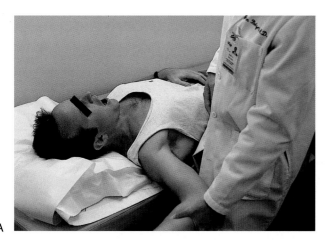
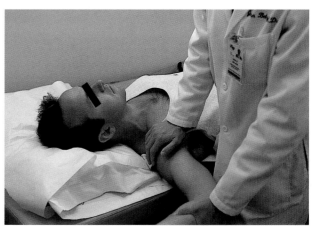

A   B

FIG. 29. Apprehension/apprehension suppression test. **A:** The patient's shoulder is positioned in 90 degrees of abduction and then maximally externally rotated. In patients with symptomatic anterior instability, the patient will experience apprehension that the shoulder will dislocate. **B:** A gentle posterior force is then applied to the anterior humerus, reducing the humeral head into the glenoid and suppressing the patient's apprehension.

of the assessment of the unstable shoulder. The purpose of this portion of the examination is to determine the direction and magnitude of instability. Many stability tests have been described, including the sulcus test, the drawer test, the shift and load test, and testing of anterior and posterior translation with the patient supine or lateral.

The sulcus test assesses inferior translation of the glenohumeral joint and determines the inferior component of multidirectional instability.

In the drawer test, the patient is seated with the patient's arm dangling comfortably at the side to prevent muscular guarding. The examiner stands behind the patient and grasps the humeral head with one hand while the other hand stabilizes the scapula. The examiner then applies an axial load to the humerus, compressing the glenohumeral articulation, centering the humeral head in the glenoid fossa. The examiner then applies an anteriorly directed force to the posterior aspect of the humeral head. In normal patients, a firm end point should be reached without evidence of the humeral head translating over the anterior lip of the glenoid. A posteriorly directed force is then applied to the anterior humerus and the posterior translation is determined. Posterior translation of up to one half of the humeral head diameter is considered normal.

The limitation of the drawer test is that it is an evaluation of the shoulder stability in a position in which instability is rarely problematic. For example, patients with traumatic anteroinferior instability of the shoulder sustain an injury to the anteroinferior glenohumeral ligament-labral complex (1,12,13,33). This ligament has been shown to provide stability to the glenohumeral articulation when the shoulder is abducted and externally rotated (34,35). Thus, evaluation of shoulder stability with the arm in neutral abduction is of relatively little use in evaluating patients with this type of instability because the injured anteroinferior glenohumeral ligament is not stressed in neutral abduction. An evaluation that is performed with the arm in 90 degrees of abduction with rotation applied to discriminate between normal ligamentous laxity and pathologic instability represents a more effective examination technique.

Shoulder stability testing with the arm in abduction with applied rotation can be performed with the patient in either a supine (Fig. 30) or lateral position. For testing patients in the lateral position, the patients are asked to lie comfortably on their side with their back toward the examiner at the edge of the examination table. The examiner grasps the patient's extremity at the level of the elbow with one hand and abducts the patients arm to 90 degrees. The other hand grasps the humeral head between the thumb and index finger while stabilizing the scapula between the heel of the hand and the remaining three fingers. With varying degrees of external rotation applied by the examiner to the patient's humerus, an anteriorly directed force is applied to the posterior humeral head. A clunk or dislocation may be felt. Subsequently, with varying degrees of internal rotation, a posteriorly directed force is applied to the anterior humeral head (Fig. 31).

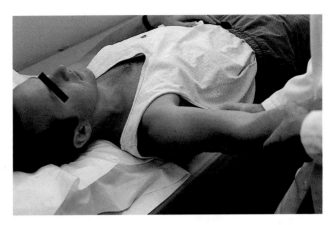

FIG. 30. The load and shift test. Axial compression is placed on the abducted extremity, centering the humeral head in the glenoid. An anterior or posterior shift is then performed by the examiner to assess the level of instability.

Alternatively, rather than grasping the humeral head and scapula, the examiner may position the more proximal hand on the shaft of the humerus and apply an axial load to center the humeral head in the glenoid. An anterior or posterior force is then applied by the more proximal hand while varying the rotation with the other hand. This method of examination is easier to perform, but has the disadvantage of losing the stabilizing effect of the examiner's proximal hand on the scapula. Additionally, more subtle translation may not be appreciated without the examiner's fingers located near the joint line. In either case, both shoulders should be examined to determine a side-to-side discrepancy.

The examination may be performed in a similar fashion with the patient in the supine position. The primary advantage of supine testing is the ability to compare the afflicted shoulder with the contralateral side without having to reposition the patient. This is important when the examination is performed in the operating room under anesthesia (36,37). Examination under anesthesia of instability may be necessary in clarifying shoulder instability because stability testing of the shoulder in the office setting may cause patient discomfort, resulting in guarding and a less sensitive examination.

Instability is graded by the amount of translation of the humeral head on the glenoid (37). Grade 1 is no translation, grade 2 is translation that is not sufficient for the humeral head to rise up on the rim of the glenoid, grade 3 is translation of the humeral head to but not over the rim of the glenoid, and grade 4 is dislocation of the glenohumeral articulation.

Superior Labrum–Anterior to Posterior Lesions

With the advent of arthroscopy of the shoulder, orthopedists have gained a more thorough understanding of the shoulder joint and pathologic anatomy that may result in painful symptoms. Lesions of the superior labrum–biceps

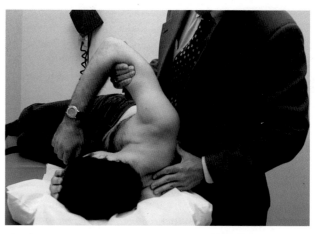
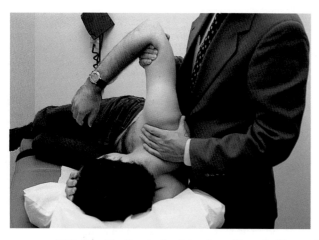

A

B

FIG. 31. Testing in the lateral position. **A:** The patient's glenohumeral articulation is reduced by allowing the weight of the arm to center the humeral head in the glenoid. **B:** A posterior force applied to the humerus results in posterior dislocation of the glenohumeral joint in this patient with symptomatic traumatic posterior instability.

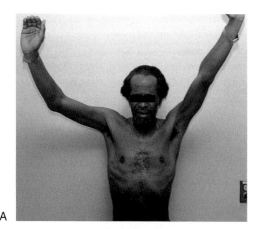
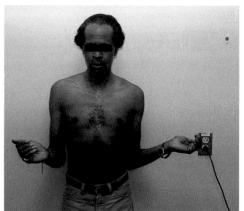

A

B

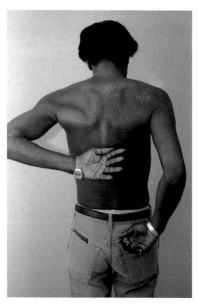

C

FIG. 32. Physical findings in patients with adhesive capsulitis include limitations in forward elevation **(A)**, external rotation **(B)**, and internal rotation **(C)**.

tendon complex, otherwise known as superior labrum-anterior to posterior, or SLAP, lesions, have been identified and classified arthroscopically, and have been implicated as a previously overlooked source of shoulder symptoms (21,38–42). Although this lesion has been observed in 6% to 12% of patients undergoing arthroscopy for shoulder symptoms, a classical history or reproducible physical finding to identify these lesions more effectively preoperatively has not been distinguished (40,41).

Three mechanisms that lead to SLAP lesions have been proposed. In Snyder and colleagues' series, the most common mechanism of injury was a fall onto the outstretched arm (31%). However, traction injuries (14%), such as those that result from lifting a heavy weight from a dead lift or overhead racquet sports, and glenohumeral dislocations (16%) have also been documented as mechanisms leading to the development of SLAP lesions (40,41). The primary consistent complaint in all patients in Snyder's series was pain. An additional component of mechanical symptoms was noted in half of the patients in the study group.

On physical examination, no finding or specific test has been reported to reproducibly indicate underlying anterior labral conditions. Snyder reported that only 34% of patients had symptoms referable to the long head of the biceps, evaluated by biceps tension testing (Speed's test). Crepitus suggestive of labral conditions was noted in 22% of patients. Most patients had findings relative to their associated findings. These signs were indicative of underlying impingement, rotator cuff tears, AC joint arthritis, and glenohumeral instability (40,41).

EXAMINATION FOR MISCELLANEOUS PROBLEMS

Adhesive Capsulitis (Frozen Shoulder)

Adhesive capsulitis (frozen shoulder) is a pathologic process that is unique to the shoulder. It is often misdiagnosed as impingement or rotator cuff disease, and therefore careful attention to the physical findings associated with this disease process is necessary to direct treatment. The patient generally complains of the idiopathic onset of shoulder pain followed by weakness or stiffness. In most cases, the patient can recall a minor injury that may or may not be related to the onset of the process.

The most dramatic physical finding in adhesive capsulitis is the loss of normal shoulder range of motion. This finding is often attributed by the examining physician to pain in the shoulder as a result of rotator cuff impingement or tendinopathy. This diagnosis may lead to worsening of the limited range of motion because patients are frequently instructed to rest the shoulder for several weeks resulting in further capsular contracture and joint stiffness.

The most common restriction of motion is in external rotation tested in both 0 and 90 degrees of abduction, although all planes of motion are usually involved to some degree.

Controversy exists over the exact diagnostic criteria for adhesive capsulitis. In general, a loss of approximately 50% of external rotation with limitation of combined forward elevation of 135 degrees or combined abduction of 90 degrees have all been considered criteria for the diagnosis of adhesive capsulitis (10), although patients with motion slightly better than that noted above are likely to be experiencing the same pathologic process (Fig. 32).

Specific Shoulder Disorders/Extrinsic

Extrinsic sources of shoulder pain include cervical radiculopathy, brachial plexopathy, postural pain, and neoplasm. These should be considered in all patients with shoulder complaints. This is especially true in patients in whom symptoms are not consistent with primary shoulder conditions or in patients with a history of cervical spine disease (18).

REFERENCES

1. Rowe CR, Patel D, Southmayd WW. The Bankart procedure. A long-term end-result study. *J Bone Joint Surg* 1978;60-A(1):1–16.
2. Altchek DW, Warren RF, Wickiewicz TL, et al. Arthroscopic acromioplasty. Technique and results. *J Bone Joint Surg* 1990;72-A(8):1198–1207.
3. Ellman H. Diagnosis and treatment of incomplete rotator cuff tears. *Clin Orthop Rel Res* 1990;254:64.
4. Constant CR, Murley AHG. A clinical method of functional assessment of the shoulder. *Clin Orthop* 1987;214:160.
5. Richards RR, An K-N, Bigliani LU, et al. A standardized method for the assessment of shoulder function. *J Shoulder Elbow Surg* 1994;3(6):347–352.
6. Hawkins RJ, Chris T, Bokor D, et al. Failed anterior acromioplasty. A review of 51 cases. *Clin Orthop Rel Res* 1989;243:106–111.
7. Rowe CR. Recurrent anterior transient subluxation of the shoulder. The "dead arm" syndrome. *Orthop Clin North Am* 1988;19(4):767–772.
8. Neer CS II. Impingement lesions. *Clin Orthop Rel Res* 1983;173:70.
9. Nevaiser JS. Adhesive capsulitis and the stiff and painful shoulder. *Orthop Clin North Am* 1980;11:327.
10. Murnaghan JP. Frozen shoulder. In: Rockwood CA Jr, Matsen FA III, eds. *The shoulder*. Philadelphia: WB Saunders, 1990:837–862.
11. Nevaiser RJ. Painful conditions affecting the shoulder. *Clin Orthop* 1983;173:63.
12. Bankart ASB. Recurrent or habitual dislocation of the shoulder joint. *BMJ* 1923;2:1132.
13. Bankart ASB. The pathology and treatment of recurrent dislocation of the shoulder joint. BMJ 1938;26:23.
14. Fronek J, Warren RF, Bowen M. Posterior subluxation of the glenohumeral joint. *J Bone Joint Surg* 1989;71-A:205.
15. Matsen FA III, Thomas SC, Rockwood CA Jr. Glenohumeral instability. In: Rockwood CA Jr, Matsen FA III, eds. *The shoulder*. Philadelphia: WB Saunders, 1990:526–622.
16. Pollock RG, Bigliani LU. Recurrent posterior shoulder instability: diagnosis and treatment. *Clin Orthop Rel Res* 1993;291:85–96.
17. Glockner SM. Shoulder pain: a diagnostic dilemma. *Am Fam Phys* 1995;51:1677.
18. Zuckerman JD, Mirabello SC, Newman D, et al. The painful shoulder: Part I. Extrinsic disorders. *Am Fam Phys* 1991;43(1):119–128.
19. Hawkins RJ, Bokor DJ. Clinical evaluation of shoulder problems. In: Rockwood CA Jr, Matsen FA III, eds. *The shoulder*. Philadelphia: WB Saunders, 1990:149–177.
20. Inman VT, Saunders JB, Abbott LC. Observation of the function of the shoulder joint. *J Bone Joint Surg* 1944;26-A:1–30.
21. Schulte KR, Warner JJP. Uncommon causes of shoulder pain in the athlete. *Orthop Clin North Am* 1995;26(3):505–528.
22. Lyons AR, Tomlinson JE. Clinical diagnosis of tears of the rotator cuff. *J Bone Joint Surg* 1992;74-B(3):414–415.
23. Wiener BD, Rossario EJ, Feldman AJ. A comparison between physical

examination and MRI in the detection of rotator cuff tears confirmed with arthroscopy. In: *American Shoulder and Elbow Surgeons.* Thirteenth Open Meeting at the American Academy of Orthopaedic Surgeons Annual Meeting, San Francisco, CA, 1997.

24. Neer CS II. *Shoulder reconstruction.* Philadelphia: WB Saunders, 1990.
25. Hoppenfeld S. Physical examination of the spine and extremities. East Norwalk, CT: Appleton-Century-Crofts, 1976.
26. Gerber C, Krushell RJ. Isolated rupture of the tendon of the subscapularis muscle. *J Bone Joint Surg* 1991;73-B:389–394.
27. Yergason RM. Supination sign. *J Bone Joint Surg* 1931;13:160.
28. Hawkins RJ, Hobeika P. Physical examination of the shoulder. *Orthopedics* 1983;6(10):1270–1278.
29. Jobe FW, Kvitne RS. Shoulder pain in the overhand throwing athlete: the relationship of anterior instability and rotator cuff impingement. *Orthop Rev* 1989;18:963.
30. Kvitne RS, Jobe FW. The diagnosis and treatment of anterior instability in the throwing athlete. *Clin Orthop Rel Res* 1993;291:107–123.
31. Rowe CR. Prognosis in dislocations of the shoulder. *J Bone Joint Surg* 1956;38-A:957–977.
32. Rowe CR, Pierce DS, Clark JG. Voluntary dislocation of the shoulder. A preliminary report on a clinical, electromyographic, and psychiatric study of 26 patients. *J Bone Joint Surg* 1973;55-A:445.
33. Reeves B. Experiments on the tensile strength of the anterior capsular structures of the shoulder in man. *J Bone Joint Surg* 1968;50-B(4):858–865.

34. O'Connell PW, Nuber GW, Mileski RA, et al. The contribution of the glenohumeral ligaments to anterior stability of the shoulder joint. *Am J Sports Med* 1990;18:579–584.
35. Turkel SJ, Panio MW, Marshall JL, et al. Stabilizing mechanisms preventing anterior dislocation of the glenohumeral joint. *J Bone Joint Surg* 1981;63-A:1208–1217.
36. Cofield RH, Irving JF. Evaluation and classification of shoulder instability—with special reference to examination under anesthesia. *Clin Orthop Rel Res* 1987;223:32.
37. Cofield RH, Nessler JP, Weinstabl R. Diagnosis of shoulder instability by examination under anesthesia. *Clin Orthop Rel Res* 1993;291:45–53.
38. Andrews JR, Carson WG, McLeod WD. Glenoid labrum tears related to the long head of the biceps. *Am J Sports Med* 1985;13:337.
39. Snyder SJ, et al. SLAP lesions of the shoulder. *Arthroscopy* 1990;6:274–279.
40. Snyder SJ, Banas MP, Karzel RP. An analysis of 140 injuries to the superior glenoid labrum. *J Shoulder Elbow Surg* 1995;4(4):243–248.
41. Snyder SJ, Banas MP, Belzer JP. Arthroscopic evaluation and treatment of injuries to the superior glenoid labrum. In: Pritchard DJ, ed. *Instructional Course Lectures.* Rosemont, IL: American Academy of Orthopaedic Surgeons, 1996:65–70.
42. Maffet MW, Gartsman GM, Moseley B. Superior labrum-biceps tendon complex lesions of the shoulder. *Am J Sports Med* 1995;23(1) 93–98.

Shoulder Magnetic Resonance Imaging,
edited by Lynne S. Steinbach, et al.
Lippincott–Raven Publishers, Philadelphia © 1998.

CHAPTER 6

Rotator Cuff Disease

Lynne S. Steinbach

The rotator cuff tendons are important stabilizers of the shoulder. These tendons provide 80% of the external rotation force and up to half of the abduction mechanism. Injury to the rotator cuff leads to shoulder pain and dysfunction. Identification of the problem and the origin of the disease can often be benefited by the use of magnetic resonance imaging (MRI). This chapter focuses on abnormalities associated with rotator cuff disease, including impingement and tear, with important considerations regarding the rotator cuff when interpreting an MRI study.

Rotator cuff disease can be related to a number of factors. Impingement within the coracoacromial outlet, primary degeneration of the rotator cuff tendons, aging, trauma, overuse associated with athletic and occupational activities, underlying disorders that weaken the tendon, and instability contribute to rotator cuff pathology (Table 1).

L. S. Steinbach: Department of Radiology, University of California, San Francisco, San Francisco, California 94143

IMPINGEMENT

Definition of Impingement

The impingement syndrome is a common, progressively painful compression of the supraspinatus tendon, subacromial-subdeltoid bursa, and long head of the biceps tendon between the humeral head and the coracoacromial arch. The coracoacromial arch is comprised of the undersurface of the anterior third of the acromion, the coracoacromial ligament, the anterior third of the coracoid process, the acromioclavicular (AC) joint, and the distal clavicle. The pain occurs when the arm is raised into a position of abduction and external rotation or is elevated forward and internally rotated (1).

Impingement is common in young athletes, especially those who engage in sports that involve overhead arm movement such as tennis, football, and baseball. It is also seen in persons whose occupations require overhead motion and in older individuals with degenerative changes of the coracoacromial arch.

TABLE 1. *Causes of rotator cuff tear*

Impingement
Aging and degeneration
Acute trauma
Overuse
Arthritides
    Rheumatoid arthritis
    Calcium pyrophosphate dihydrate crystal deposition disease
Other systemic disorders that weaken tendons
    Diabetes
    Renal disease
    Steroid use
    Smoking
Instability

TABLE 3. *Stages of impingement of the supraspinatus tendon (neer classification)*

I Reversible edema and hemorrhage (usually seen in patients younger than 25 years of age)
II Fibrosis and tendinitis resulting from chronic trauma
III Degeneration and rupture of the supraspinatus tendon, often associated with osseous changes (usually seen in patients older than 40 years of age)

There are several forms of impingement (Table 2). Classic primary extrinsic type of impingement results from entrapment of the supraspinatus tendon by the coracoacromial arch, which is caused by variations in the architecture of the coracoacromial arch, including one or more of the following: a subacromial enthesophyte, anteriorly hooked acromion, downsloping or low-lying acromion, inferior AC joint osteophytes, os acromiale, or a thickened coracoacromial ligament. Secondary extrinsic impingement can be caused by inferior narrowing of the coracoacromial outlet from glenohumeral or scapulothoracic instability. Posterior-superior impingement is an internal form of impingement that can produce shoulder pain and can lead to partial thickness tears of the undersurface of the rotator cuff. Supraspinatus muscle hypertrophy and a prominent greater tuberosity can also lead to narrowing of the coracoacromial outlet with subsequent impingement.

Stages of Impingement

In 1972, Neer described the technique of anterior acromioplasty to relieve the symptoms of impingement (1). He hypothesized that abnormalities of the anterior third of the acromion and excessive traction by the coracoacromial ligament result in a progression of degenerative changes of the supraspinatus tendon.

The area of the tendon that is most frequently affected by impingement is called the critical zone, a region first described by Codman (2). This is an area approximately 1 cm from the tendon insertion on the greater tuberosity. It is believed that mechanical impingement to the critical zone leads

TABLE 2. *Causes of supraspinatus tendon impingement*

Primary extrinsic impingement
Secondary extrinsic impingement
    Glenohumeral instability
    Scapulothoracic instability
Internal impingement
    Posterosuperior glenoid impingement
Supraspinatus muscle hypertrophy
Callus around greater tuberosity fracture
Prominent greater tuberosity

to inflammatory tendinitis that represents the first stage of the degenerative process.

Neer subsequently described three stages of impingement involving the critical zone of the supraspinatus tendon (3) (Table 3). The first stage is that of reversible edema and hemorrhage usually seen in patients younger than 25 years of age. The second stage is fibrosis and tendinitis resulting from chronic trauma, and the third stage is degeneration and rupture of the supraspinatus tendon, often associated with osseous changes and usually seen in patients older than 40 years of age. Neer also demonstrated that a laterally placed or shallow bicipital groove caused the long head of the biceps tendon to undergo impingement by the anterior one third of the acromion, resulting in eventual tendinitis and rupture.

Neer postulated that up to 95% of rotator cuff tears result from chronic impingement (3). Other researchers believe that degeneration with aging is perhaps the most important (2,4), followed by impingement, acute trauma, overuse, and chronic inflammatory disease (see Table 1).

Clinical Assessment of Impingement

An impingement-injection test, first described by Neer, is a tool to assess the presence of impingement (3). The examiner elevates the humerus of the patient with one hand while preventing scapular rotation with the other. Pain is produced when the greater tuberosity of the humeral head impinges against the acromion. The pain is relieved by injection of an anesthetic agent into the subacromial space. Caution should be taken when using this test alone for the diagnosis of impingement, because other causes for the pain may also be relieved by the injection. See Chapter 5 for a more complete review of this topic.

Imaging Workup of Impingement and Rotator Cuff Tear

Different imaging techniques are available for evaluation of impingement and rotator cuff abnormalities: conventional radiographs, sonography, arthrography, and MRI. Each technique has advantages and disadvantages.

Conventional Radiographs

Early diagnosis and treatment of impingement syndrome may prevent progression of soft tissue abnormalities, especially rotator cuff tears. Conventional radiography and arthrography have been disappointing in the early diagnosis of impingement. Surrounding osseous changes such as a subacromial enthesophyte, laterally downsloping or low-lying acromion, and AC joint undersurface osteophytes can be identified; however, these can also be present in the absence of rotator cuff disease.

An anteroposterior radiograph obtained with 30 degrees of caudal angulation of the central ray best demonstrates anterior acromial enthesophytes (5). A modified transscapular lateral view obtained at 10 to 15 degrees of caudal angulation, termed the *supraspinatus outlet view,* is often used to show the anterior inferior aspect of the acromion (6,7). Fluoroscopy can also be helpful for detection of subacromial enthesophytes (8). They are best seen on spot films obtained with the patient standing and leaning forward toward the image intensifier.

The conventional radiograph is somewhat limited in evaluation of the rotator cuff. It can be pathognomonic for a chronic tear if there is elevation of the humeral head with either acromiohumeral articulation or an acromiohumeral distance of less than 7 mm, but this is not commonly seen in patients with acute rotator cuff tear. Concavity of the undersurface of the acromion as a result of molding by the humeral head is also suggestive of a rotator cuff tear. Well-circumscribed lytic lesions and sclerosis of the greater tuberosity occur frequently with rotator cuff tears, but these findings are nonspecific.

Arthrography

Glenohumeral joint arthrography is an invasive study limited to demonstration of partial thickness undersurface and full-thickness tears of the rotator cuff and does this with high sensitivity and specificity (9). It cannot demonstrate partial thickness tears in the substance or superior surface of the tendon and cannot directly evaluate important soft tissue structures in and around the glenohumeral joint that may be causing or contributing to the symptomatic shoulder, including labrocapsular abnormalities, bursitis, and paralabral cysts (10,11). Furthermore, arthrography does not allow for evaluation of the muscles of the rotator cuff or marrow abnormalities.

Ultrasound

Ultrasound is an operator-dependent technique that can demonstrate abnormalities of the rotator cuff, bursa, and long head of the biceps tendon (12–18). It allows for noninvasive evaluation of the muscles and tendons of the rotator cuff. Ultrasound can be used with high sensitivity and specificity when scanned and interpreted by a highly experienced sonographer using state-of-the-art ultrasound equipment. Several groups have published results that demonstrate diagnostic sensitivity and specificity above 90% for detecting partial and full-thickness rotator cuff tears (19–22). Ultra-

sound has not been as successful in the hands of less experienced radiologists. Changes in the tendon with shoulder motion can be directly assessed using ultrasound. Ultrasound is not able to evaluate many abnormalities of the shoulder that might be causing a rotator cuff tear or contributing to shoulder pain, including lesions associated with instability such as labral and capsular disruption. It has been shown to demonstrate greater tuberosity fractures (23) but is limited in its evaluation of the deeper osseous structures. A normal ultrasound in a patient with impingement symptoms should be followed up with further imaging examinations to detect changes associated with the osseous structures of the coracoacromial arch and secondary causes of impingement, including lesions of the labrum and glenohumeral ligaments associated with instability.

Magnetic Resonance Evaluation of Impingement

MRI is able to demonstrate osseous and soft tissue abnormalities of the shoulder in any plane with high soft tissue contrast. The status of the tendons, muscles, marrow, and labrocapsular structures can be assessed. Normal tendons and those with a full-thickness tear are easily identified on routine noncontrast MR studies. The most sensitive and specific study, especially for partial undersurface tears of the rotator cuff, is one obtained with some native fluid, saline, or contrast in the joint. The study may be limited for this evaluation if fluid is not present in the glenohumeral joint.

Brief Anatomic Review

The rotator cuff is composed of the supraspinatus, infraspinatus, teres minor, and subscapularis tendons (Fig. 1). These tendons are important stabilizers of the glenohumeral joint. The first three of these tendons insert on the superior and posterior aspect of the greater tuberosity, whereas the subscapularis attaches anteriorly on the lesser tuberosity. There is a space between the supraspinatus and subscapularis tendons called the *rotator interval.* The coracohumeral ligament, long head of the biceps tendon, and coracoid lie in this region.

The rotator cuff tendons, subacromial bursa, and the long head of the biceps tendon lie within the coracoacromial outlet (Fig. 2). The superior aspect of this outlet, the coracoacromial arch, includes the acromion, which is an anterolateral extension of the scapular spine, the anterior third of the coracoid, the coracoacromial ligament, which spans from the coracoid to the anterior-inferior aspect of the acromion, the distal clavicle, and the AC articulation. The coracoacromial ligament restricts anterior and superior movement of the humeral head and related structures.

On axial MR images, the supraspinatus tendon is seen superiorly on sections just below the acromion and clavicle (Fig. 3). The scapular spine lies posterior to the supraspinatus. More caudally, the infraspinatus (Fig. 4), and then the teres minor may be identified immediately adjacent to the

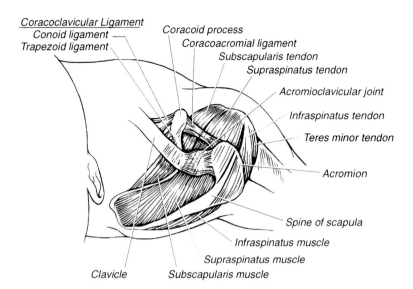

Coracoclavicular Ligament
  Conoid ligament —
  Trapezoid ligament
    Coracoid process
    Coracoacromial ligament
    Subscapularis tendon
    Supraspinatus tendon
    Acromioclavicular joint
    Infraspinatus tendon
    Teres minor tendon
    Acromion
    Spine of scapula
  Infraspinatus muscle
  Supraspinatus muscle
Clavicle   *Subscapularis muscle*

FIG. 1. Overhead schematic view of the rotator cuff. The supraspinatus tendon lies under the coracoacromial arch and inserts on the greater tuberosity of the humerus along with the more posterior and inferior infraspinatus and teres minor tendons. The subscapularis muscle and tendon originate in front of the scapula and insert on the lesser tuberosity of the humerus.

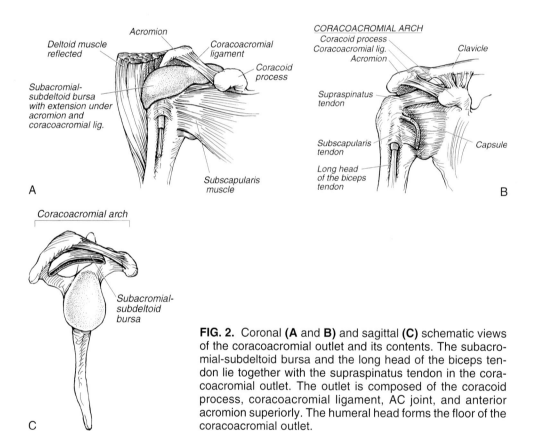

FIG. 2. Coronal **(A** and **B)** and sagittal **(C)** schematic views of the coracoacromial outlet and its contents. The subacromial-subdeltoid bursa and the long head of the biceps tendon lie together with the supraspinatus tendon in the coracoacromial outlet. The outlet is composed of the coracoid process, coracoacromial ligament, AC joint, and anterior acromion superiorly. The humeral head forms the floor of the coracoacromial outlet.

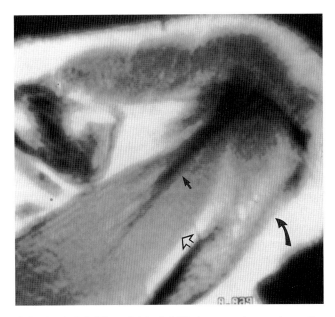

FIG. 3. Axial T1-weighted MR image shows how the supraspinatus muscle *(open arrow)* and tendon *(black arrow)* lie anterior to the scapular spine *(curved arrow)*. The main central tendon axis lies approximately 10 degrees anterior to the axis of the muscle.

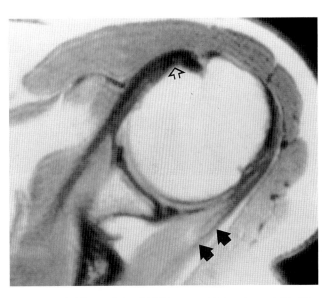

FIG. 4. Axial T1-weighted MR image obtained caudal to Fig. 3 at the level of the infraspinatus muscle and tendon *(solid arrows)*. The subscapularis muscle lies anteriorly with the tendon extending laterally to attach on the lesser tuberosity of the humerus *(open arrow)*.

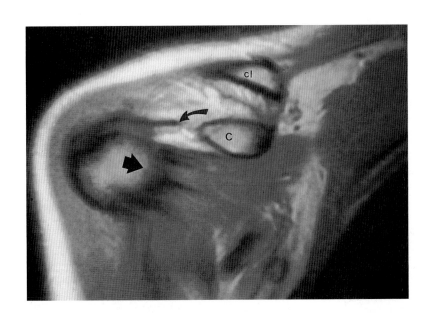

FIG. 5. Oblique coronal T1-weighted MR image anterior at the level of the coracoid *(c)*. The subscapularis muscle lies below the coracoid with multiple tendon slips inserting on the lesser tuberosity of the humerus *(arrow)*. The distal clavicle *(cl)* lies superiorly. The coracohumeral ligament is also identified *(curved arrow)*.

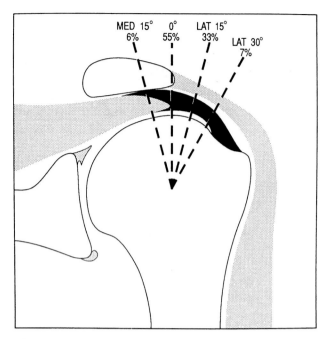

FIG. 6. Diagram showing the percentage of each location of the supraspinatus musculotendinous junction (the most distal point where muscle is visualized) in asymptomatic individuals. This junction usually lies at approximately 12-o'clock position above the humeral head. (From ref. 76, with permission.)

posterior surface of the scapula, below the scapular spine. The last tendon, the subscapularis, arises from the anterior aspect of the scapula and inserts on the lesser tuberosity anterolateral to the glenohumeral joint (see Fig. 4).

The coracoid serves as an anterior marker in the oblique coronal plane, which should be oriented along the long axis of the supraspinatus tendon. The subscapularis muscle runs under the coracoid with multiple tendon slips inserting on

the lesser tuberosity (Fig. 5). The coracohumeral ligament also may be seen on anterior oblique coronal images (see Fig. 5). Further posterior, the supraspinatus tendon runs above the humeral head. The musculotendinous junction of the supraspinatus usually lies near the 12-o'clock position above the humeral head (Fig. 6). The subacromial-subdeltoid (SA-SD) bursa lies above the supraspinatus muscle and tendon. It can contain a few milliliters of fluid in some asymptomatic shoulders, but is usually not directly visualized. A rim of fat may line the inferior aspect of the bursa and this fat can be seen in many symptomatic and asymptomatic shoulders (Fig. 7A). The infraspinatus and teres minor tendons are seen more posteriorly below the long axis of the scapular spine (see Fig. 7B).

On sagittal images, the muscles and tendons of the rotator cuff are seen in cross section (Fig. 8). The supraspinatus, infraspinatus, and teres minor course superior and posterior to the humeral head, respectively. The biceps tendon lies anterior and superior in an area known as the *rotator interval,* which lies between the supraspinatus and subscapularis tendons. It contains the biceps tendon, superior glenohumeral ligament and the coracohumeral ligament and can tear with trauma. The glenohumeral ligaments, which are part of the anterior capsule of the shoulder, lie anterior to the humeral head, and the subscapularis tendon is anterior and inferior. The low signal intensity coracoacromial ligament is often seen on more medial sagittal views. This ligament limits anterior and superior migration of the humeral head during abduction. Some researchers believe that thickening of the coracoacromial ligament may play a role in impingement syndrome as discussed later.

The acromion is viewed on images obtained lateral to the AC joint (Fig. 9). On these images, the shape and orientation of the acromion are evaluated and the clinician looks for the presence of anterior hooking and osteophytes, which can

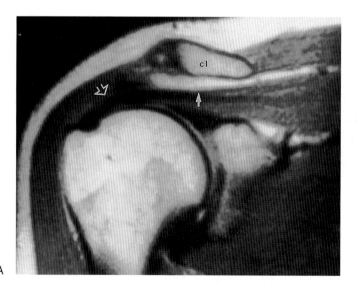

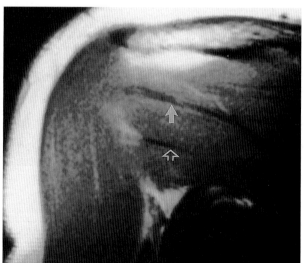

A   B

FIG. 7. A: Normal supraspinatus tendon *(open arrow)* on a oblique coronal T1-weighted MR image. There is some fat below the distal clavicle *(cl)* and acromioclavicular joint *(solid arrow)*. This fat is intermittently present in asymptomatic individuals with normal rotator cuffs. **B:** Oblique coronal MR image obtained posterior to **(A)** now demonstrates the infraspinatus tendon underneath the scapular spine *(solid arrow)* and the teres minor below *(open arrow)*.

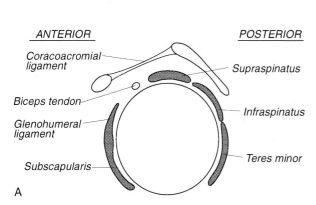

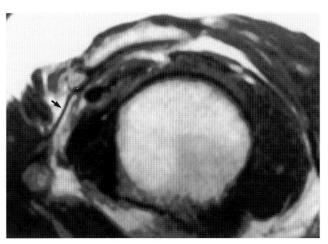

FIG. 8. A: Sagittal schematic view of the rotator cuff muscles and tendons medially at the level of the coracoacromial ligament. **B:** Corresponding oblique sagittal T1-weighted MR image shows the normal coracoacromial ligament *(arrow)* attaching to the anterior acromion (this acromion has an os acromiale). The muscles and tendons of the rotator cuff and the tendon of the long head of the biceps are seen in cross section.

lead to impingement of the rotator cuff tendons. The most lateral oblique sagittal images show the low signal intensity tendons in cross section. The osseous coracoacromial arch is no longer seen (Fig. 10).

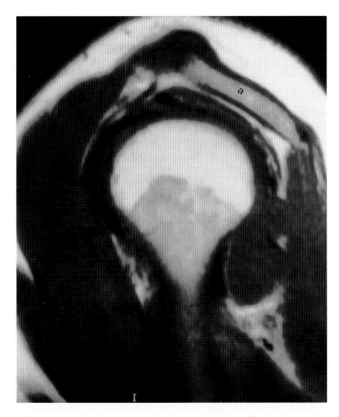

FIG. 9. This oblique sagittal T1-weighted MR image is obtained lateral to the acromioclavicular joint. This is one of several sagittal sections in which acromial shape and slope are assessed. This acromion *(a)* has a flat *(type I)* undersurface and slopes upward posteroanteriorly. The rotator cuff muscles are beginning to thin out with more cross sectional area being occupied by the tendons.

Specific Technical Aspects Regarding Magnetic Resonance Imaging of the Rotator Cuff

Many different MR pulse sequences have been used to evaluate the tendons of the rotator cuff. Standard dual-echo spin-echo images with proton-density and T2-weighted technique, gradient echo sequences, FSE T2-weighted sequences with or without fat saturation, and short tau inversion recovery (STIR) imaging have all been used. Each of these sequences has different strengths and weaknesses, as outlined in the chapter on technique. Our routine noncontrast shoulder MR protocol begins in the axial plane with images extending from the top of the acromion through the inferior

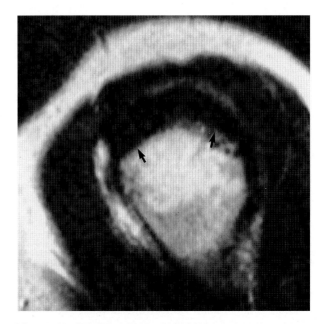

FIG. 10. Far lateral oblique sagittal image shows a crescent of low signal intensity rotator cuff tendons on top of the humeral head *(arrows)*.

margin of the glenoid. The subscapularis, infraspinatus, and teres minor tendons are particularly well seen in this plane. Routinely, an axial T1-weighted scout sequence is followed by a gradient echo sequence in this plane (700/15; flip angle, 40 degrees). This portion of the study is used predominantly for evaluation of lesions associated with instability. The rotator cuff tendons and muscles are also well seen in the axial plane.

Cursors are placed along the axis of the central supraspinatus tendon on T1-weighted scout axial images to define the plane for oblique coronal images. It is important to angle the coronal images along the supraspinatus axis, so that the tendon can be seen in continuity. Both T1-weighted and T2-weighted FSE sequences in the oblique coronal plane are obtained. Frequency-selective fat saturation is used to aid in differentiating fat from fluid when using the FSE T2-weighted sequence; however, the fat may not be completely saturated. When this happens, it is helpful to compare this sequence with the T1-weighted sequence, in which fat is routinely high signal intensity.

An oblique sagittal plane is then selected perpendicular to the oblique coronal images and parallel to the glenoid rim. It is important to obtain this sequence with T2-weighting to further evaluate the cuff muscles and tendons in cross section. I use the T2-weighted FSE sequence with fat saturation for this purpose. Further out into the periphery, the cuff tendons form a dark crescent over the humeral head. An increase in signal intensity representing degeneration, inflammation, or a tear is appreciated on images obtained with this orientation. Rotator interval tears are also well seen in this plane. In addition, oblique-sagittal images provide excellent visualization of the acromion and SA-SD bursa.

Fat-saturated FSE T2-weighted images have been shown to significantly improve specificity for identification of an intact rotator cuff without significantly altering the sensitivity (24). The FSE T2-weighted sequence has the advantage of increased spatial resolution, improved signal-to-noise ratio, and decreased imaging time when compared to routine spin-echo images (25). As mentioned, occasionally, there is incomplete fat suppression when using the frequency-selective fat saturation in conjunction with the FSE sequence because of the bulk susceptibility artifact/magnetic field inhomogeneity related to the curved external surface of the shoulder. If this occurs, alternative sequences include T2-weighted FSE with an echo time (TE) = 160 ms without fat suppression, conventional T2-weighted spin-echo imaging, or a fast inversion recovery sequence, which does not rely on frequency selective fat-saturation.

Although it is invasive, is time-consuming, and requires fluoroscopy for needle placement, MR arthrography can be helpful when no native joint fluid is seen on MRI in a patient with equivocal full-thickness or partial thickness undersurface rotator cuff tears. For the gadolinium study, a solution of dilute gadolinium in saline, which is high signal intensity on T1-weighted fat-saturated images, can be used. For this type of study, I draw up 0.1 cc of gadolinium in a tuberculin syringe and add it to 20 cc of saline. With fat saturation, there is decreased signal from fat, but the signal intensity of gadolinium remains high. Direct injection of saline rather than gadolinium diluted in saline is an alternative to direct MR arthrography with gadolinium. One limitation of the saline MR study, however, is that native joint fluid is not differentiated from injected joint fluid, and this could interfere with diagnosis of abnormalities such as a full-thickness rotator cuff tear or bursitis.

Many investigators are also exploring the role of intravenous gadolinium administration for diagnosis of rotator cuff and labral abnormalities (26). Winalski et al. (27) were able to produce an arthrographic effect of contrast enhancement of joint effusion in the knee 15 minutes following intravenous gadolinium administration and this effect persisted for up to 1 hour. This technique involves a standard intravenous dose of gadolinium contrast agent followed by 10 minutes of exercise of the shoulder. T1-weighted spin-echo images are then obtained in all three routine planes using frequency-selective fat saturation with an additional FSE T2-weighted sequence in the coronal and/or sagittal planes. There is potential for this technique to outline and demonstrate tears of the rotator cuff and labrum that might be difficult to identify on conventional MR images. This technique is also less cumbersome than the intraarticular gadolinium injection technique. It does not require fluoroscopy for joint injection and is less time-consuming. On the other hand, it does not allow for capsular distention and therefore does not provide as complete a study as a direct MR arthrogram. The usefulness of this method remains to be seen.

Preliminary studies suggest that specialized positioning of the shoulder during MRI may facilitate evaluation of certain specific shoulder disorders. For example, oblique axial images of the glenohumeral joint can be obtained with the patient's palm resting under the head, resulting in the dislocation position of abduction and external rotation (ABER) position, previously discussed in Chapter 2 (Fig. 11). This position places traction on the inferior glenohumeral ligamentous complex and may cause distraction of an otherwise unrecognized tear involving the insertion of the anterior band of this complex on the anteroinferior labrum, that is, a Bankart lesion (28). This position has also been demonstrated to be of value in the evaluation of patients with posterosuperior glenoid impingement and of patients with partial thickness tears of the humeral surface of the rotator cuff (29).

Osseous Abnormalities Seen on Magnetic Resonance Imaging in Association with Primary Extrinsic Impingement

MRI can aid in detecting osseous and soft tissue abnormalities that may predispose to or be the result of rotator cuff impingement (30,31). The soft tissue abnormalities in the supraspinatus tendon and subacromial bursa are discussed in the next section. The osseous lesions include morphologic abnormalities of the acromion and AC joint (Table 4). Many of these anatomic features may be present in asymptomatic

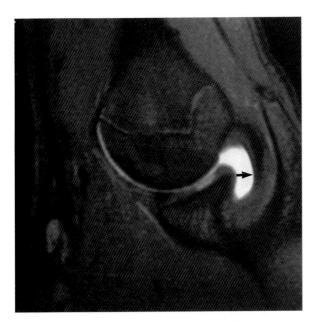

FIG. 11. Normal T1-weighted fat-saturated gadolinium MR arthrogram obtained with the abduction and external rotation (ABER) position. The smooth undersurface of the rotator cuff tendons is well seen adjacent to the high signal intensity gadolinium *(arrow).*

TABLE 4. *Osseous abnormalities that may be associated with supraspinatus tendon impingement*

Acromion
   Subacromial enthesophyte
   Anterior hooking
   Anterior inferior downsloping
   Inferolateral downsloping
   Low position with respect to the distal clavicle
   Os acromiale
   Paget's disease of the acromion
AC joint
   Inferior acromioclavicular joint osteophytes or callus
Greater tuberosity
   Greater tuberosity fracture with posttraumatic remodeling
   Prominent greater tuberosity

shoulders, and clinical correlation is imperative (30–34). Additionally, the diagnosis of impingement is based on clinical criteria, and therefore should not be made from static MRI studies.

Acromion and Acromioclavicular Joint

Osseous changes that can lead to primary extrinsic impingement include subacromial enthesophytes, and osteophytes and capsular hypertrophy along the inferior aspect of the AC joint (1,35). Anteriorly hooked, anteroinferior and inferolaterally downsloping, and low-lying acromions are believed by some researchers to predispose to impingement by narrowing the acromiohumeral distance (36,37). An os acromiale can also predispose to impingement (38).

The subacromial enthesophyte can be definitively diagnosed on MRI if downward projection of marrow signal is seen below the expected location of the cortex (Fig. 12). If the enthesophyte contains mostly cortical bone, it will be low signal intensity. This type of enthesophyte is more difficult to distinguish from the low signal intensity deltoid tendon (39) (Fig. 13) and the coracoacromial ligament, which insert on the inferolateral and inferomedial acromion, respectively. It is helpful to correlate the MR findings with conventional radiographs when the diagnosis is uncertain.

In 1986, Bigliani et al. (40) studied the shape of the acromion in 140 cadaver shoulders to determine the relationship of acromial configuration to full-thickness rotator cuff tears. They defined three different acromial shapes: A type I configuration with a flat undersurface was present in 18.6% of cases; 42% had a type II acromion with a curved undersurface; and 38.6% had a type III acromion with an an-

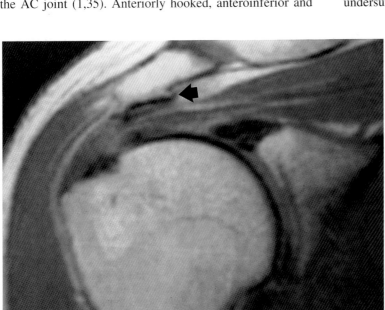

FIG. 12. Note the downward extension of marrow into a subacromial enthesophyte *(arrow)* on a T1-weighted oblique coronal MR image.

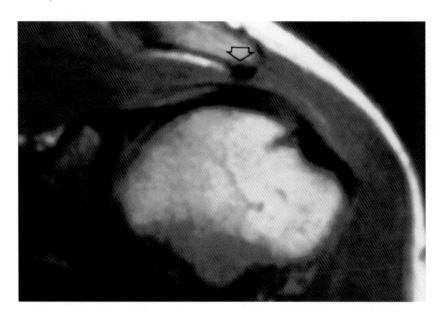

FIG. 13. Low signal intensity structure under the distal acromion represents the normal insertion of the deltoid tendon *(arrow)*. This can be mistaken for an enthesophyte.

terior hook (Fig. 14). Recently, a fourth type of acromial shape with a convex inferior surface has been discovered (41). This configuration is relatively uncommon and there is potential for narrowing the osseous acromial outlet near the mid posterior portion of the distal acromion rather than at the anterior portion of the acromion near the AC joint. There has yet been no definite correlation between this type IV acromion and impingement.

The hooked acromion can be congenital or acquired (36,40). Some researchers believe that the type III anteriorly hooked configuration increases in frequency with increasing age (42) and that this shape can develop as a result of calci-

fication of the acromial attachment of the coracoacromial ligament. Others have found no relationship between acromial type and age (43). The latter group also showed that the type III acromion is more common in males. They found that acromial morphology was symmetric in 70.7% of 191 pairs of cadaveric acromions and that there was an increased incidence of subacromial enthesophytes in patients with type II and type III acromions.

Supraspinatus tendon tears are frequently associated with the anteriorly hooked (type III) acromion. In studies correlating acromial shape to surgical or arthrographic results, Morrison and Bigliani demonstrated that 70% and 80%, re-

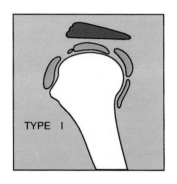

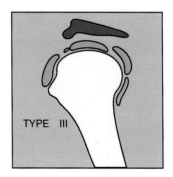

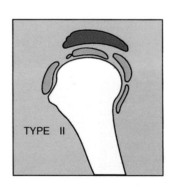

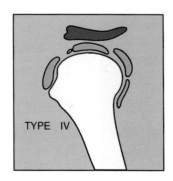

FIG. 14. Schematic demonstration of the four acromial shapes that have been described and are seen on oblique sagittal MR images obtained lateral to the acromioclavicular joint. The first three types were described by Bigliani et al. The type I acromion has a flat undersurface and no significant relationship to impingement. (Adapted with permission from Farley TE, Neumann CH, Steinbach LS, Petersen SA. The coracoacromial arch: MR evaluation and correlation with rotator cuff pathology. *Skeletal Radiology* 1994;23:641–645.)

spectively, of the rotator cuff tears were associated with type III acromions (36,40). The remaining patients with rotator cuff tear had a type II acromion. Only 3% of type I acromions were associated with a rotator cuff tear.

The shape of the acromion can be determined on oblique sagittal MR images located lateral to the AC joint (Fig. 15). In one study that looked at acromial morphology on oblique sagittal MR images, patients with rotator cuff tear had a significantly increased prevalence of hooked acromion compared with control patients (62% versus 13%, $p<0.001$) and there was a greater prevalence of hooked acromions in the group with impingement (30%, $p=0.17$) (44). Farley et al. (41) also found a correlation between the anteriorly hooked acromion seen on MRI and the presence of clinical impingement.

Several studies have found MR assessment of acromial shape to be confusing. Haygood et al. (45) showed significant variability between MR readers in identifying a particular acromial morphology. These investigators did not use a routine location for assessment of acromial shape. A more recent study by Peh et al. (46) concluded that apparent acromial shape is sensitive to minor changes in MR section viewed. There was poor correlation between morphology identified during radiographic and MR assessment.

An acromion that slopes anteroinferiorly or inferolaterally or is low-lying with respect to the distal clavicle has potential to narrow the coracoacromial outlet (31,37,47). The lateral aspect of the normal acromion is nearly horizontal or upward sloping from posterior to anterior. If the anterior acromion is more caudal in relation to the posterior portion,

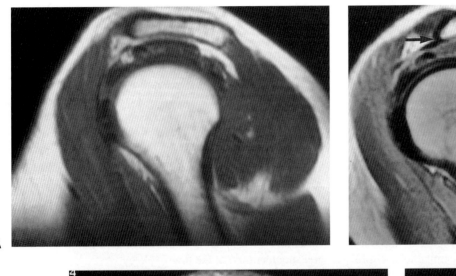

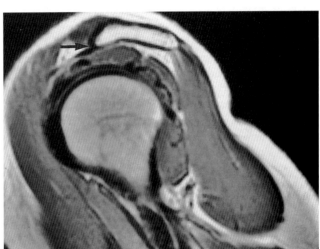

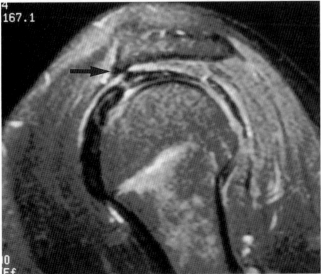

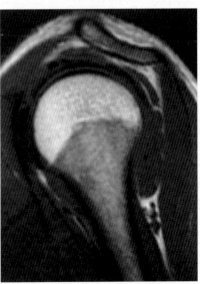

A B C D

FIG. 15. MR images of several types of acromial shapes. **A:** The type II acromion has a curved undersurface and occasionally contributes to impingement. **B and C:** The type III acromion has an anterior hook *(arrow)* and predisposes to impingement. **D:** The fourth type of acromion, recently described in the radiological literature, is convex and has not been shown to contribute to impingement.

Regular A-C Joint   Downsloping A-C Joint

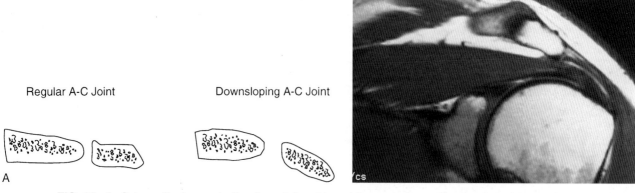

A   B

FIG. 16. A: Schematic demonstrating the relationships of the acromion to the distal clavicle on oblique coronal images. **B:** Laterally downsloping acromion on a T1-weighted coronal-oblique MR image. Some researchers believe that a laterally downward sloping acromion may narrow the distance between the acromion and humeral head, resulting in impingement of the supraspinatus tendon.

some researchers believe that there is greater risk of symptomatic anterior acromial impingement (47). This type of configuration would produce impingement primarily on the midportion of the supraspinatus tendon in the area of the critical zone. In one study, however, there was lack of association between this type of inferiorly sloping acromion on the oblique coronal sequence and the presence of rotator cuff tear (41). Such downward sloping of the acromion also may cause impingement of the superior aspect of the subscapularis tendon (48,49). An inferior-laterally sloping acromion appears to be associated with lateral supraspinatus injury near the greater tuberosity insertion, especially in patients who perform forceful abduction of the shoulder, such as pitchers, divers, and swimmers (50) (Fig. 16).

Osteophytes and osseous or fibrous callus under the AC joint from degenerative change can predispose to impingement (1,35) (Fig. 17). The mechanism is similar to sawing a log, with the supraspinatus tendon simulating a log and the osteophytes cutting the tendon, especially when the patient abducts the shoulder. AC joint osteoarthrosis is not specific for impingement and can be seen with high prevalence in asymptomatic individuals (51).

The os acromiale is an accessory ossification center along the outer aspect of the acromion that has failed to fuse to the acromion by the age of 25 years. It is seen in 1% to 15% of the population but it is not known how many of these are symptomatic (52–55). The unfused segment can be united to the remaining acromion via an articulation composed of fibrous tissue, cartilage (synchondrosis), periosteum, or synovium (38,52). The os acromiale is classified as a pre-, meso-, meta- or basi-acromion based on its regions of articulation with the acromion (38) (Fig. 18). The meta-acromion is the most proximal center and the meso- and pre-acromion are progressively more distal. Most are of the meso- or meta-acromial type (56). Os acromiales are seen in the contralateral shoulder 60% of the time (57).

An os acromiale is more mobile than an acromion without accessory ossification centers. Motion is increased at the del-

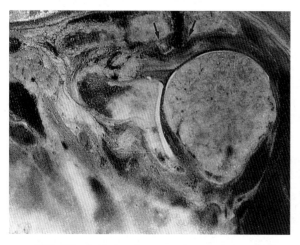

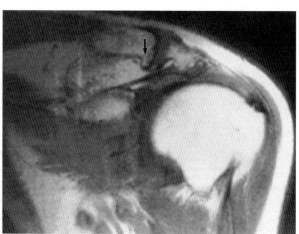

A   B

FIG. 17. A: Osteophytes project underneath the acromioclavicular joint in a cadaver shoulder *(arrows).* **B:** A corresponding oblique coronal T1-weighted MR image obtained from a patient reveals an osteophyte along the undersurface of the acromioclavicular joint *(arrow).* This patient also has a chronic supraspinatus tendon tear with tendon retraction and severe fatty atrophy of the muscle.

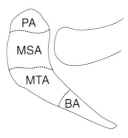

FIG. 18. Axial diagram of the acromion demonstrating the potential regions of attachment of an os acromiale to the acromion. PA, pre-acromion; MSA, meso-acromion; MTA, meta-acromion; BA, basi-acromion.

toid tendon insertion along the lateral inferior aspect of the ossification center. Contraction of the deltoid muscle can pull down on the lateral aspect of the acromion, creating a hinge effect that narrows the subacromial outlet with resultant impingement and tears of the rotator cuff. The coracoacromial ligament also commonly attaches to the unfused segment. Hyperostosis may develop along the undersurface of the os acromiale at its site of failed union, leading to impingement and eventual tear of the supraspinatus tendon (38,54,56). Surgical and radiologic literature has confirmed the association between os acromiale and impingement and rotator cuff pathology (38,56,58). Simply identifying the os acromiale does not implicate it as the source of shoulder pain or rotator cuff disease.

Careful preoperative imaging evaluation is necessary to exclude the presence of an os acromiale. This ossification center may be difficult to find on conventional radiographs (52,54,55,59). It is best seen on an axillary view that displays the long axis of the acromion (Fig. 19A). It can also be seen on an axial computed tomography (CT) or on an MR study, in which it is important to include high axial sections that demonstrate the entire acromion (Fig. 19B). The os acromiale is easiest to identify in the axial plane, although it

can usually be noticed in all three planes, especially if it is larger (Fig. 20). The clinician should be careful not to miss the synchondrosis, which can have an appearance similar to the neighboring AC joint (Fig. 21). This is especially easy to do on the oblique sagittal images. MRI has an advantage over conventional radiographs and CT in that it can reveal underlying, frequently associated rotator cuff tendon abnormalities.

It is important to report the presence of an os acromiale, especially in patients who are being considered for subacromial decompression for impingement (56). The os acromiale has the potential for even more mobility and there can be further weakening of the synchondrosis after this procedure, leading to more impingement (1,56). I have seen several patients months to years following subacromial decompression with previously undiagnosed os acromiale who have done poorly. Small ossification centers are often excised with reattachment of the deltoid; larger or unstable ones may be fused to the rest of the acromion.

I have seen several cases of Paget's disease of the acromion, a rare cause of impingement (Fig. 22). Paget's disease can produce enlargement of the acromion, resulting in narrowing of the coracoacromial outlet. The enlargement of the acromion and occasional abnormal signal intensity of the marrow can aid in diagnosis on MRI. Other bones may also be involved (see Fig. 22). A conventional radiograph should be consulted in such cases to identify pagetoid characteristics and confirm the diagnosis.

Soft Tissue Abnormalities Associated with Impingement

Some of the soft tissue abnormalities associated with impingement are listed in Table 5. Secondary injury that affects the supraspinatus tendon and subacromial bursa from abnormalities of the coracoacromial arch are best evaluated with MRI. Analysis of signal intensity changes in the supraspina-

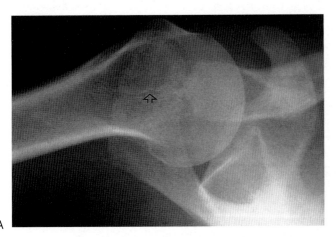
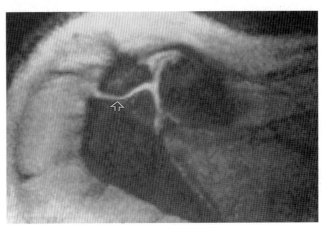

A   B

FIG. 19. Os acromiale is best seen in the axial plane. **A:** The os acromiale is demonstrated on the axillary view of conventional radiographs *(arrow).* **B:** A routine high axial gradient-echo T2* image is obtained through the acromion, best demonstrating the os acromiale *(arrow).*

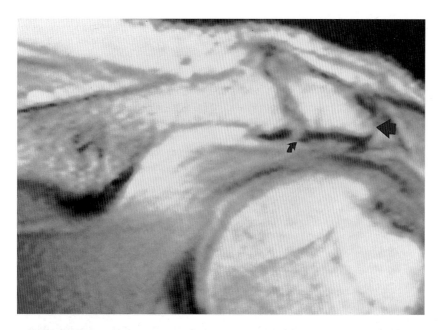

FIG. 20. A large os acromiale attached at the basiacromion is well seen on a oblique coronal T1-weighted image obtained posteriorly at the level of the scapular spine *(arrow)*. A small osteophyte projects inferiorly *(curved arrow)*. This can cause impingement on the underlying tendons.

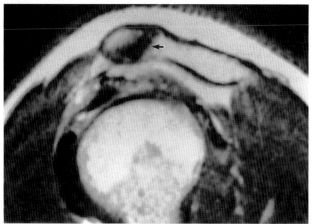

A

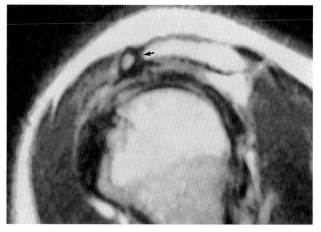

B

FIG. 21. An os acromiale may be mistaken for an acromioclavicular joint. Careful scrutiny of all images avoids this pitfall. Oblique sagittal images in the same patient extending from **A**, the acromioclavicular joint *(arrow)*, to **B**, where there is an os acromiale of the pre-acromial type *(arrow)*.

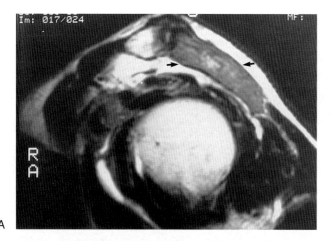

A

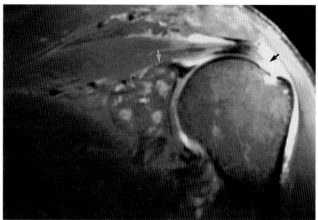

B

FIG. 22. Paget's disease of the acromion producing impingement and rotator cuff tear. **A:** An oblique sagittal T2-weighted MR image shows the expanded acromion with abnormal low signal intensity *(arrows)*, which is one of many presentations of Paget's disease on MRI. **B:** An oblique coronal T1-weighted fat-saturated MR image obtained following intravenous administration of gadolinium reveals the high signal intensity supraspinatus tendon tear *(black arrow)*. The scapula is also involved with Paget's disease *(white arrow)*.

TABLE 5. *Soft tissue abnormalities that can be associated with impingement*

Supraspinatus tendon
  Tendinosis
  Partial thickness tear
  Full-thickness tear
Thickened coracoacromial ligament
Subacromial bursitis
Hypertrophied supraspinatus muscle
Biceps tendon abnormalities

tus tendon should be correlated with clinical findings. Focal regions of intermediate or high signal intensity may be seen in asymptomatic individuals because of degeneration rather than inflammation or partial thickness tear (60–62). The MR appearance of these soft tissue abnormalities are discussed in the section on Rotator Cuff Tendon Evaluation by Magnetic Resonance.

A thickened coracoacromial ligament has been associated with the impingement syndrome (63) (see Fig. 15B). Some believe that it is a cause of impingement (64), whereas others postulate that it is thickened as a result of alteration of the soft tissue structures from the impingement process (65). The criteria for thickening of the ligament on MRI is somewhat subjective. In one study, the coracoacromial ligament was considered to be thickened when the major part of the ligament was smoothly or irregularly enlarged or thicker than 2.0 mm (33). This definition was arbitrarily chosen by the study's authors based on clinical experience. There was a statistically significant association between a thickened coracoacromial ligament and rotator cuff tear in that study. An anatomic study of the coracoacromial ligament demonstrated that the subacromial thickness can vary from 2 to 5.6 mm with an average measurement of 3.9 mm (66). Posttraumatic calcification or ossification of the coracoacromial ligament is a another rare cause of impingement (67).

Neer has shown that a shallow or laterally placed bicipital groove exposed the long head of the biceps tendon to impingement by the anterior third of the acromion, resulting in inflammation or rupture of the intraarticular portion of the tendon. Disorders of the biceps tendon are discussed in Chapter 8. A brief discussion of this subject follows.

Fluid in the biceps tendon sheath is often seen in asymptomatic individuals because this structure communicates with the glenohumeral joint. Paratenonitis (also called tenosynovitis) can be diagnosed when the amount of fluid in the tendon sheath is out of proportion to that in the glenohumeral joint. Mild paratenonitis is not detected using this more specific criteria. With tendinosis, the tendon may be increased in size and may concomitantly or alternatively demonstrate internal high signal intensity on T2 weighting. Partial thickness tears may be difficult to distinguish from tendinosis if the tendon is not thinned, split, or irregular. The full-thickness biceps tendon rupture is seen with discontinuity of the tendon and several axial MR images showing an empty intertubercular groove.

Treatment of Primary Extrinsic Impingement

Findings on MRI can be used as a basis for planning conservative treatment and surgical repair. Criteria based on the type of impingement and severity of tendon disease may be developed for prophylactic coracoacromial arch decompression before the development of irreversible cuff disease. Decisions should be based on careful evaluation of the MR findings with close clinical correlation.

Classic primary extrinsic impingement without rotator cuff tear is usually treated conservatively with injection of steroids or other antiinflammatory medication. If this fails, then decompression in the form of acromioplasty, resection of the distal clavicle, or coracoacromial ligament release is performed. This alleviates anatomic or mechanical elements and provides the supraspinatus tendon and other soft tissue structures a larger space in which to function (68). Tendon repair is attempted when tears are seen in the rotator cuff.

Other Causes of Impingement

Other causes of impingement syndrome include secondary extrinsic impingement (resulting from an unstable glenohumeral joint), posterosuperior glenoid impingement, supraspinatus muscle hypertrophy, posttraumatic remodeling of the proximal humerus (following greater tuberosity fracture), and a prominent greater tuberosity (69–74). These secondary forms of impingement must be treated in a different manner than primary extrinsic impingement with attention directed toward the primary problem rather than the coracoacromioclavicular structures. Secondary extrinsic impingement may be treated with rotator cuff strengthening and avoidance of activities that cause instability or, when severe, may result in repair of underlying labral and capsular abnormalities related to instability.

Secondary extrinsic impingement varies from primary extrinsic impingement in that there is no morphologic abnormality of the coracoacromial arch. This form of impingement is produced in the setting of glenohumeral instability, which produces narrowing of the coracoacromial outlet owing to abnormal superior migration of the humeral head (69). It can also result from scapulothoracic instability and posterosuperior glenoid impingement. It is more common in younger patients and athletes who perform repetitive overhead or throwing motions. In one study, 68% of patients with anterior or multidirectional shoulder instability had impingement signs in addition to apprehension and capsular laxity (75).

The following is the cascade of events that leads to secondary extrinsic impingement. Chronic instability is accompanied by weakening of the capsule and glenohumeral ligaments (the static stabilizers). In this situation, the dynamic stabilizers of the shoulder (the rotator cuff tendons) must play a greater role in preventing subluxation and dislocation. This can produce wear and fatigue of these tendons, allowing for excessive humeral head translation. The humeral head glides along the undersurface of the tendons and pushes up on them, which produces narrowing of the coracoacromial outlet. This results in undersurface impingement with eventual tendon degeneration and tear.

Scapulothoracic instability results from abnormal scapular motion during throwing. Stability and positioning of the scapulothoracic articulation is dependent on a delicate balance between scapulothoracic muscles (trapezius, serratus anterior, rhomboids, and latissimus dorsi). Abnormalities in the biomechanics of this articulation can result in malpositioning of the glenoid articular fossa. This may produce superior positioning of the humeral head with respect to the glenoid with narrowing of the coracoacromial outlet, leading to impingement.

Posterior superior impingement of the glenoid rim can produce shoulder pain and can lead to partial thickness tears of the undersurface of the rotator cuff. This form of internal impingement was first described by Walch (71) and then Liu

(72) and their coworkers in overhead athletes; more recently it has been recognized in nonathletes who frequently rotate the shoulder into the extremes of abduction and external rotation (70). The mechanism that leads to this form of impingement involves superior or posterosuperior angulation of the humerus with respect to the glenoid. In this syndrome, the articular side of the rotator cuff tendons and the greater tuberosity are compressed against the posterosuperior glenoid labrum, resulting in partial thickness tendon tears, especially of the posteroinferior supraspinatus and the infraspinatus, a degenerative tear of the posterior surface of the posterior superior labrum or underlying glenoid, and an osteochondral compression fracture in the region of the greater tuberosity of the humeral head (which can simulate a Hill-Sachs lesion) (Fig. 23). The inferior glenohumeral ligament and adjacent labrum can also be injured. The tears can be well seen on MR arthrograms obtained in the ABER position

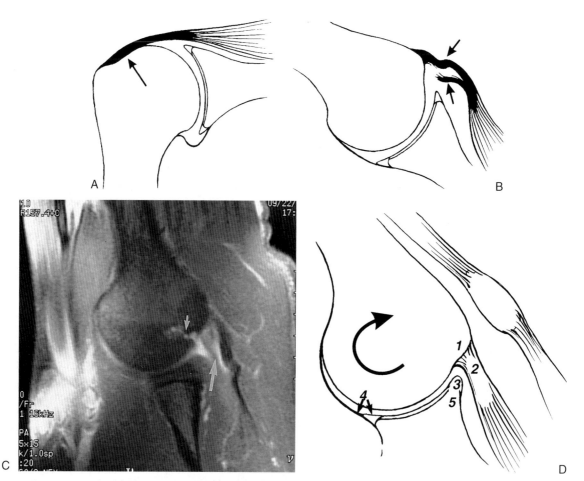

FIG. 23. Posterosuperior glenoid impingement. **A:** Schematic showing how an undersurface tear can be missed on routine oblique coronal images, even during an MR arthrogram. **B:** The ABER position opens up the undersurface of the supraspinatus and infraspinatus tendons, allowing for demonstration of some tears not seen in the adducted position. **C:** Oblique axial T1-weighted MR arthrogram with gadolinium obtained with the ABER position reveals high signal intensity gadolinium extending into a lesion in the humeral head near the greater tuberosity (*small arrow*). Gadolinium also fills a flap tear located along the undersurface of the infraspinatus tendon (*large arrow*). **D:** Schematic demonstrating the potential regions of the joint that can be affected by this disorder. 1, humeral head; 2, undersurface of the supraspinatus and infraspinatus tendons; 3, posterosuperior glenoid labrum; 4, inferior glenohumeral ligament and anteroinferior labrum; 5, posterosuperior glenoid.

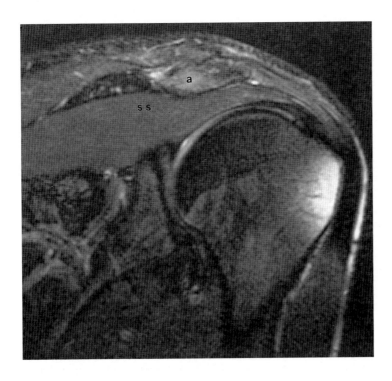

FIG. 24. The acromion *(a)* indents this hypertrophied supraspinatus muscle *(ss)* on an oblique coronal T2-weighted FSE image obtained with fat saturation. This phenomenon could lead to impingement.

(29). Treatment is aimed at controlling extremes of shoulder elevation and abduction external rotation by exercise or surgery and at repair of the injured structures.

Supraspinatus muscle hypertrophy is an intrinsic form of impingement of the supraspinatus muscle (Fig. 24). It is common in athletes such as weight-lifters and swimmers who perform forceful overhead arm movements. This form of impingement can be seen in the presence of a normal coracoacromial arch (50). Patients tend to be most symptomatic when carrying heavy objects with the arms at the sides and when sleeping. In this condition, there is deformation of the supraspinatus musculotendinous junction beneath the AC joint and anterior acromion on oblique coronal MR images. Supraspinatus muscle hypertrophy can be treated by reduction in overhead activity.

Callus around a healed greater tuberosity fracture can also lead to impingement of the supraspinatus tendon between the remodeled prominent greater tuberosity and the lateral acromion. A prominent greater tuberosity can lead to impingement of the supraspinatus tendon by the same mechanism.

ROTATOR CUFF TENDON EVALUATION BY MAGNETIC RESONANCE

Causes for Elevated Signal Intensity in the Supraspinatus Tendon on Short TE Images (T1-Weighted, Proton Density, and Some Gradient Echo Sequences)

There has been difficulty in distinguishing between the various causes of focal or diffuse increased signal intensity in the tendons of the rotator cuff when there is no morphologic disruption (Table 6). The pattern of focally increased signal intensity in the tendon on short TE images that does not increase in signal intensity on T2 weighting is generally believed to represent an artifact, partial volume averaging, or a clinically less significant abnormality. Moderate increase in signal intensity in the distal supraspinatus tendon should not be considered a definite rotator cuff abnormality (34,39,76,77).

Intermediate signal intensity muscle slips can lie between various tendinous components (78). Clinicians must also be careful in interpreting signal intensity within the tendons on short TE MR images because there is angular anisotropy also termed the "magic angle" phenomenon that produces increased signal intensity in normal tendons at a 55-degree an-

TABLE 6. *Causes for elevated signal intensity on short TE images*

Without increase in signal intensity on T2-weighted or STIR images
Partial volume averaging with adjacent tissues (muscle, fascia, fat)
"Magic angle" phenomenon
Overriding of infraspinatus tendon in internal rotation
Partial volume averaging with humeral head cartilage
Artifacts
Tendinosis
Fibrosis and granulation tissue in rotator cuff tear (10% of tears)
With increase in signal intensity on T2-weighted or STIR images
Fluid in biceps tendon sheath
Tendinosis
Tendinitis (plus or minus calcium)
Partial thickness tear
Full-thickness tear
Immediate postoperative period
Recent injection
Metallic artifact from surgery

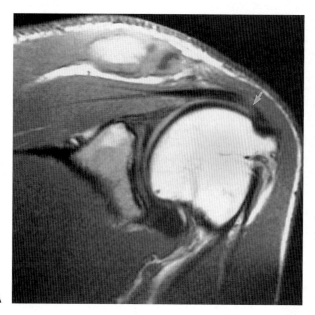

A

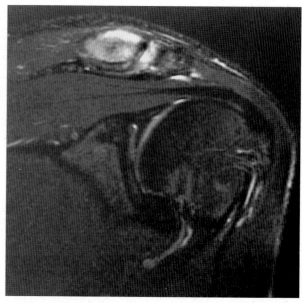

B

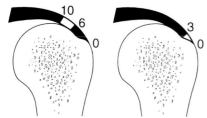

C

FIG. 25. A: Intermediate signal intensity created by the magic angle phenomenon frequently occurs in the critical zone of the supraspinatus tendon *(arrow)* on short TE sequences such as this T1-weighted oblique coronal image (TR = 600; TE = 16). **B:** This signal disappears on a fat-saturated FSE T2-weighted MR image obtained with a longer TE. **C:** The location and size of intermediate signal intensity related to the magic angle can change when the shoulder is repositioned in the magnet, as demonstrated on this schematic of the same shoulder imaged in two different positions. The white area is the region of the magic angle phenomenon. (Adapted with permission from ref. 81.)

gle from the static magnetic field on short TE sequences including spin-echo T1-weighted and some gradient echo (MPGR) sequences (79–81) (Fig. 25). The signal intensity decreases on images obtained with a longer TE. The magic angle phenomenon tends to occur in the area of the critical zone, approximately 1 cm from the insertion of the

supraspinatus tendon on the greater tuberosity. Coincidentally, this is the region that is prone to impingement and rotator cuff tears. Another potential cause of elevated signal intensity within the rotator cuff on short TE images is overriding of the infraspinatus tendon over the supraspinatus tendon, seen with internal rotation of the shoulder (82). In-

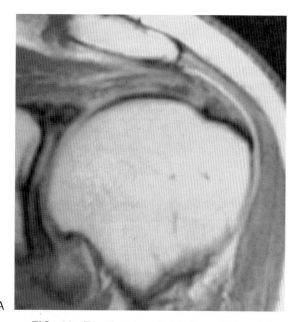

A

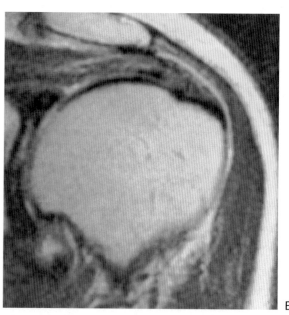

B

FIG. 26. Tendinosis reflected as diffuse intermediate signal intensity scattered throughout the supraspinatus tendon on proton density (TR = 1800; TE = 30) **(A)** and T2-weighted (TR = 1800; TE = 80) **(B)** oblique coronal MR images.

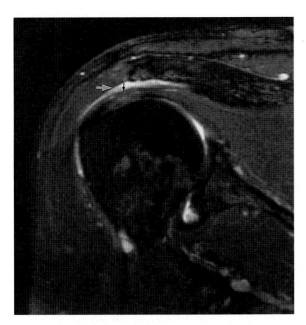

FIG. 27. Tendinosis of the supraspinatus tendon. There is diffuse high signal intensity and thickening within the critical zone of the tendon on this oblique coronal fat-saturated fast spin echo T2-weighted image *(black arrow)*. This patient also has subacromial-subdeltoid bursitis *(white arrow)*.

termediate signal intensity may be seen in the supraspinatus tendon when there is partial volume averaging of the hyaline cartilage overlying the humeral head with the rotator cuff. Degenerative or inflammatory changes in the tendon (tendinosis) usually do not usually increase in signal intensity on

T2-weighted images; however, they can occasionally result in high signal intensity, more diffuse and less intense than a tear (60). Fibrosis or granulation tissue within a tear may keep the signal intensity from being elevated on a T2-weighted MR image (61).

Fluid in the biceps tendon sheath can become partial volume averaged with the critical zone of the supraspinatus tendon on T2-weighted oblique coronal images, creating a pseudotear. Clinicians can avoid this pitfall by checking the T2-weighted oblique sagittal images and noticing the lack of signal in the tendon at this location. Other causes for elevated signal intensity in an intact supraspinatus tendon include motion artifact of the vessels, breathing, or the patient, producing increased signal intensity from ghosting; chemical shift misregistration artifact between the rotator cuff and fat; recent injection of medication; recent surgical repair of the cuff; and metallic artifacts from prior surgery.

Tendinosis, Tendinopathy, and Tendinitis

When a tendon has a signal intensity abnormality without focal disruption or associated findings to suggest a partial thickness tear, the terms "tendinosis" or "tendinopathy" have been used to signify an underlying tendon degeneration or inflammation (60). These terms suggest that there is a chronic, often preexisting, degenerative process. In general, the signal intensity of the lesion is not as marked as that of a tear on T2 weighting (Figs. 26 and 27). There is usually some thickening of the tendon (the normal thickness of the supraspinatus tendon is between 2 and 4 mm, with a mean of 3.2 mm) (77).

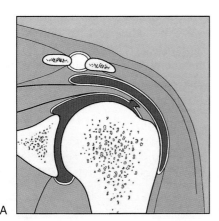

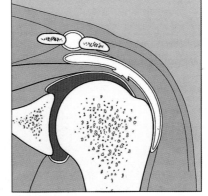

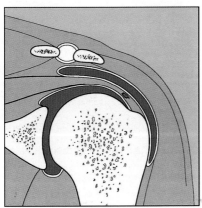

FIG. 28. Schematic diagrams showing the different types of partial thickness tears. **A:** Partial thickness tear of the articular surface of the tendon. **B:** Partial thickness tear on the bursal surface of the tendon. **C:** Partial intrasubstance tear. Bursal and articular surface tears can extend into the midsubstance of the tendon.

TABLE 7. *Abnormalities seen on magnetic resonance image in association with partial thickness rotator cuff tear*

Increased signal intensity extending through a portion of the tendon (with rare exception)
Nonretracted tendon
Irregularity, thinning, and/or thickening of tendon[a]
Fluid in subacromial subdeltoid bursa[a]
Intra-articular fluid[a]

[a]Occasional.

Use of the word *tendinitis* is reserved for those cases when a definite relationship to tendon inflammation can be substantiated. This is the result of experience with histopathologic correlation of tendons with presumed inflammation or tendinitis based on shoulder MRI studies that were shown to have degenerative changes (60). The term *tendinitis* has been used loosely to describe signal intensity alterations in the rotator cuff tendons that may represent degeneration, edema, or inflammation. The presence of tendinous enlargement and an inhomogeneous signal pattern that demonstrates increased signal intensity on T1 weighting with a further increase in signal intensity on T2 weighting is seen in patients with tendinitis (32,61,83,84), but cannot be used to make the diagnosis from an MR study. This same appearance could represent severe degeneration. Close clinical correlation is needed. I recommend that the term *tendinitis* not be used in the MR report, because it can have certain underlying false connotations, influencing treatment and remunerative decisions, including those made in Worker's Compensation or personal injury cases.

Partial Thickness Tears

Partial thickness tears of the rotator cuff can be seen inferiorly at the articular surface, superiorly at the bursal surface, or within the tendon substance (Fig. 28). Tears at the articular surface are the most common type of partial thickness tears (85). These are the only types of partial thickness tears demonstrated by conventional shoulder arthrography.

There are several abnormalities seen on MRI in association with partial thickness rotator cuff tears (Table 7). Focal increased signal intensity extending through a portion of a nonretracted tendon is suggestive of a partial thickness tear (Figs. 29 through 33). Partial thickness rotator cuff tears can also present with irregularity, thinning, or thickening within a nonretracted tendon without abnormal signal intensity. These tears may occasionally be difficult to distinguish from tendinosis or nondisplaced full-thickness tears if they are elevated in signal intensity on all imaging sequences (see Fig. 32). Routine MRI can miss a significant number of partial tears (24,61,62,86). Because of increased lesion conspicuity, FSE T2-weighted images with fat suppression tend to have a higher sensitivity for the diagnosis of partial thickness tears of the rotator cuff than a comparable sequence without fat suppression (87). Detection of partial thickness tears is more difficult than full-thickness tears using both techniques (24). The use of higher resolution techniques may improve the sensitivity of MR imaging for detecting partial-thickness tears. Fluid accumulation in the SA-SD bursa, common with full-thickness rotator cuff tears, may also be seen in patients with all types of partial thickness tears. Increased intraarticular fluid may also be found in the setting of a partial or full-thickness rotator cuff tear.

MR arthrography has been shown to be more accurate than conventional MRI for evaluation of partial tears, especially those located on the undersurface of the rotator cuff (88–90). Additional detection and characterization of undersurface tears can be obtained if the arm is in the ABER position during the MR examination (29) (see Figs. 23 and 31). Abduction of the arm allows the undersurface to be depicted

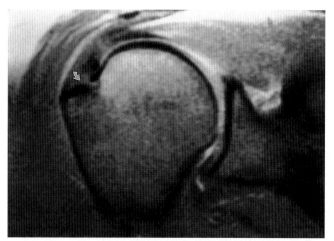
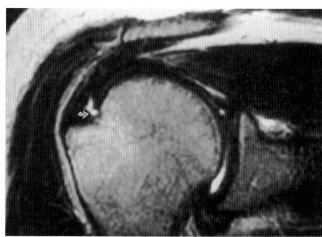

A   B

FIG. 29. Partial undersurface tear of the supraspinatus tendon. **A:** The tear presents as a subtle region of intermediate signal intensity that takes up intravenous gadolinium *(arrow)* on this fat-saturated T1-weighted oblique coronal image. **B:** The corresponding fat-saturated fast spin echo T2-weighted image reveals high signal intensity through the tear *(arrow)*.

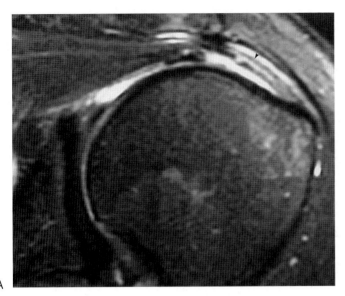
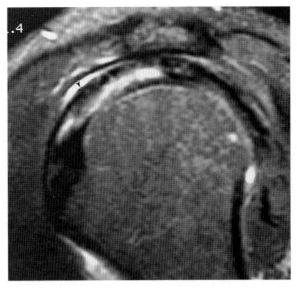

A

B

FIG. 30. Partial undersurface tear of the supraspinatus tendon. The tendon is thinned and has high signal intensity within its substance with sparing of the superior fibers *(arrowheads)* on oblique coronal **(A)** and oblique sagittal **(B)** fat-saturated fast spin echo T2-weighted MR images.

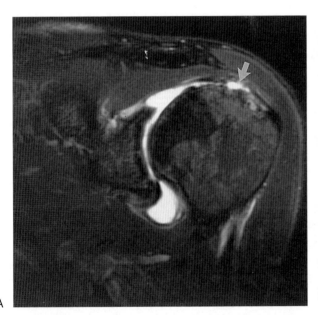
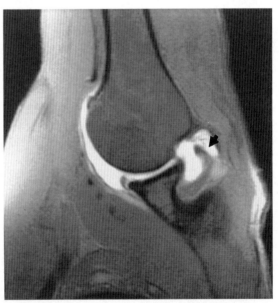

A

B

FIG. 31. A: Partial undersurface tear of the supraspinatus produces thinning and irregularity of the tendon on this oblique coronal T1-weighted fat-saturated image from an MR arthrogram *(arrow)*. **B:** The tear is even more evident *(arrow)* on an oblique axial T1-weighted fat-saturated image obtained in the ABER position.

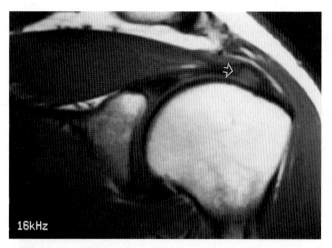

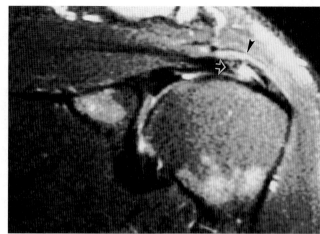

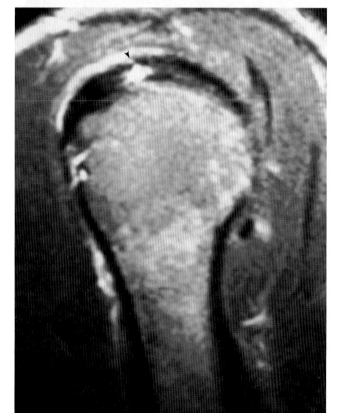

FIG. 32. Extensive partial undersurface tear of the supraspinatus tendon *(arrows)* on oblique coronal T1-weighted **(A)** and fat-saturated fast spin echo T2-weighted **(B)** images. There is some fluid in the subacromial-subdeltoid bursa *(arrowhead).* **C:** A small strand of tendon still crosses the superior aspect *(arrowhead)* on this oblique sagittal T2-weighted fast spin echo image.

free from the superior surface of the humerus and also promotes spreading of the frayed and torn edges of the inferior surface (29,71).

Full-Thickness Tears

A full-thickness rotator cuff tear involves a complete disruption of the tendon from the articular to the bursal surface

(Fig. 34). MR findings in full-thickness rotator cuff tears include one or more of the following signs: disruption of the low signal intensity tendon by an area of high signal intensity on T1- and T2- or T2*-weighted images, tendon retraction, muscle atrophy and fatty replacement, absence of the tendon, acromiohumeral articulation, and fluid in the SA-SD bursa (Figs. 35 through 40 and Table 8).

It has been shown, however, that up to 10% of partial and full-thickness tears do not demonstrate high signal intensity

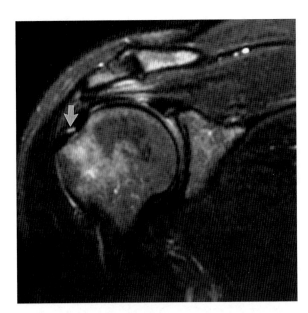

FIG. 33. Focal intrasubstance tear of the supraspinatus tendon is revealed on this oblique coronal fast spin echo T2-weighted MR image *(arrow)*.

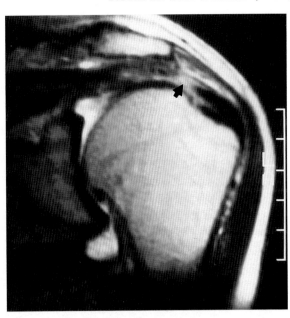

FIG. 35. Full-thickness supraspinatus tear. The high signal intensity tear extends through the entire substance of the supraspinatus tendon *(arrow)* and there is fluid in the subacromial-subdeltoid bursa on this oblique coronal T2-weighted MR image.

on long TE (T2-weighted) images (61). This may be due in part to the fact that chronic tears fill in with fibrous or granulation tissue that is low signal intensity on T2 weighting. In such cases, the clinician can look for abnormal tendon morphology such as attenuation or irregularity of the rotator cuff (61).

Full-thickness tears of the rotator cuff tendons can be accurately identified using conventional nonarthrographic MRI with high sensitivity and specificity (15,33,39,62,83). Increased signal intensity extending from the inferior to the superior surface of the tendon on all imaging sequences is an accurate sign of a full-thickness rotator cuff tear (60). Use of fat-saturation technique can improve detection of both full-thickness and partial thickness tears compared to standard

spin-echo imaging techniques (24). In one study, the fat-saturation technique increased sensitivity for detection of full-thickness tears from 80% to 100% (24).

Tendon retraction is a specific sign of full-thickness rotator cuff tear (33). The musculotendinous junction, that is the point where muscle is no longer seen, should lie no further medial than 15 degrees from a line drawn through the 12-o'-clock position of the humeral head (33) (see Fig. 6). Severe muscle atrophy and fatty replacement is common in patients with large rotator cuff tears (31,84,91) (see Figs. 38 and 39). The muscle size decreases and there is often fatty replacement characterized by high signal intensity on T1-weighted images. Muscle atrophy was 97% specific for a rotator cuff tear in one series (33). This type of information can be useful for decisions regarding conservative versus operative repair and type of operative repair (cuff substitute or muscle

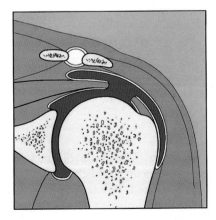

FIG. 34. Schematic diagram demonstrating how a full-thickness tear extends from the glenohumeral joint through the superior tendon surface and communicates with the subacromial subdeltoid bursa *(all in blue)*.

TABLE 8. *Abnormalities seen on magnetic resonance image in association with full-thickness rotator cuff tear*

Increased signal intensity extending from the inferior to the superior surface of the tendon on all imaging sequences (with rare exception)
Tendon retraction[a]
Muscle atrophy[a]
Absence of the tendon[a]
Acromiohumeral articulation[a]
Fluid in the subacromial-subdeltoid bursa[a]
Intraarticular fluid[a]
Loss of peribursal fat[a]

[a]Occasional.

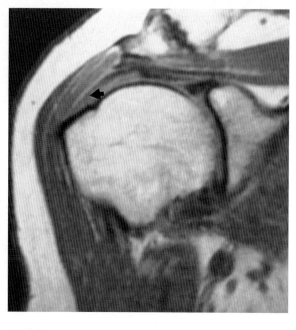

A

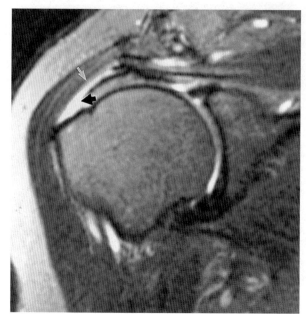

B

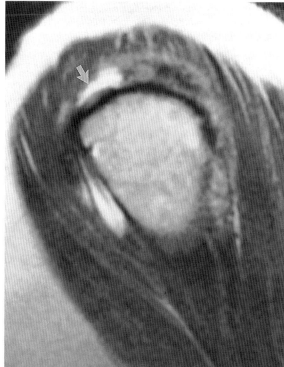

C

FIG. 36. Full-thickness supraspinatus tear at the distal attachment *(arrows)* on oblique coronal T1-weighted **(A)** and fat-saturated fast spin echo T2-weighted **(B)** MR images. There is fluid in the subacromial subdeltoid bursa *(white arrow)*. **C:** The high signal intensity tear is well seen on a far lateral oblique sagittal fat-saturated fast spin echo T2-weighted MR image *(arrow)*.

transfer), and when providing a postoperative prognosis (92). Additional causes of muscle atrophy and fatty replacement such as denervation, myositis, muscle trauma, and disuse should be considered if the tendon itself appears intact.

Absence of the tendon and acromiohumeral articulation are signs of a chronic rotator cuff tear (see Fig. 40). The conventional radiograph is useful for identifying acromio-

humeral articulation. When the distance between the acromion and the humeral head is less than 7 mm, a rotator cuff tear is likely. There is no need to perform other studies to exclude a tear in this situation. However, additional studies such as MRI would be indicated if the referring clinician desires information about other structures in and around the glenohumeral joint.

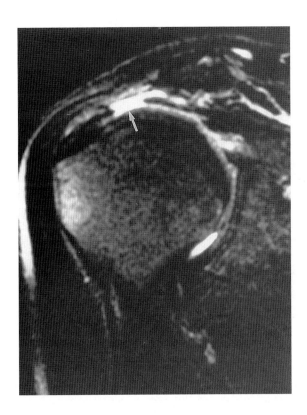

FIG. 37. Large high signal intensity full-thickness supraspinatus tear *(arrow)* with musculotendinous retraction is well seen on this oblique coronal fat-saturated fast spin echo T2-weighted MR image.

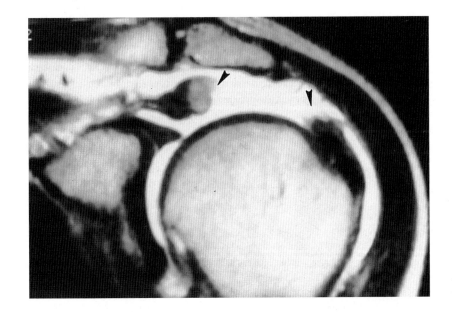

FIG. 38. Massive supraspinatus tear *(arrowheads)* with musculotendinous retraction is demonstrated on a T2-weighted oblique coronal MR image.

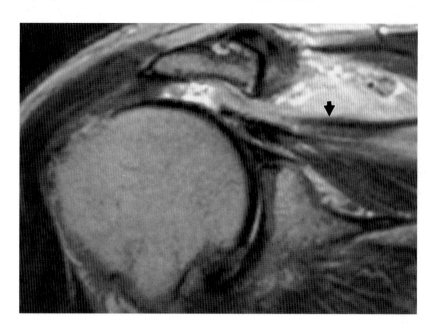

FIG. 39. There is significant musculotendinous retraction and atrophy of the supraspinatus muscle *(arrow)* on this oblique coronal fat saturated fast spin echo T2-weighted MR image.

Fluid in the SA-SD bursa is a sensitive, but relatively nonspecific finding in patients with rotator cuff tears (33). The fluid escapes from the glenohumeral joint through the articular surface tear into the bursa that lies above the superior surface of the tear. Small amounts of fluid in the bursa can be seen as an isolated finding (32,34,39,76,77,93). Cases of isolated SA-SD bursitis without rotator cuff tear can be seen following trauma and in association with inflammatory disorders such as rheumatoid arthritis or infection. SA-SD bursitis is also common with impingement syndrome. A small amount of fluid may also be seen in the bursa in asymptomatic patients (76,77). Previous injection of a local anesthetic or steroid preparation may cause difficulty in interpretation of the rotator cuff tendons and bursa (30). The area of

injection is high signal intensity on MRI and can mimic a bursitis, tendinopathy, or tear. It is important for the referring physician to know of this phenomenon and request an MR study prior to injection or to delay the MR examination for a few months if such treatment has been performed. The patient should be questioned and counseled about recent injections at the time of the MR appointment. The interpreting radiologist needs to be aware of such injections and their date of administration when evaluating the MR study.

If there is any question concerning the distinction of a full- and partial thickness tear, MR arthrography is recommended, particularly if the abnormal signal intensity extends from the undersurface of the tendon (90). When gadolinium is injected into the glenohumeral joint, it fills a defect in the

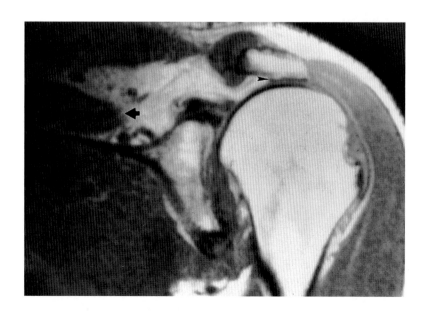

FIG. 40. This patient has acromiohumeral articulation from a long-standing full-thickness supraspinatus tear depicted on an oblique coronal T1-weighted MR image. The tendon is absent and the muscle is severely retracted and atrophic *(arrow)*. Fat fills in the space that the supraspinatus muscle and tendon used to occupy. An enthesophyte projects from the undersurface of the acromion *(arrowhead)*.

rotator cuff that extends to the articular surface, including partial thickness undersurface tears. It does not demonstrate a partial tear in the substance or at the superior surface of the rotator cuff tendons. The gadolinium may be imbibed at frayed, friable tendon margins. If the tear is full thickness, the contrast enters the SA-SD bursa. The SA-SD bursa must be carefully evaluated for the presence of contrast in patients with equivocal full-thickness tears. It is important to use fat-suppression to decrease the signal from fat without affecting the high signal intensity of the gadolinium on T1-weighted images (90).

Ancillary Findings in Rotator Cuff Tears

Preservation of the extrasynovial fat that lies under the SA-SD bursa is a useful sign because it usually indicates that the rotator cuff is normal (33,51). Focal obliteration of the peribursal fat plane has often been described in asymptomatic individuals (31,32,39,61,76,77,94) and this finding has not been shown to be a good indicator of disease (34).

Large glenohumeral joint effusions are often seen with advanced rotator cuff abnormalities (51). Humeral head cysts and an irregular surface of the greater tuberosity are occasionally seen in association with rotator cuff disease, but they are rather nonspecific.

The presence of a fluid-filled mass above the AC joint should prompt a search for a rotator cuff tear (95,96). AC joint cysts are rare but usually occur when there is a communication between the glenohumeral and AC joints in patients with full-thickness rotator cuff tears (Fig. 41). It is believed that there is chronic friction between the high-riding humeral head and the AC joint, leading to mechanical wear and tearing of the inferior articular capsule of the AC joint.

This leads to passage of fluid from the glenohumeral joint through the rotator cuff tear and the subacromial bursa into the AC joint (96). The AC joint capsule dilates, resulting in a superior cystic mass. Simple aspiration of the cyst should be avoided, because recurrence is likely in the presence of a rotator cuff tear. Nonsurgical treatment is performed if the patient is elderly with acceptable function and without shoulder pain. In patients with functional impairment or chronic shoulder pain, the rotator cuff is repaired and the cyst removed. If the tear is massive and cannot be repaired, it is recommended that the cyst be excised, accompanied by acromioplasty and distal clavicular resection. Alternatively, humeral head arthroplasty has been recommended as a treatment by some orthopedists (97).

Infraspinatus, Teres Minor, and Subscapularis Tears

An isolated tear of the infraspinatus tendon is rare (98). An increasing role is being placed on this tendon as a source of symptoms (99). Tears of the infraspinatus are more common in younger athletes who use overhead motion. This tendon may also be affected by the posterosuperior glenoid impingement syndrome. Tears of this tendon are well seen in all three imaging planes (Figs. 42 and 43).

Subscapularis tendon tears are uncommon and usually are seen in middle-aged and older patients with recurrent shoulder dislocation or in association with massive tears of the other rotator cuff tendons (100–102). Tears may also be seen following direct trauma to the anterior aspect of the shoulder joint and with hyperextension or external rotation of the adducted arm (103). In the latter case, the patient experiences pain and weakness when the arm is used below shoulder level. Downward sloping of the coracoid also can cause impingement and eventual tear of the superior aspect of the

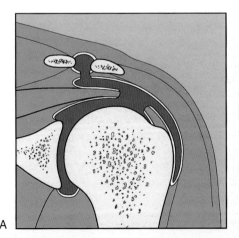
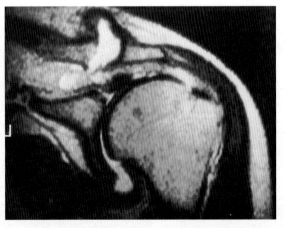

A   B

FIG. 41. Schematic diagram **(A)** and T2-weighted oblique coronal MR image **(B)** demonstrate an acromioclavicular joint cyst in association with full-thickness tears of the rotator cuff. The fluid escapes from the glenohumeral joint through the tendon tear into the subacromial subdeltoid bursa and then into the broken capsule of the acromioclavicular joint, acquired as a result of friction of the humeral head against its undersurface.

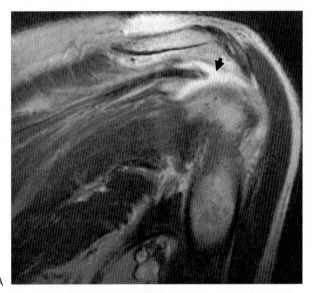
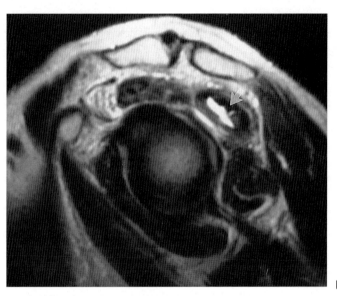

FIG. 42. Isolated infraspinatus tear. **A:** The infraspinatus tendon is medially retracted with a lateral high signal intensity gap on this oblique coronal fat saturated fast spin echo T2-weighted MR image *(arrow).* **B:** The tear is localized to the region of the supraspinatus on this T2-weighted oblique sagittal image *(arrow).*

subscapularis tendon (48,49). A portion of the coracoid can be excised in such cases.

On MRI, subscapularis tendon tears can be identified as areas of abnormal high signal intensity on T2- or T2*-weighted images and/or poor tendon definition (104). The tendon is often medially retracted (Figs. 44 and 45). In one study of 149 patients with MR evidence of rotator cuff tears, nine patients (6%) had primary tears of the subscapularis tendon (104). Only one of those patients had a history of dislocation; the rest suffered direct anterior trauma to the shoulder, usually from a fall. Perhaps the patients suffered anterior dislocation but were unaware of this event. Fluid was not

commonly seen in the SA-SD bursa in these patients (four of nine). There was associated abnormality in the long head of the biceps tendon in seven of these patients, including five with medial tendon dislocation. The tendon may sublux or dislocate out of the intertubercular groove (see Fig. 45 and Fig. 46). Occasionally, it may lie in front of the glenohumeral joint. This is because an extension of the subscapularis tendon, the transverse humeral ligament, is a major stabilizer of the long bicipital tendon and disruption of this ligament and the adjacent tendon allow the tendon to escape the bicipital groove (105,106). This is further discussed in Chapter 8.

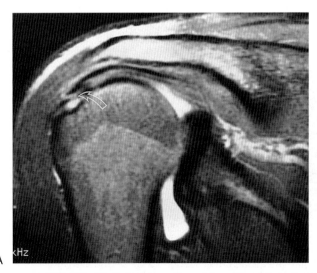
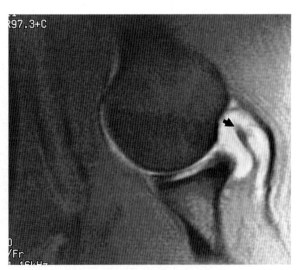

FIG. 43. Partial undersurface tear of the infraspinatus tendon is demonstrated by MR arthrography on an oblique coronal fat-saturated fast spin echo T2-weighted MR image **(A)** and a T1-weighted fat-saturated MR image **(B)** obtained in the ABER position *(arrows).*

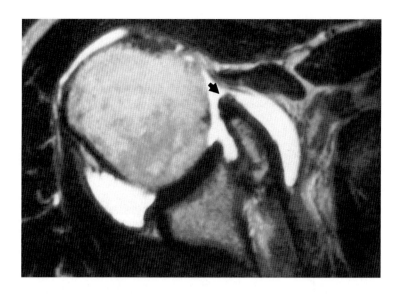

FIG. 44. Subscapularis tendon tear with medial retraction of the tendon and escape of fluid into the anterior soft tissues is demonstrated on this axial T2-weighted MR image *(arrow)*.

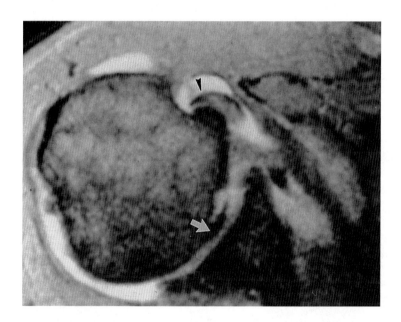

FIG. 45. Subluxed biceps tendon in association with a subscapularis tendon tear is shown on this axial gradient echo MR image *(arrowhead)*. This patient also has osteoarthrosis of the glenohumeral joint with an inferomedial osteophyte projecting from the humeral head *(white arrow)*.

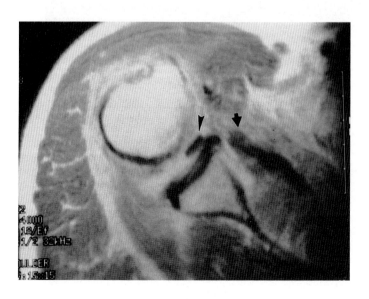

FIG. 46. The biceps tendon has dislocated into the glenohumeral joint *(arrowhead)* in association with a subscapularis tendon tear *(arrow)* on this axial fast spin echo proton density MR image.

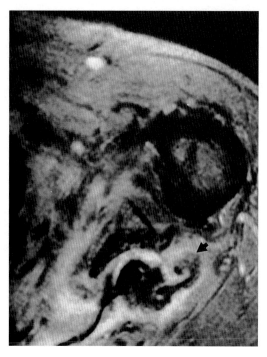

FIG. 47. There is medial retraction of the teres minor tendon following a full-thickness tear seen on this axial gradient echo MR image *(arrow)*.

Teres minor tendon tears are rare (Fig. 47). Posterior dislocation is a common predisposing mechanism. It is important for the clinician to check the posterior labrocapsular structures for abnormalities when such a tear is present. Teres minor muscle strains may also be an important clue to underlying posterior glenohumeral instability (Fig. 48).

Rotator Interval Tears

Another type of tear that should not be overlooked involves the rotator interval. The rotator interval refers to the ligamentous region between the anterior fibers of the supraspinatus and the superior fibers of the subscapularis tendons (see Fig. 8). The coracoid protrudes into this area. The coracohumeral ligament lies superficially and the biceps tendon more deeply in this region. It is seen at the anterosuperior convexity of the humeral head. The superior glenohumeral ligament also lies in this region. This is often the region that surgeons use to enter the joint for an arthrotomy.

Lesions of the rotator interval are most commonly associated with enlargement or tearing from a shoulder dislocation; however, some individuals with abnormalities in the region do not have glenohumeral instability (107). The supraspina-

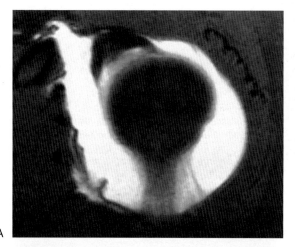

A

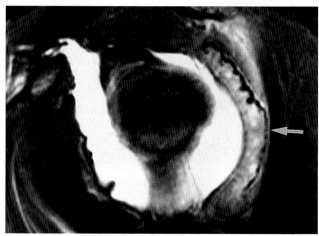

B

C

FIG. 48. This patient had a posterior dislocation with an associated strain of the teres minor muscle. Oblique sagittal T1-weighted MR image with fat saturation **(A)** does not demonstrate the muscle abnormality that is readily apparent on an oblique sagittal fat-saturated fast spin echo T2-weighted MR image **(B)** *(arrow).* **C:** This patient also had a reverse Hill-Sachs lesion along the anterior humeral head as a result of the posterior dislocation *(arrow).*

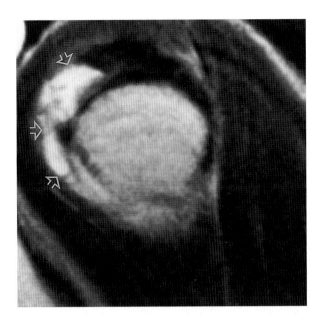

FIG. 49. An oblique sagittal T2-weighted MR image shows a high signal intensity rotator cuff tear extending from the supraspinatus above through the rotator interval and into the region of the subscapularis *(arrows)*.

tus and subscapularis tendons may be torn in association with the rotator interval tear (Fig. 49). Isolated tears of the rotator cuff interval are thin and longitudinal, and are not associated with muscle retraction (108) (Fig. 50). A tear of the rotator interval produces communication with the SA-SD bursa, and fluid or intraarticularly injected contrast may be seen in this bursa (see Fig. 50). T2-weighted oblique sagittal MR images are particularly useful for demonstrating these tears as a region of high signal intensity often in association with biceps tendon and coracohumeral ligament abnormalities. It must be remembered that synovium and capsule can herniate into this space in asymptomatic individuals in the absence of a tear, which may produce a pitfall consisting of high signal intensity fluid in this region on T2-weighted images (Fig. 51).

Statistical Considerations Regarding Magnetic Resonance Imaging of Rotator Cuff Tears

Conventional MRI has been shown to be variably sensitive, specific, and accurate for the diagnosis of full-thickness

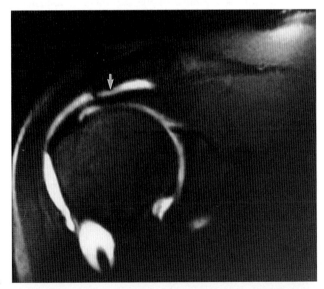

A

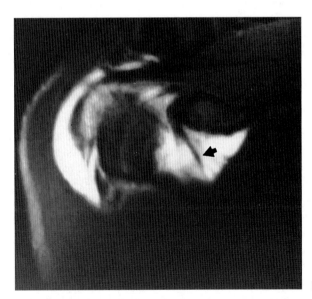

B

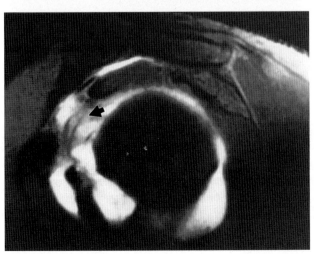

C

FIG. 50. Rotator interval tear demonstrated on fat-saturated T1-weighted MR images following an intraarticular injection of gadolinium. **A:** This coronal MR image from an MR arthrogram shows the high signal intensity contrast in the glenohumeral joint and biceps tendon sheath as expected. There is also contrast in the subacromial subdeltoid bursa *(arrow)* surrounding an intact supraspinatus tendon. All of the tendons were intact. **B:** The mystery is solved on this anterior section of an oblique coronal MR image, which shows a tear of the coracohumeral ligament *(arrow)* **C:** The contrast escapes through the rotator interval on the oblique sagittal MR image *(arrow)*.

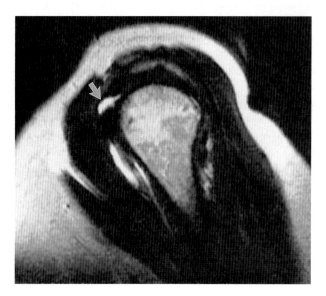

FIG. 51. Normal capsular herniation through the rotator interval on a sagittal T2-weighted MR image *(arrow)*.

rotator cuff tears (15,33,91,109,110). In a study by Zlatkin et al. (109), which evaluated MR findings in shoulders of 40 patients with surgical and arthrographic correlation, MR was 91% sensitive, 88% specific, and 89% accurate for demonstrating all types of rotator cuff tears. Another study that looked at arthroscopic or surgical correlation in full-thickness cuff tears in 91 patients found that MRI had a sensitivity of 100% and a specificity of 95% (91). Burk et al. (15) reported a similar sensitivity of 92% for MRI and arthrography for the diagnosis of rotator cuff tears. In an investigation by Rafii et al. (61) of 80 patients with shoulder pain and surgical evaluation, 47 of whom had either full- or partial thickness tears, MRI was 95% and 84% accurate in demonstrating full-thickness and partial thickness tears, respectively. For full-thickness tears, of which there were 37 in the study, there was a sensitivity of 97% and specificity of 94%. In a different study, MR scans of 87 consecutive patients with arthroscopic correlation showed a sensitivity of 91% and specificity of 95% for full-thickness tears and a sensitivity of 74% and specificity of 87% for partial thickness tears using combined spin-echo and T2*-weighted gradient echo MR imaging (111). A study by Quinn et al. (110) evaluated fat-suppressed MRI with arthroscopic correlation in 100 patients. With data combined for complete and partial tears of the rotator cuff, MRI had an accuracy of 93%, a sensitivity of 84%, and a specificity of 97%. A recent study by Singson shows a 100% sensitivity for full-thickness tears. Reinus et al. (24) have shown that using the fat-saturation technique with conventional MRI improves detection of both full-thickness and partial thickness tears compared with standard spin-echo imaging techniques (24). They also found that detection of partial thickness tears was poor with both techniques. A recent study by Sonin et al. (25) on 26 patients with surgical correlation showed a sensitivity of 89%, a

specificity of 94%, and a diagnostic accuracy of 92% using FSE T2-weighted sequences.

Treatment of Partial and Full-Thickness Rotator Cuff Tears

Treatment planning can be influenced by the type of rotator cuff abnormality seen on MRI and other associated abnormalities, including those that are the result of shoulder instability. Decisions should be based on careful evaluation of the MR findings with close clinical correlation, especially because rotator cuff repair surgery usually requires 6 to 9 months of rehabilitation.

Many factors are used to decide whether a tear should be treated conservatively, with a primary repair, or with a subacromial decompression or distal clavicular resection. Treatment philosophies also vary between institutions. Initial treatment of a symptomatic rotator cuff with tendinosis or a partial tear is usually conservative without surgical intervention. However, at some centers, a partial thickness tear is explored and debrided or repaired. Partial intrasubstance tears can be difficult if not impossible to identify during surgery. Preoperative knowledge of the existence of intrasubstance partial tears gained from an MRI can alter the surgical approach leading to a probe of the undersurface of the rotator cuff in the region of the intrasubstance tear. The surgeon may then enter the tear and debride it, often with successful results.

Distinction between a high-grade partial thickness tear and a small full-thickness tear may not be necessary, because both are usually treated in a similar fashion (87). A full-thickness tear may be repaired depending on different circumstances including the patient's age, level of activity, and the degree of retraction and muscle atrophy. It is possible for an arthroscopist to underdiagnose a full-thickness tear of the cuff if only one side of the cuff is directly visualized (24). If the patient has an underlying lesion related to shoulder instability, which may lead to or exacerbate a rotator cuff tear, the lesions relating to instability can be addressed.

CALCIFIC TENDINITIS

Calcific tendinitis is characterized by deposition of hydroxyapatite crystals within the rotator cuff. The deposits are frequently asymptomatic, but they can result in chronic shoulder pain in 30% to 45% of patients. The pain is caused by inflammation and is frequent with resorption of the apatite deposits (112). This condition is most common in the region of the critical zone of the supraspinatus tendon (113,114). As previously discussed, this area has altered vascularity and it is also a site of mechanical pressure which may predispose to hydroxyapatite deposition. Fibrocytes may be transformed to chondrocytes with resultant enchondral ossification. With degeneration of these chondrocytes,

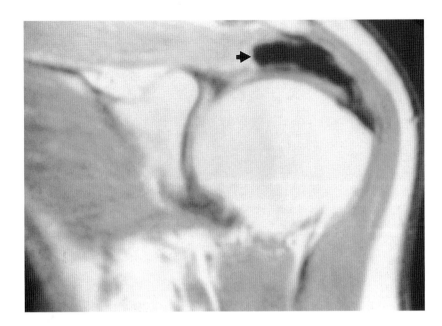

FIG. 52. Calcific tendinitis presents as an amorphous low signal intensity mass in the supraspinatus tendon on this oblique coronal T1-weighted MR image *(arrow)*.

hydroxyapatite mineral deposits can form. There is often localized hyperemia of the tendon and in the supraspinatus, this may lead to impingement.

It is always important to obtain conventional radiographs with the shoulder in external and internal rotation in patients with shoulder pain to exclude calcific tendinitis. The calcification is easy to identify on CT, but may be difficult to distinguish from the low signal intensity tendon on MRI. It can be detected on MRI when it is large or if there is surrounding high signal intensity edema or inflammation on T2- or T2*-weighted images (Figs. 52 and 53). A blooming effect

is often produced by the calcium on T2* images (see Fig. 53). The surrounding edema and occasional reactive bursal fluid has the potential to mimic a rotator cuff tear on MRI. It is important in such cases to look for the focal region of low signal intensity calcification and to correlate this with conventional radiographs.

The treatment of this condition is variable. The calcific deposits may resorb on their own (112). Rest, local steroid injections, and inflammatory compounds may alleviate symptoms. The apatite deposits can also be removed surgically or with needle aspiration.

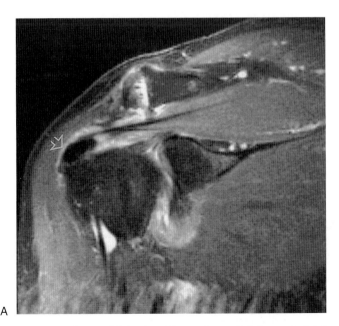
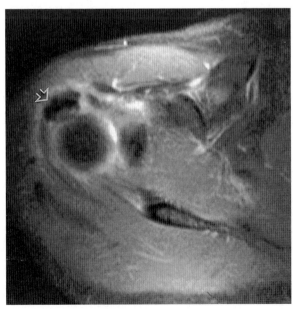

A

B

FIG. 53. High signal intensity gadolinium administered intravenously outlines a clump of calcific tendinitis *(arrow)* on these oblique coronal **(A)** and axial **(B)** fat-saturated T1-weighted MR images.

REFERENCES

1. Neer CS. Anterior acromioplasty for the chronic impingement syndrome in the shoulder. *J Bone Joint Surg* 1972;54A:41–50.
2. Codman EA. The shoulder. Rupture of the supraspinatus tendon and other lesions in or about the subacromial bursa. Brooklyn, NY: G. Miller, 1934.
3. Neer CS. Impingement lesions. *Clin Orthop Rel Res* 1983;173:70.
4. Ozaki J, Fujimoto S, Nakagawa Y, Masuhara K, Tamai S. Tears of the rotator cuff of the shoulder associated with pathological changes in the acromion. A study in cadavers. *J Bone Joint Surg* 1988;70A: 1224–1230.
5. Cone RO III, Resnick D, Danzig L. Shoulder impingement syndrome: radiographic evaluation. *Radiology* 1984;150:29–33.
6. Neer CS, Poppen NK. Supraspinatus outlet. *Orthop Trans* 1987;11: 234.
7. Kilcoyne RF, Reddy PK, Lyons F, Rockwood CA. Optimal plain film imaging of the shoulder impingement syndrome. *Am J Roentgenol* 1989;153:795–797.
8. Newhouse KE, El-Khoury GY, Nepola JV, et al. The shoulder impingement view: a fluoroscopic technique for the detection of subacromial spurs. *Am J Roentgenol* 1988;151:539–541.
9. Mink JH, Harris E, Rappaport M. Rotator cuff tears: evaluation using double-contrast shoulder arthrography. *Radiology* 1985;157:621–623.
10. Sullivan T. Rotator cuff disease [Letter to the Editor]. *Am J Roentgenol* 1995;165:1554–1555.
11. Freiberger R. Best test for detection of rotator-cuff tear [Answer to Question]. *Am J Roentgenol* 1995;164:1018–1019.
12. Middleton WD. Sonographic detection and quantification of rotator cuff tears. *Am J Roentgenol* 1993;160:109–110.
13. Wiener SN, Seitz WH. Sonography of the shoulder in patients with tears of the rotator cuff. *Am J Roentgenol* 1993;160:103–107.
14. Bretzke CA, Crass JR, Craig EV. Ultrasonography of the rotator cuff: normal and pathologic anatomy. *Invest Radiol* 1985;20:311–315.
15. Burk DL Jr, Karasick D, Mitchell DG, et al. Rotator cuff tears: prospective comparison of MR imaging with arthrography, sonography, and surgery. *Am J Roentgenol* 1989;152:87–92.
16. Soble MG, Kaye AD, Guay RC. Rotator cuff tear: clinical experience with sonographic detection. *Radiology* 1989;173:319–321.
17. Drakeford MK, Quinn MJ, Simpson SL, Pettine KA. A comparative study of ultrasonography and arthrography in evaluation of the rotator cuff. *Clin Orthop Rel Res* 1990;253:118–122.
18. Mack LA, Matsen FA III. US evaluation of the rotator cuff. *Radiology* 1985;157:205–209.
19. van Holsbeeck MT, Kolowich PA, Eyler WR, et al. US depiction of partial-thickness tear of the rotator cuff. *Radiology* 1995;197: 443–446.
20. Mack LA, Gannon MK, Kilcoyne RF. Sonographic evaluation of the rotator cuff: accuracy in patients without prior surgery. *Clin Orthop* 1988;234:21–27.
21. Crass JR, Craig EV, Bretzke CA. Ultrasonography of the rotator cuff. *RadioGraphics* 1985;5:941–953.
22. Middleton WD, Reinus WR, Totty WG, Melson CL, Murphy WA. Ultrasonographic evaluation of the rotator cuff and biceps tendon. *J Bone Joint Surg* 1986;68A:440–450.
23. Patten RM, Mack LA, Wang KY, Lingel J. Nondisplaced fractures of the greater tuberosity of the humerus: sonographic detection. *Radiology* 1992;182:201–204.
24. Reinus WR, Shady KL, Mirowitz SA, Totty WG. MR diagnosis of rotator cuff tears of the shoulder: value of using T2-weighted fat-saturated images. *Am J Roentgenol* 1995;164:1451–1455.
25. Sonin AH, Peduto AJ, Fitzgerald SW, Callahan CM, Bresler ME. MR imaging of the rotator cuff mechanism: comparison of spin-echo and turbo spin-echo sequences. *Am J Roentgenol* 1996;167:333–338.
26. Vahlensieck M, Peterfy CG, Wischer T, et al. Indirect MR arthrography: optimization and clinical applications. *Radiology* 1996;200 249–254.
27. Winalski CS, Aliabadi P, Wright RJ, Shortkroff S, Sledge CB, Weissman BN. Enhancement of joint fluid with intravenously administered gadopentetate dimeglumine: technique, rationale, and implications. *Radiology* 1993;187:179–185.
28. Tirman PFJ, Bost FW, Steinbach LS, et al. MR arthrographic depiction of tears of the rotator cuff: benefit of abduction and external rotation of the arm. *Radiology* 1994;192:851–856.
29. Tirman PFJ, Bost F, Garvin GJ, et al. Posterosuperior glenoid impingement of the shoulder: findings at MR imaging and MR arthrography with arthroscopic correlation. *Radiology* 1994;193:431–436.
30. Kieft GJ, Bloem JL, Rozing PM, Obermann WR. Rotator cuff impingement syndrome: MR imaging. *Radiology* 1988;166:211–214.
31. Seeger LL, Gold RH, Bassett LW, Ellman H. Shoulder impingement syndrome: MR findings in 53 shoulders. *Am J Roentgenol* 1988;150: 343–347.
32. Chandnani V, Ho C, Gerharter J, et al. MR findings in asymptomatic shoulders: a blind analysis using symptomatic shoulders as controls. *Clin Imaging* 1992;16:25–30.
33. Farley TE, Neumann CH, Steinbach LS, Jahnke AJ, Petersen SS. Full-thickness tears of the rotator cuff of the shoulder: diagnosis with MR imaging. *Am J Roentgenol* 1992;158:347–351.
34. Liou JTS, Wilson AJ, Totty WG, Brown JJ. The normal shoulder: common variations that simulate pathologic conditions at MR imaging. *Radiology* 1993;186:435–441.
35. Watson M. Rotator cuff function in the impingement syndrome. *J Bone Joint Surg* 1989;71-B:361–366.
36. Morrison DS, Bigliani LU. The clinical significance of variations in acromial morphology. *Orthop Trans* 1986;11:234.
37. Edelson JG, Taitz C. Anatomy of the coraco-acromial arch. Relation to degeneration of the acromion. *J Bone Joint Surg* 1992;74B:589.
38. Mudge MK, Wood VE, Frykman GK. Rotator cuff tears associated with os acromiale. *J Bone Joint Surg* 1984;66-A:427–429.
39. Kaplan PA, Bryans KC, Davick JP, Otte M, Stinson WW, Dussault RG. MR imaging of the normal shoulder: variants and pitfalls. *Radiology* 1992;184:519–524.
40. Bigliani LU, Morrison DS, April EW. The morphology of the acromion and its relationship to rotator cuff tears. *Orthop Trans* 1986;10:228.
41. Farley TE, Neumann CH, Steinbach LS, Petersen SA. The coracoacromial arch: MR evaluation and correlation with rotator cuff pathology. *Skeletal Radiology* 1994;23:641–645.
42. Edelson JG. The "hooked" acromion revisited. *J Bone Joint Surg* 1995;77-B:284–287.
43. Getz JD, Recht M, Piraino DW, et al. Acromial morphology: relation to sex, age, symmetry, and subacromial enthesophytes. *Radiology* 1996;199:737–742.
44. Epstein RE, Schweitzer ME, Frieman BG, Fenlin JM, Mitchell DG. Hooked acromion: prevalence on MR images of painful shoulders. *Radiology* 1993;187:479–481.
45. Haygood TM, Langlotz CP, Kneeland JB, Iannotti JP, Williams GR Jr, Dalinka MK. Categorization of acromial shape: interobserver variability with MR imaging and conventional radiography. *Am J Roentgenol* 1994;162:1377–1382.
46. Peh WCG, Farmer THR, Totty WG. Acromial arch shape: assessment with MR imaging. *Radiology* 1995;1995:501–505.
47. Aoki M, Ishii S, Usui M. The slope of the acromion and rotator cuff impingement. *Proc Am Shoulder Elbow Surg* 1986.
48. Dines DM, Warren RF, Inglis AE, Pavlov H. The coracoid impingement syndrome. *J Bone Joint Surg* 1990;72-B:314–316.
49. Gerber C, Terrier F, Ganz R. The role of the coracoid process in the chronic impingement syndrome. *J Bone Joint Surg* 1985;67B:703.
50. Crues JV, Fareed DO. Magnetic resonance imaging of shoulder impingement. *Topics Magn Res Imaging* 1991;3(4):39–49.
51. Needell SD, Zlatkin MB, Sher JS, Murphy BJ, Uribe JW. MR imaging of the rotator cuff: peritendinous and bone abnormalities in an asymptomatic population. *Am J Roentgenol* 1996;166:863–867.
52. Liberson F. Os acromiale: a contested anomaly. *J Bone Joint Surg* 1937;19:683–689.
53. Norris TR, Fischer J, Bigliani LU, Neer CS II. The unfused acromial epiphysis and its relationship to impingement syndrome. *Orthop Trans* 1983;7:505–506.
54. Edelson JG, Zuckerman J, Hershkovitz I. Os acromiale: anatomy and surgical implications. *J Bone Joint Surg* 1993;74-B:551–555.
55. Andrews JR, Byrd TJW, Kupferman SP, Angelo RL. The profile view of the acromion. *Clin Orthop* 1991;263:1991.
56. Hutchinson MR, Veenstra MA. Arthroscopic decompression of shoulder impingement secondary to os acromiale. *Arthroscopy* 1993;9(1):28–32.
57. Gold RH, Seeger LL, Yao L. Imaging shoulder impingement. *Skeletal Radiol* 1993;22:555–561.

58. Park JG, Lee JK, Phelps CT. Os acromiale associated with rotator cuff impingement: MR imaging of the shoulder. *Radiology* 1994;193:255–257.

59. McClure JG, Raney RB. Anomalies of the scapula. *Clin Orthop* 1975;110:22–31.

60. Kjellin I, Ho CP, Cervilla V, et al. Alterations in the supraspinatus tendon at MR imaging: correlation with histopathologic findings in cadavers. *Radiology* 1991;181:837–841.

61. Rafii M, Firooznia H, Sherman O. Rotator cuff lesions: signal patterns at MR imaging. *Radiology* 1990;177:817–823.

62. Robertson PL, Schweitzer ME, Mitchell DG, et al. Rotator cuff disorders: interobserver and intraobserver variation in diagnosis with MR imaging. *Radiology* 1995;1995:831–835.

63. Watson M. Major ruptures of the rotator cuff. *J Bone Joint Surg* 1985;67B:618.

64. Burns WC, Whipple TL. Anatomic relationships in the shoulder impingement syndrome. *Clin Orth Rel Res* 1993;(294):96–102.

65. Sarkar K, Taine W, Uhthoff HK. The ultrastructure of the coracoacromial ligament in patients with chronic impingement syndrome. *Clin Orth Rel Res* 1990;(254):49–54.

66. Gallino M, Battiston B, Annartone G, Terragnoli F. Coracoacromial ligament: a comparative arthroscopic and anatomic study. *Arthroscopy* 1995;11(5):564–567.

67. Morimoto K, Mori E, Nakagawa Y. Calcification of the coracoacromial ligament. A case report of the shoulder impingement syndrome. *Am J Sports Med* 1988;16:80.

68. Neviaser RJ, Neviaser TJ. Observations on impingement. *Clin Orth Rel Res* 1990;(254):60–63.

69. Jobe FW, Kvitne RS. Shoulder pain in the overhand or throwing athlete: the relationship of anterior instability and rotator cuff impingement. *Orthop Review* 1989;18:963.

70. Jobe CM. Posterior superior glenoid impingement: expanded spectrum. *Arthroscopy* 1995;11(5):530–536.

71. Walch G, Boileau P, Noel E, Donell ST. Impingement of the deep surface of the supraspinatus tendon on the posterosuperior glenoid rim: an arthroscopic study. *Shoulder Elbow Surg* 1992;1:238–245.

72. Liu SH, Boynton E. Posterior superior impingement of the rotator cuff on the glenoid rim as a cause of shoulder pain in the overhead athlete. *Arthroscopy* 1993;9:697–699.

73. Miniaci A, Fowler PJ. Impingement in the athlete. *Clin Sports Med* 1993;12:91–110.

74. Wolf WB. Shoulder tendinoses. *Clin Sports Med* 1992;11:871–890.

75. Warner JJP, Micheli LJ, Arsianian L, Kennedy J, Kennedy R. Patterns of flexibility, laxity, and strength in normal shoulders and shoulders with instability and impingement. *Am J Sports Med* 1990;18:366.

76. Neumann CH, Holt RG, Steinbach LS, Jahnke AH, Petersen SA. MR imaging of the shoulder: appearance of the supraspinatus tendon in asymptomatic volunteers. *Am J Roentgenol* 1992;158:1281–1287.

77. Mirowitz SA. Normal rotator cuff: MR imaging with conventional and fat-suppression techniques. *Radiology* 1991;180:735–740.

78. Vahlensieck M, Pollack M, Lang P, Grampp S, Genant HK. Two segments of the supraspinatus muscle: cause of high signal intensity at MR imaging. *Radiology* 1993;186:449–454.

79. Erickson SJ, Cox IH, Hyde JS, Carrera GF, Strandt JA, Estkowski LD. Effect of tendon orientation on MR imaging signal intensity: a manifestation of the "magic angle" phenomenon. *Radiology* 1991;181:389–392.

80. Erickson SJ, Prost RW, Timins ME. The "magic angle" effect: background physics and clinical relevance. *Radiology* 1993;188:23–25.

81. Timins ME, Erickson SJ, Estkowski LD, Carrera GF, Komorowski RA. Increased signal in the normal supraspinatus tendon on MR imaging: diagnostic pitfall caused by the magic-angle effect. *Am J Roentgenol* 1995;164:109–114.

82. Davis SJ, Teresi LM, Bradley WG, Ressler JA, Eto RT. Effect of arm rotation on MR imaging of the rotator cuff. *Radiology* 1991;181:265–268.

83. Tsai JC, Zlatkin MB. Magnetic resonance imaging of the shoulder. *Radiol Clin North Am* 1990;28:279–291.

84. Zlatkin MB, Dalinka MK, Kressel HY. Magnetic resonance imaging of the shoulder. *Magnetic Reson Q* 1989;5:3–22.

85. Tamai K, Ogawa K. Intratendinous tears of the supraspinatus tendon exhibiting winging of the scapula. *Clin Orthop Rel Res* 1985;194:159.

86. Traughber PD, Goodwin TE. Shoulder MRI: arthroscopic correlation with emphasis on partial tears. *J Computer Assist Tomogr* 1992;16(1)129–133.

87. Singson RD, Hoang T, Dan S, Friedman M. MR evaluation of rotator cuff pathology using T2-weighted fast spin-echo technique with and without fat suppression. *Am J Roentgenol* 1996;166:1061–1065.

88. Hodler J, Kursunoglu-Brahme S, Snyder SJ, et al. Rotator cuff disease: assessment with MR arthrography versus standard MR imaging in 36 patients with arthroscopic confirmation. *Radiology* 1992;182:431–436.

89. Flannigan B, Kursunoglu-Brahme S, Snyder S, et al. MR arthrography of the shoulder: comparison with conventional MR imaging. *Am J Roentgenol* 1990;155:829–832.

90. Palmer WE, Brown JH, Rosenthal DI. Rotator cuff: evaluation with fat-suppressed MR arthrography. *Radiology* 1993;1993:683–687.

91. Ianotti JP, Zlatkin MB, Esterhai JL, et al. Magnetic resonance imaging of the shoulder. *J Bone Joint Surg* 1991;73-A:17–29.

92. Nakagaki K, Ozaki J, Tomita Y, Tamai S. Function of supraspinatus muscle with torn cuff evaluated by magnetic resonance imaging. *Clin Orth Rel Res* 1995;(318):144–151.

93. Mitchell MJ, Causey G, Berthoty DP, Sartoris DJ, Resnick D. Peribursal fat plane of the shoulder: anatomic study and clinical experience. *Radiology* 1988;168:699–704.

94. Zlatkin MB, Reicher MA, Kellerhouse LE, McDade W, Vetter L, Resnick D. The painful shoulder: MR imaging of the glenohumeral joint. *J Comput Assist Tomogr* 1988;12(6):995–1001.

95. Craig EV. The acromioclavicular joint cyst: An unusual presentation of a rotator cuff tear. *Clin Orthop* 1986;202:189.

96. Postacchini F, Perugia D, Gumina S. Acromioclavicular joint cyst associated with rotator cuff tear. *Clinical Orthop Rel Res* 1993;(294):111–113.

97. Groh GI, Badwey TM, Rockwood CA. Treatment of cysts of the acromioclavicular joint with shoulder hemiarthroplasty. *J Bone Joint Surg* 1993;75-A(12):1790–1794.

98. Bryan W, Wild J. Isolated infraspinatus atrophy. *Am J Sports Med* 1989;17:130–133.

99. Ferrari JD, Ferrari DA, Coumas J, Pappas AM. Posterior ossification of the shoulder: the Bennett lesion. *Am J Sports Med* 1994;22(2):171–176.

100. Symeonides PP. The significance of the subscapularis muscle in the pathogenesis of recurrent anterior dislocation of the shoulder. *J Bone Joint Surg (Br)* 1972;54:476–483.

101. Neviaser RJ, Neviaser TJ, Neviaser JS. Concurrent rupture of the rotator cuff and anterior dislocation of the shoulder in the older patient. *J Bone Joint Surg* 1988;70-A(9):1308–1311.

102. Neviaser RJ, Neviaser TH, Neviaser JS. Anterior dislocation of the shoulder and rotator cuff rupture. *Clin Orthop Rel Res* 1993;(291):103–106.

103. Gerber C, Krushell RJ. Isolated rupture of the tendon of the subscapularis muscle. *J Bone Joint Surg* 1991;73-B:389–394.

104. Patten RM. Tears of the anterior portion of the rotator cuff (the subscapularis tendon): MR imaging findings. *Am J Roentgenol* 1994;162:351–354.

105. Chan TW, Dalinka MK, Kneeland BJ, Chevrot A. Biceps tendon dislocation: evaluation with MR imaging. *Radiology* 1991;179:649–652.

106. Cervilla V, Schweitzer ME, Ho C, Mott A, Kerr R, Resnick D. Medial dislocation of the biceps brachii tendon: appearance at MR imaging. *Radiology* 1991;180:523–526.

107. Nobuhara K, Hitoshi I. Rotator interval lesion. *Clin Orthop Rel Res* 1987;223:44.

108. Seeger LL, Lubowitz J, Thomas BJ. Case report 815. *Skeletal Radiol* 1993;22:615–617.

109. Zlatkin MB, Iannotti JP, Roberts MC, et al. Rotator cuff tears: Diagnostic performance of MR imaging. *Radiology* 1989;172:223–229.

110. Quinn SF, Sheley RC, Demlow TA, Szumowski J. Rotator cuff tendon tears: evaluation with fat-suppressed MR imaging with arthroscopic correlation in 100 patients. *Radiology* 1995;195:497–501.

111. Tuite MJ, Yandow DR, DeSmet AA, Orwin JF, Quintana FA. Diagnosis of partial and complete rotator cuff tears using combined gradient echo and spin echo imaging. *Skeletal Radiol* 1994;23:541–546.

112. Uhthoff HK, Sarkar K. Calcifying tendinitis: its pathogenetic mechanism and a rationale for its treatment. *Int Orthop* 1978;2:187–193.

113. Bosworth BM. Calcium deposits in the shoulder and subacromial bursitis. *JAMA* 1941;116:2477.

114. Plenk HP. Calcifying tendonitis of the shoulder. *Radiology* 1952;59:384.

Shoulder Magnetic Resonance Imaging,
edited by Lynne S. Steinbach, et al.
Lippincott–Raven Publishers, Philadelphia © 1998.

CHAPTER 7

Glenohumeral Instability

Phillip F.J. Tirman

Glenohumeral instability refers to the humeral head slipping out of the glenoid socket and causing symptoms. This is a relatively common abnormality in that the shoulder is considered to be the most unstable joint in the body (1,2). The humeral head can sublux part of the way out or dislocate all the way out of the joint. Although the humeral head may normally move (translate) to a small degree within the glenoid socket during daily activities, movement causing pain resulting from spasm or capsular stretching is what is thought of as glenohumeral instability. The situation is analogous to gastroesophageal reflux: Most people experience minor reflux to a degree, probably every day, but when it causes heartburn, it becomes a clinically apparent problem.

A number of qualifying terms can be added to glenohumeral instability to further define the abnormality. Continuing instability resulting from a single traumatic dislocation is referred to as "posttraumatic" or even "posttraumatic recurrent instability" and is involuntary. Instability resulting from congenital ligamentous laxity is often referred to as "atraumatic instability." Some patients are able to freely sublux or even dislocate their shoulders at will without causing symptoms. This is not considered glenohumeral instability and these patients are not generally surgical candidates.

CLINICAL CLASSIFICATION SCHEMES

Instability can be classified according to temporal relationship of antecedent trauma (acute first time versus recurrent) and degree (subluxation versus dislocation). Orthopedists often refer to instability with respect to direction: unidirectional (e.g., anterior-inferior or posterior); multidirectional (e.g., gross instability). Additionally, orthopedists often classify patients into two broad clinical categories of instability. One group who has suffered a traumatic dislocation resulting in unidirectional anteroinferior instability with a Bankart lesion is referred to by the acronym TUBS—*t*raumatic, *u*nidirectional, *B*ankart, *s*urgical. The other group is characterized by *a*traumatic, *m*ultidirectional, *b*ilateral recurrent *i*nstability referred to as AMBRI (3–5). TUBS patients are often surgical candidates if the dislocation is recurrent, whereas AMBRI patients are usually not (3–5).

The usual dislocation occurs during a fall on the outstretched (externally rotated, abducted) arm. This often results in a trip to the emergency department where the dislocation is documented and a routine reduction is performed. These patients fit into the TUBS category and usually have a Bankart or Bankart variant lesion. (These are defined further on in this chapter.) Imaging beyond plain films is rarely required because the patients are initially treated conservatively. Many traumatic episodes occur in which the patients feel that their shoulder popped out (dislocated) and self-reduced but the dislocation is difficult to document clinically and is not documented radiographically. Some of these

P. F.J. Tirman: Department of Radiology; San Francisco Magnetic Resonance Center–St. Francis Memorial Hospital, University of California, San Francisco, San Francisco, California 94118-1944

episodes represent true dislocations and some are severe subluxations (4). Imaging may be required in these patients to document the damage done and to plan further therapy. This is especially true in the older patient because the spectrum of resultant lesions are generally quite different than a typical Bankart lesion (6,7).

The lesions resulting in recurrent dislocation are varied and are discussed in detail in this chapter. The anatomic causes of atraumatic instability are under debate, and these patients are often not currently candidates for imaging. The cause may be hypermobility or laxity, perhaps because of stretching of the supporting structures from overuse and because reliable standards of normal have not yet been defined with imaging.

WHY IMAGE INSTABILITY?

The concept of glenohumeral instability and resulting clinical pain and disability is still being defined. A number of abnormalities that may lead to clinical instability have been described, primarily because of the proliferation of arthroscopy. The most important reason to image is to diagnose the anatomic lesion leading to the problem. Additionally, unless a clear distinct history of anterior dislocation is received by the treating physician, more minor forms of injury leading to instability can present in a confusing manner, necessitating diagnostic testing. A spectrum of lesions, which is partially age dependent, results from glenohumeral dislocation. For optimal operative planning, an accurate preoperative diagnosis is necessary, especially in those cases that are clinically confusing. Some lesions resulting from an-

terior dislocation, for example, nondisplaced greater tuberosity fracture in an older patient, may respond very well to conservative management.

TECHNICAL CONSIDERATIONS

The choice of the type of magnetic resonance imaging (MRI) study depends on the clinical history. In the younger patient with chronic, recurrent instability, MR arthrography is the method of choice. The spectrum of lesions resulting in continued instability can often be subtle owing to the results of partial healing, which add to the difficulty of diagnosis (8–13). Typically, at conventional, nonarthrographic MRI, a paucity of joint fluid leads to the close apposition of structures of similar signal intensity, which makes it difficult to distinguish between the structures (Fig. 1). This is especially true in the anteroinferior portion of the joint where the anterior capsule folds on itself in the neutral position and becomes closely applied to the anterior labrum. Additionally, the "magic angle" artifact affects the collagenous tissues present in the shoulder joint where those tissues are oriented at 55 degrees to the static external magnetic field (14,15) (Fig. 2). This results in a diffuse increase in signal intensity on short TE sequences (T1, proton density, gradient echo), thus potentially obscuring a distinct linear tear of the labrum or capsule by masking the tear. The magic angle artifact affects a portion of the capsule, labrum, and adjacent tendon in the anteroinferior portion of the joint, anterior and posterior superior portion of the joint, and to some degree the posteroinferior portion of the joint. Many abnormalities leading to continued subluxation or dislocation are located in the an-

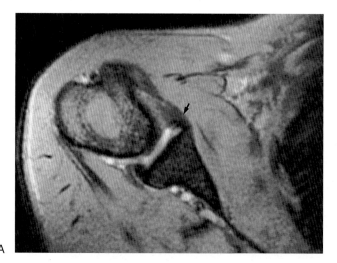
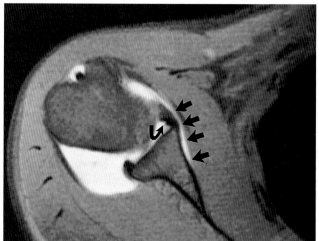

A   B

FIG. 1. Benefit of arthrography: pseudostripping of the capsule. **A:** Axial gradient echo image through the inferior portion of the joint demonstrates the inferior glenohumeral labral ligamentous complex as a thick, predominantly decreased signal intensity structure *(arrow)*. **B:** After the administration of intraarticular contrast material, this axial T1-weighted image with fat saturation demonstrates the inferior glenohumeral labral ligamentous attachment to the glenoid to better advantage *(curved arrow)*. Note the interligamentous recess *(small thick arrows)* adjacent to the inferior glenohumeral ligament mimicking stripping of the capsule. At surgery for posterior labral abnormality not shown, the anterior labrum and capsule were defined as normal.

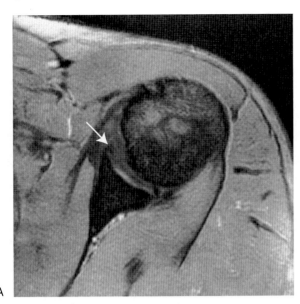 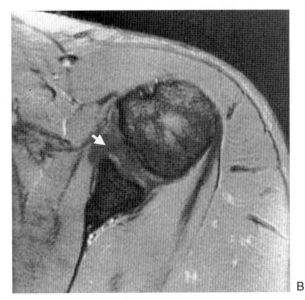

FIG. 2. Magic angle anteroinferior labrum. **A:** Axial gradient echo image demonstrates decreased signal intensity triangular anterior glenoid labrum *(arrow)*. **B:** One image inferior to **(A)** demonstrates diffuse increased signal intensity *(arrow)* within the anterior glenoid labrum caused by the magic angle artifact in this asymptomatic volunteer.

teroinferior quadrant, so accurate depiction of the anatomy is essential and best accomplished by arthrography. If partial healing or complete healing of a capsulolabral injury occurs, the abnormality may go undetected with conventional MRI (16). The joint may resynovialize the injury, making it potentially occult both at surgery and imaging (9,16). Placing stress on the stabilizing structures of the shoulder may bring out an otherwise undetected lesion (16). Therefore, I recommend standard position MR arthrography coupled with imaging in the abducted externally rotated (ABER) position for adequate visualization of this region (Fig. 3). This is true anteriorly and inferiorly with the use of the ABER position. ABER stresses the inferior glenohumeral labral-ligamentous complex and "opens up" some partially healed or healed and incompetent labral ligamentous attachments to the underlying glenoid (16) (Fig. 4).

In the older patient, the spectrum of abnormalities resulting in continued instability is different and, in general, conventional technique is satisfactory.

ANATOMIC CONSIDERATIONS

There are two main categories of stabilizers of the shoulder: the rotator cuff muscles and the labral ligamentous complex (8,17–20). The rotator cuff muscles are referred to as *dynamic stabilizers* and the labral ligamentous complex as *static stabilizers*. This is best understood when considering the full range of motion allowed by the shoulder joint. It is the synchronous action of the rotator cuff muscles that keep the humeral head within the glenoid socket during active motion, especially in the mid range. When the arm is moving throughout various ranges of motion, synergistic actions of the muscles keep the humeral head within the glenoid socket—a dynamic process. The labral ligamentous complex, on the other hand, acts as a check rein, as is discussed in Chapter 4, and prevents the humeral head from moving excessively once the end range of motion has been reached.

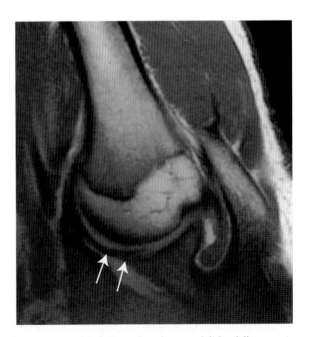

FIG. 3. Normal inferior glenohumeral labral ligamentous attachment on the abduction and external rotation (ABER) view. T1-weighted arthrographic image obtained in ABER demonstrates a normal attachment site of the inferior glenohumeral ligament to the anteroinferior labrum *(arrows)*.

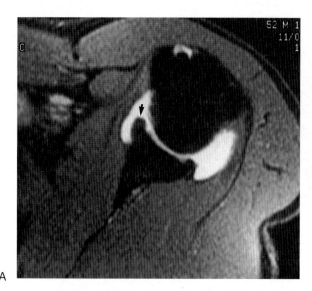
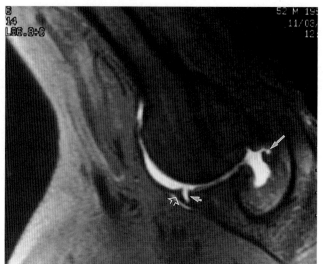

FIG. 4. Perthes lesion. Benefit of imaging in the abduction and external rotation (ABER) position. **A:** Axial gradient echo arthrographic image demonstrates a normal-appearing, albeit somewhat rounded, anteroinferior labrum *(arrows).* **B:** ABER image demonstrates detachment of the inferior glenohumeral labral ligamentous complex *(open arrow)* from the underlying glenoid *(short arrow).* A small undersurface tear of the rotator cuff *(long arrow)* was also found at surgery.

In other words, the labral ligamentous complex stops the humeral head from moving entirely out of the joint. In ABER, the position of risk for suffering an anterior dislocation, the inferior labral ligamentous complex becomes tightened and prevents the humeral head from dislocating out of the joint anteroinferiorly. Thus, the labral ligamentous complex acts in a static stabilizing form. Of the dynamic stabilizers, the subscapularis is the anteriormost muscle and is thought of as an anterior stabilizer by its location.

The glenohumeral ligaments represent a condensation of the shoulder capsule and are variable in appearance when imaging (Fig. 5). The ligaments act to strengthen the joint capsule and course from the humerus to their glenoid attachments (21). The inferior glenohumeral ligament complex (IGHLC) originates laterally at the region of the anatomic neck of the humerus and inserts on the inferior portion of the glenoid inserting onto the labrum (22). The anteroinferior, inferior, and posteroinferior labrum represents a fibrous thickening of the IGHLC at its attachment to the glenoid rim (22). The IGHLC is a complex structure composed of collagenous thickenings at its anterior and posterior margin referred to as the *anterior* and *posterior bands.* In the neutral position, the IGHLC forms the axillary pouch inferiorly, seen best in the distended state on oblique coronal images and filled with contrast at plain film arthrography (Fig. 6). Visualization of the site of insertion of the anterior band of the inferior glenohumeral ligament is important for instability evaluation. It is often at this site where damage occurs after dislocation or subluxation, leading to recurrent instability. When the patient is imaged in the conventional neutral (arm by side) position, this insertion site can be quite inferior in location and difficult to assess properly without a joint effusion (Fig. 7).

Imaging in the ABER position draws the IGHLC taut, placing stress on the ligament and helping to rid magic angle artifact (Fig. 8).

The middle glenohumeral ligament is congenitally variable and can be absent in 8% to 30% of individuals (1,23,24). On MR images, the ligament is seen as a decreased signal intensity structure coursing between the humerus and glenoid and can be "cordlike" or "sheetlike." When cordlike, it inserts in conjunction with the superior glenohumeral ligament at the base of the biceps insertion onto the superior glenoid (Fig. 9).

When sheetlike, the ligament can insert onto the tip of the anterosuperior glenoid or medially onto the scapular neck. The ligament functions as a secondary restraint to both inferior and anterior instability and is a primary stabilizer for anterior stability at 45 degrees of abduction (25).

The superior glenohumeral ligament blends with the superior portion of the labrum and biceps tendon anchor. It can often be seen coursing obliquely across the superior portion of the joint near the coracoid process on sagittal images (Fig. 10). Many authors believe it has little role in anterior instability and mainly functions to limit external rotation when the shoulder is adducted (25).

The labrum is an important structure for joint stability (8,17,19,22,26–28). As discussed, it is the attachment of the inferior glenohumeral ligament to the anterior, inferior, and posterior portions of the glenoid. The labrum deepens the shallow glenoid fossa, increasing the contact area for the humeral head. The intact labrum may also act as a pressure seal, allowing negative pressure to occur within the glenoid fossa during shoulder motion. It also acts as a bumper, thus partially stabilizing the joint during the mid range of motion and, so to a degree, is a dynamic stabilizer (26, 29). The in-

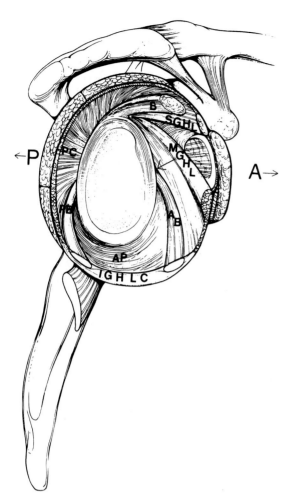

FIG. 5. Shoulder capsular anatomy. Sagittal view with the humerus taken away. Note that the inferior glenohumeral ligament (IGHLC) inserts onto the anterior inferior portion of the labrum *(arrow)*. In this patient, the middle glenohumeral ligament (MGHL) is cordlike and inserts along with the superior glenohumeral ligament (SGHL) at the base of the biceps (b). (a), anterior; (p), posterior; ap, axillary pouch; ab, anterior band of the IGHL; pb, posterior band; pc, posterior capsule. (From ref. 10, with permission.)

creasing understanding of the functional significance of the labrum has led to increased importance of the evaluation of its integrity in clinical medicine.

The anterior labrum is usually triangular in shape (see Fig. 1); however, numerous variations have been demonstrated (30–32). This is especially true anterosuperiorly where the labrum can be detached or absent as a variation of normal.

An opening in the anterior joint communicating with the subscapularis recess (bursa) can occur in many different locations (33) This bursa often serves as an accumulation site for normal joint fluid and can be seen resting on top of the subscapularis tendon or even "saddlebagging" over the tendon as a variation of normal (Fig. 11). This recess normally fills during arthrography and may rupture, commonly leading to contrast extravasation.

Characterizing capsular anatomy with imaging can be dif-

ficult. This is especially true in light of the changes in understanding of what constitutes normal shoulder anatomy. For instance, variations in labral anatomy, especially anterosuperiorly, are considered normal variations rather than pathology as was the case before the early 1990s (34–36). Also, correlation between imaging and arthroscopy is somewhat difficult, primarily because the shoulder joint is viewed in different ways using the two different techniques. It is important to understand the differences in visualization to understand the potential discrepancy in how some lesions may appear to the surgeon and how they may appear at imaging. Capsular stripping is one example. Radiologists and orthopedists have for some time described variations in capsular insertion on the glenoid as predisposing to glenohumeral instability and laxity (37). This is difficult to prove because the clinical definition of laxity varies among surgeons. Between the inferior glenohumeral ligament and the other glenohumeral ligaments, the joint capsule is often redundant because the capsule is capacious, allowing the wide range of motion of the shoulder. Sometimes, capsular stripping perceived by the radiologist actually represents visualization of these interligamentous recesses, because they are often closely applied to the scapula as they curve around anterolaterally to insert on the labrum (see Fig. 1). Also, when the middle glenohumeral ligament is sheetlike, it may actually insert medially on the scapula. In addition, there is a wide variation in the appearance of the subscapularis bursa, which is often mistaken for medial insertion of the capsule or capsular stripping. The thin portions of the capsule that make up the interligamentous recesses may also become disrupted during arthrography and allow extravasation of contrast, thereby adding to the confusion and to the pathologic appearance of the anterior joint, allowing consideration of a posttraumatic injury related to the patient's symptoms rather

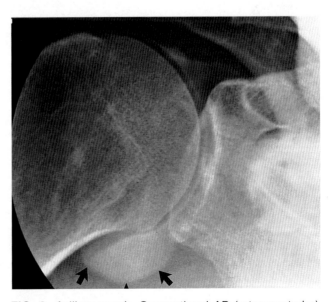

FIG. 6. Axillary pouch. Conventional AP (arteroposterior) view of the shoulder during arthrography demonstrates distention of the axillary pouch *(arrows)*, which is made up of the inferior glenohumeral ligament.

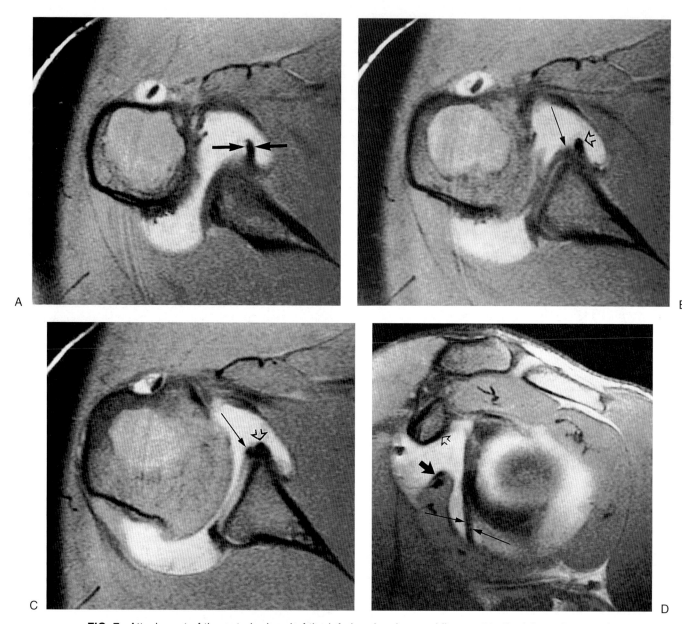

FIG. 7. Attachment of the anterior band of the inferior glenohumeral ligament to the labrum in a surgically proven normal patient. **A:** Axial arthrographic image of the inferiormost portion of the joint demonstrates the anterior band of the inferior glenohumeral ligament *(arrows)* coursing up to insert onto the labrum. **B:** Axial arthrographic image obtained 4 mm superior to **(A)** further demonstrates the ligament coursing superior *(open arrow)* to attach onto the labrum *(long arrow)*. **C:** Axial arthrographic image 4 mm more superior than **(B)** demonstrates the attachment of the inferior glenohumeral ligament *(open arrow)* to the labrum *(long arrow)*. This should not be mistaken for an ALPSA lesion as the labral ligamentous complex is not displaced medially. **D:** Sagittal arthrographic image from the same patient demonstrates the anterior band of the inferior glenohumeral ligament *(long thin arrows)*, which is quite inferior in location. Without the use of intraarticular contrast material, the actual insertion of the anterior band would have been difficult to visualize on axial images. Note the subscapularis tendon *(thick arrow)* and the coracoid process *(open arrow)* for orientation purposes.

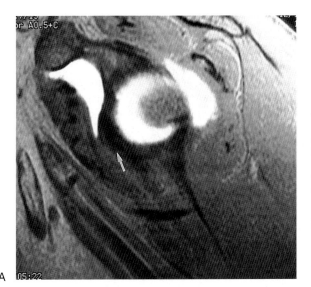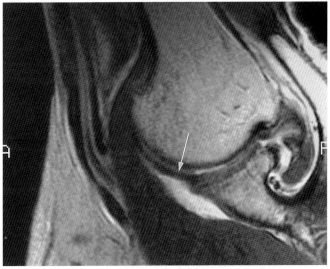

A   B

FIG. 8. A: Nonvisualization of the inferior glenohumeral ligament ligamentous attachment. Even with arthrography, sometimes the ligamentous insertions are difficult to see. This sagittal arthrographic image demonstrates close apposition of the anterior structures not allowing separate identification of the ligaments *(arrow)*. **B:** Normal inferior glenohumeral labral ligamentous attachment in the abduction and external rotation (ABER) view. Oblique axial fast spin-echo T2-weighted images obtained with the patient in ABER shows normal inferior glenohumeral ligament *(arrow)* labrum complex attaching to the glenoid *(arrow)*.

than an iatrogenic occurrence. When surgeons refer to capsular stripping, they are, in general, referring to stripping of the inferior glenohumeral labral ligamentous complex from the glenoid as the result of a traumatic event. This means that the labral ligamentous complex is in effect torn from the glenoid. During arthroscopic evaluation, the arm is often abducted from the body at approximately 30 degrees and traction is placed on the joint. This "draws up" the inferior glenohumeral labral ligamentous complex and this complex can be seen in the mid portion of the joint (Fig. 12). When radiologists image the shoulder in neutral position, the inferior glenohumeral ligament becomes lax and actually drapes down inferiorly. The insertion of the anterior band is often present in the inferior portion of the joint, making it difficult to visualize. Using conventional technique in patients with a paucity of joint fluid, and considering the magic angle artifact, the region may be very difficult to visualize and true capsular stripping may be missed.

I and my colleagues (38) evaluated the role of capsular insertion type, or perceived capsular insertion type, in the typical clinical evaluation and surgical management of glenohumeral instability. We looked at capsular insertion types as described by Moseley and Overgaard and correlated this to the examination under anesthesia and surgical results (37). What we found was that there was no correlation in perceived capsular insertion type and glenohumeral instability as defined by examination under anesthesia in 48 patients or

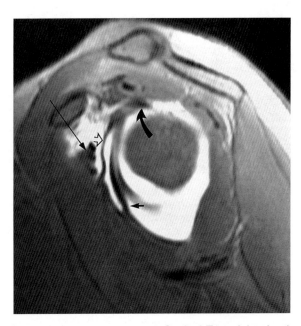

FIG. 9. Ligamentous anatomy. Sagittal T1-weighted arthrographic image with fat saturation through the joint demonstrates the inferior glenohumeral ligament coursing up and attaching onto the labrum *(small arrow)*. A cordlike middle glenohumeral ligament can be seen coursing up through the joint *(open arrow)* to attach at the insertion site for the long head of the biceps tendon *(curved arrow)*. The subscapularis tendon can be seen *(long arrow)* within the subscapularis recess.

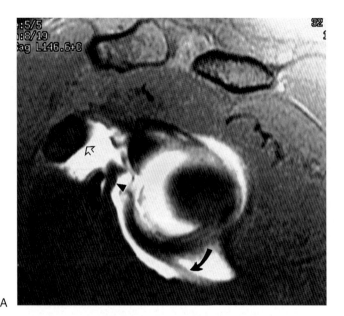

A

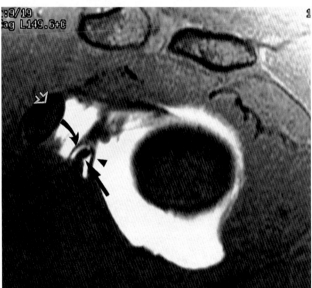

B

FIG. 10. Variation in appearance of the glenohumeral ligaments. **A:** Sagittal arthrographic image demonstrates the anterior band of the inferior glenohumeral ligament *(curved arrow)* coursing superiorly to insert onto the labrum. A cordlike middle glenohumeral ligament *(arrowhead)* is identified anterosuperiorly. The coracoid process, which indicates the anterior portion of the joint, can be seen *(open arrow).* **B:** Image 4 mm lateral to **(A)** demonstrates the cordlike middle glenohumeral ligament *(arrowhead)* and the superior glenohumeral ligament *(curved arrow)* as they course up to insert at the base of the biceps tendon. The subscapularis tendon *(long thick arrow)* can be seen between them. Note the coracoid process anterosuperiorly *(open arrow).*

as is implied by the lesions discovered at surgery. Furthermore, Palmer and Caslowitz (39) described that no correlation between capsular insertion type and glenohumeral instability existed in their patient population.

IMAGING PITFALLS—ANATOMIC VARIATIONS THAT LOOK LIKE GLENOHUMERAL INSTABILITY BUT ARE NOT

The glenoid labrum and the various capsular ligamentous insertions onto it can be variable in appearance at imaging (40). The labrum itself may be triangular in appearance or can be somewhat blunted and rounded in appearance. Small clefts may be found within the anterior labrum. It is important to appreciate the wide variation in appearance of the labrum and capsule. Perhaps the most important consideration is that the anterior superior labrum, the portion of the labrum and capsule between the glenoid notch anteriorly and the biceps anchor superiorly (Fig. 13), can be variable in appearance. The anterior labrum in this portion of the joint may be a different size than the rest of the labrum, typically being somewhat smaller. The labrum may be firmly attached or, in some patients, a recess of variable depth may be present beneath it in this quadrant of the shoulder. As a further variation, the anterosuperior labrum may be completely detached as a variation of normal and this is referred to as the sublabral hole or sublabral foramen (34,35) (Fig. 14). To further add to the confusion, the anterosuperior labrum may be completely absent. In this situation, the middle glenohumeral ligament is cordlike in appearance and the combination of the anterosuperior labral absence and cordlike middle glenohumeral ligament have been refered to as the Buford complex (34,35) (Fig. 15). The presence of this complex or the sublabral hole can be confusing to the radiologist. The sublabral hole mimics a labral detachment, and indeed it is often not possible to

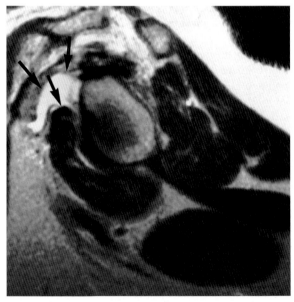

FIG. 11. The subscapularis recess. The two top arrows outline the recess. The bottom arrow points to the subscapularis muscle/tendon. The recess saddlebags over the muscle/tendon.

diagnose an isolated anterosuperior labral tear confidently in distinction to a sublabral hole. We often include both as differential possibilities based on the clinical history. Isolated injury of the anterosuperior labrum is thought to be uncommon, but may be seen in high-level throwing athletes. Clinical history coupled with basic radiologic principles can lead to confident and accurate characterization of the anterosuperior labrum. In a high-level throwing athlete in whom a sublabral hole is present, however, we offer the differential diagnosis of anterosuperior labral tear (Fig. 16). Statistically, in the general population, detachment of the anterosuperior labrum represents a sublabral hole anatomic variation (34–36,41). This means that the detachment is not associated with biceps anchor abnormality or mid and inferior labrum abnormality. If residual labral tissue is identified on the glenoid rim or the detached segment of labrum is degenerated, frayed, or further torn, we cannot confidently make the diagnosis of a sublabral hole (see Fig. 16).

With the Buford complex, the cordlike middle glenohumeral ligament stretches obliquely from the humerus to insert at the base of the biceps and is included on the image. A transaxial image through the anterosuperior portion of the joint demonstrates the absent labrum and a rounded structure away from the glenoid in the anterior joint that is often interpreted as a torn detached labrum (35). The key to making this diagnosis is identifying the cordlike middle glenohumeral ligament as a ligamentous structure, distinct and separate from the anteroinferior labrum, which appears normal. If the radiologist keeps in mind that the only things present in the anterior portion of the joint are the labrum, ligament, and subscapularis, then the radiologist can evaluate any questionable structure and more confidently identify it (Fig. 17). One particular difficulty lies in determining what defines anterosuperior as separate from anterior mid and superior. Anterosuperior is defined as that portion of the glenoid between the biceps insertion superiorly and the mid

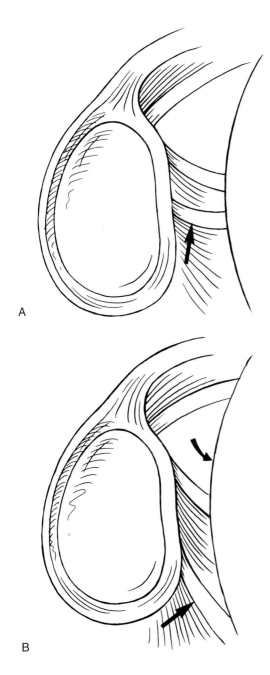

A

B

FIG. 12. Effect of arm position on the appearance of the inferior glenohumeral ligament. **A:** In the partially abducted position, as is often the case at arthroscopy, the anterior band of the inferior glenohumeral ligament *(arrow)* is drawn up more superiorly than in the neutral position. **B:** At MRI, shoulders are usually imaged in the neutral position. Anterior band of the inferior glenohumeral ligament complex is relaxed and inferior in location *(arrow)*. Humeral head *(curved arrow)*.

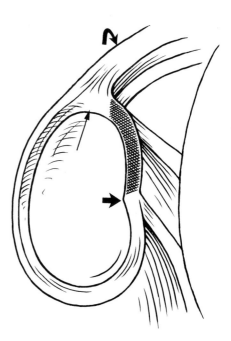

FIG. 13. Labral variations within the glenoid fossa occur between the biceps insertion superiorly *(long thin arrow)* and the mid glenoid notch inferiorly *(thick arrow)*. Curved arrow points to biceps tendon.

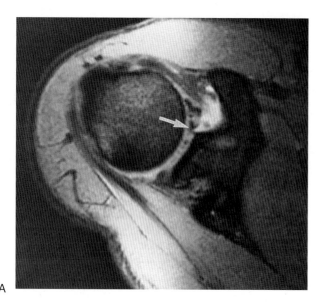
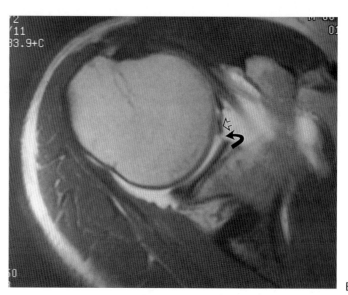

A

B

FIG. 14. Sublabral hole. **A:** Gradient echo axial image through the mid superior joint demonstrates an abnormal appearance of the anterosuperior labrum *(arrow)*. In a patient without specific traumatic history, the findings are consistent with visualization of a sublabral hole variation. **B:** Axial T1 arthrographic image through the superior portion of the joint demonstrates a detached labrum *(open arrow)*. Note the contrast material *(curved arrow)* between the labrum and the underlying glenoid.

glenoid notch inferiorly (see Fig. 13). It is often difficult to accurately identify the anterior glenoid notch. To help accurately identify a normal anatomic structure, it is important to "follow" through its entire range. The subscapularis tendon can usually be easily identified. The glenoid labrum if followed down inferiorly should be identified as distinct from the capsule and, likewise, a cordlike middle glenohumeral ligament can often be followed from the inferior portion of the joint obliquely superiorly to its insertion site and identified as a ligamentous structure. A primary point of interest is the following:

The anterosuperior labrum is variable in its imaging appearance and is easily mistaken for a labral abnormality. Accurate identification of the anatomic structures in this portion of the joint is important to avoid the false positive diagnosis of an abnormality where none may exist.

ANATOMIC LESIONS RESULTING IN GLENOHUMERAL INSTABILITY

In this section, lesions that can result in repeated subluxations or dislocations of the shoulder and their MRI appearance are discussed. Congenital laxity of the shoulder is not considered because it is difficult to define, both clinically and radiologically, and MRI standards for this diagnosis have not been developed. This is often a diagnosis of exclusion.

Subluxation

A disruption in the integrity of the rotator cuff muscles or the labral ligamentous structures can result in glenohumeral instability. This is especially true of the inferior glenohumeral labral ligamentous complex (8,22,36). The complex may become stretched and redundant as a result of chronic microtrauma, typically in the throwing athlete. This may lead to spasm and repeated subluxation. This is difficult to diagnose using imaging methods. A partial tear of the glenoid labrum at the glenohumeral ligament insertion site can result from a single traumatic event and lead to repeated subluxations, pain, and disability, but not necessarily clinical instability by physical examination. In fact, many of these patients are clinically stable and the pain and dysfunction arises from catching of the torn labrum on the moving humeral head (29). These tears are often associated with articular cartilage abnormalities and have been referred to as the GARD lesion (glenoid articular rim divot), which begins the long list of acronyms and eponyms in shoulder instability. Neviaser (42), in 1993, described the GLAD lesion (glenoid labrum articular disruption) and theorized that this lesion resulted from a forced adduction injury (Fig. 18). My colleagues and I have identified identical lesions, both at MRI and at arthroscopy that resulted from abduction external rotation injury and theorized that this may be the first abnormality in the spectrum of instability resulting from a fall on an outstretched arm as a mechanism of injury on the way

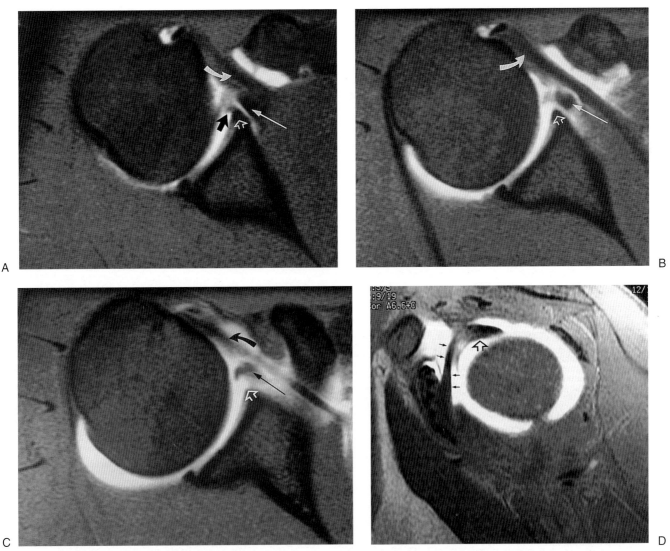

FIG. 15. Buford complex, **A:** Axial arthrographic image through the mid anterior portion of the joint demonstrates a normal-appearing anterior glenoid labrum *(open arrow)*. Note the partially visualized anterior band of the inferior glenohumeral ligament insertion onto the labrum *(black arrow)*, which appears irregular owing to volume averaging through the superiormost portion of it. The subscapularis tendon *(curved arrow)* and cordlike middle glenohumeral ligament *(long thin arrow)* are visualized anteriorly. **B:** Axial arthrographic image 4 mm superior to **(A)** demonstrates the anterior glenoid labrum *(open arrow)*, cordlike middle glenohumeral ligament *(long thin arrow)*, and subscapularis tendon *(curved arrow)* in their normal location and position. These three structures should be identified when characterizing a Buford complex. **C:** Axial arthrographic image through the superior portion of the joint demonstrates absence of the anterosuperior labrum *(open arrow)* and the cordlike middle glenohumeral ligament *(long thin arrow)* and subscapularis tendon *(curved arrow)*. **D:** Sagittal arthrographic image demonstrates the large cordlike middle glenohumeral ligament *(small arrows)* coursing up to insert at the base of the biceps tendon origin *(open arrow)*.

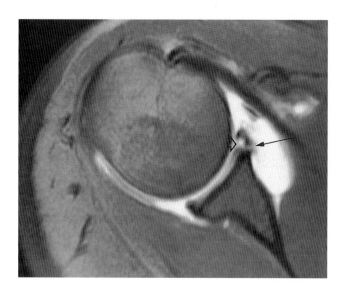

FIG. 16. Isolated anterior superior labral tear in a 25-year-old woman who fell on her partially abducted shoulder with a force from posteroinferior to anterior superior. Axial arthrographic T1-weighted image demonstrates marked irregularity of the anterior superior labrum. Note the contrast extending into the articular side of the labrum *(open arrow)*. The medial portion is partially attached. Some contrast extends through the base *(arrow)*. In many cases, it is impossible to distinguish this from a sublabral hole. The history is usually critical.

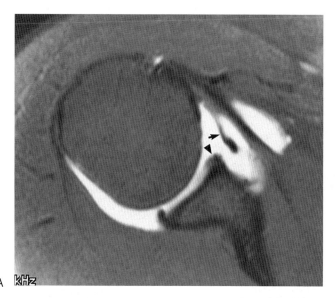

A

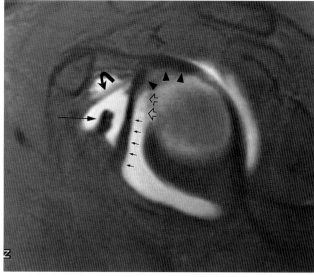

B

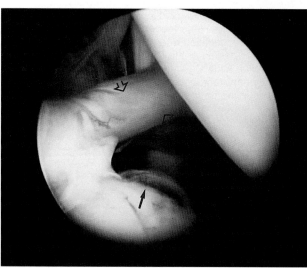

C

FIG. 17. Buford complex. **A:** Axial T1-weighted arthrographic image with fat saturation to the mid portion of the joint demonstrates a slightly irregular, but otherwise normal, anterior labrum *(arrowhead)*. A cordlike middle glenohumeral ligament *(arrow)* can be seen anterior to the labrum. **B:** Sagittal T1-weighted arthrographic image with fat saturation through the joint demonstrates an absent anterosuperior labrum *(open arrows)* and a large cordlike middle glenohumeral ligament *(small arrows)*. The subscapularis tendon *(long arrow)* can be seen projecting into the subscapularis bursa. The superior glenohumeral ligament *(curved arrow)* can be seen above the subscapularis tendon. The base of the biceps tendon insertion *(arrowheads)* serves as the attachment site for the cordlike middle glenohumeral ligament. **C:** Arthroscopic photograph of Buford complex. An arthroscopic photograph from the posterior portal viewing anteriorly demonstrates absence of the anterosuperior labrum along the anterosuperior glenoid rim *(arrow)*. The large cordlike middle glenohumeral ligament *(open arrows)* can be seen coursing up to its attachment site. The humeral head is to the right side of the image.

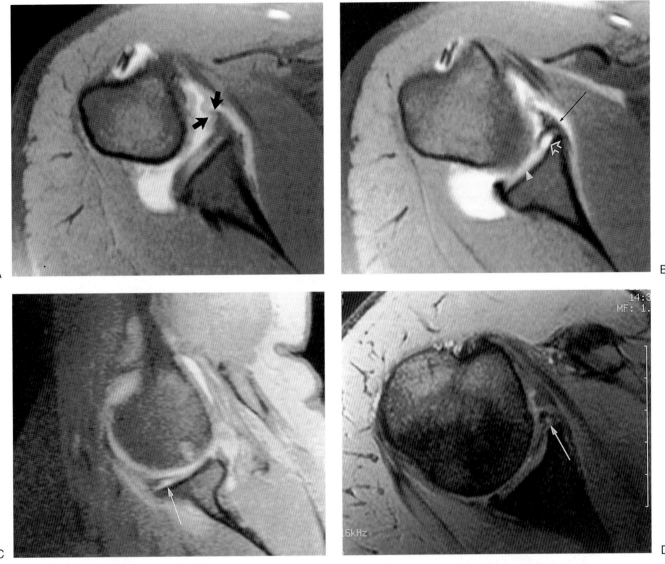

FIG. 18. GLAD lesion. **A:** Axial arthrographic T1-weighted image through the inferior joint demonstrates an intact inferior glenohumeral ligament *(arrows)* at its attachment to the labrum and underlying glenoid. **B:** Axial arthrographic T1-weighted image 4 mm higher than **(A)** demonstrates contrast extending into an articular cartilage defect *(open arrow)* adjacent to a partially detached labrum *(long arrow)*. Note the normal appearing hyaline cartilage of the glenoid *(arrowhead)*. **C:** Oblique axial ABER arthrographic T1-weighted image demonstrates the partial detachment of the labrum *(arrow)*. **D:** Partial tear of the anterior glenoid labrum. Gradient echo axial image demonstrates focus of irregular increased signal intensity within the anterior glenoid labrum *(arrow)*. This patient had a single injury to the shoulder but did not dislocate it, nor is the patient clinically unstable. Arthroscopically, a small partial tear of the mid anterior labrum was found and considered a GLAD or GARD lesion.

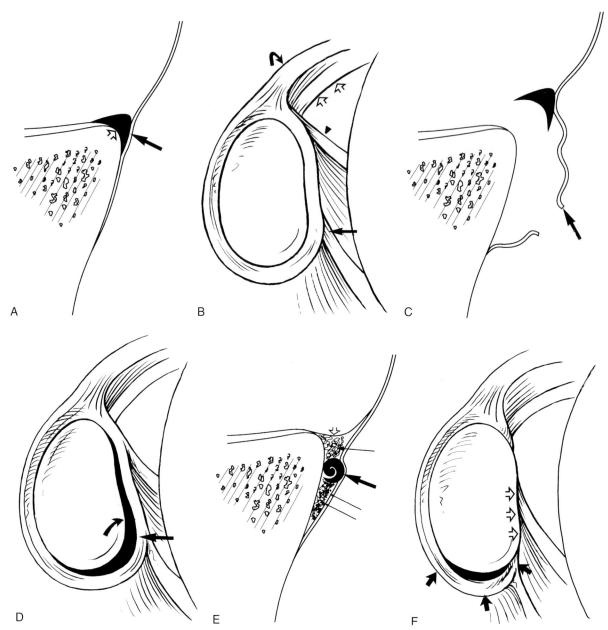

FIG. 19. Capsulolabral disruptions. **A:** Normal attachment of the inferior glenohumeral labraligamentous complex (IGHLC). Axial plane diagram through the anterior inferior joint demonstrates that the labraligamentous complex *(arrow)* inserts at the apex of the curve of the anterior glenoid *(open arrow)*. **B:** Arthroscopic diagram: note that the anterior band of the inferior glenohumeral ligamentous complex inserts onto the anterior inferior labrum, although in this diagram it is onto the lateral portion *(arrow)*. The anterior inferior labrum and inferior glenohumeral ligament are considered parts of the same structure. Long head of the biceps tendon *(curved arrow)*. Middle glenohumeral ligament (cordlike in this case) *(arrowhead)*. Superior glenohumeral ligament *(open arrows)*. **C:** Bankart lesion. Notice that the IGHLC is avulsed from the glenoid and that the scapular periosteum *(arrow)* is disrupted. **D:** Arthroscopic visualization of a Bankart lesion from the posterior portal viewing anteriorly. The inferior glenohumeral ligamentous complex *(arrow)* is avulsed away from the underlying glenoid. **E:** ALPSA lesion. The IGHLC *(thick arrow)* has rolled medially in a sleevelike fashion up the periosteum. Note that there has been fibrous tissue deposition *(long thin arrows)* around the displaced IGHLC. Synovial tissue *(open arrow)* from resynovialization (healing) sits on top of the fibrous mass. **F:** Arthroscopic visualization of an ALPSA lesion from the posterior portal viewing anteriorly. Note that the inferior glenohumeral labral ligamentous complex is displaced medially *(open arrows)* and inferiorly *(thick arrows)* with respect to the glenoid. **G:** Perthes lesion. The IGHLC *(arrow)* is resting in a relatively normal position. It may appear deceptively normal at arthroscopy. The stripped scapular periosteum *(curved arrow)* is seen medially. **H:** Detached Perthes lesion. Note the detached IGHLC is displaced anteriorly in the direction of the arrow. The stripped periosteum is shown *(curved arrow)*. *(Continued on next page.)*

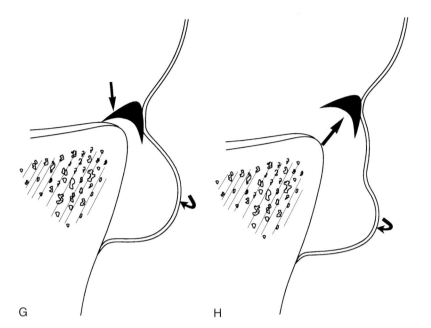

G   H   **FIG. 19.** *Continued.*

to dislocation. This type of lesion thus falls below the threshold of clinical instability evaluation demonstrating the power of MRI in identifying these subtle lesions that present with potentially confusing physical examinations and may be the progenitor of clinical instability and degenerative arthritis (see Chapter 10). Further work is needed to define the role of partial labral tears in the spectrum of clinical instability and the potential role of MRI.

Partial tears of the anterior labrum are difficult to diagnose with conventional technique. Increased sensitivity in detecting these lesions is achievable when arthrographic technique is used and the patient is imaged in ABER position. This is because the lesions may become partially healed and resynovialized, not allowing fluid to extend into the lesion in the neutral position. With abduction, the lesion is often "opened up" and thus detected (see Fig. 18). It is extremely important to consider the patient's history and mechanism of injury when considering this diagnosis. In the absence of trauma, non-degenerative tears of the glenoid labrum should not really be considered. Repeated subluxation or dislocation resulting from an initial anterior dislocation of the shoulder is referred to as *chronic posttraumatic anterior instability* (8,41). A spectrum of lesions have been described as resulting from an initial anterior dislocation. The differences in types of lesions based on the age of the patient at initial anterior dislocation are also discussed.

Younger Anterior Dislocation Patient (Teens and 20s)

Most patients who suffer an initial anterior dislocation of the shoulder in their teens or 20s suffer an avulsion of the anterior inferior labral ligamentous complex from the glenoid (8,41) (Fig. 19A–D). The injury results from excessive force against the arm in a patient whose shoulder is abducted and externally rotated. In other words, the injury usually occurs during a fall on an outstretched arm. The humeral head is levered up against the acromion and down and out of the joint anteroinferiorly, typically, and straight anteriorly in some cases.

Bankart Lesion

The most common lesion resulting from an anterior dislocation is the Bankart lesion, which is named after the British surgeon who described it (43). A Bankart lesion refers to an avulsion of the labral ligamentous complex from its attachment to the anterior and anteroinferior glenoid (Fig. 20). Oftentimes, this lesion is isolated to the anteroinferior glenoid. The lesion may be accompanied by a fracture of the anterior inferior glenoid (Fig. 21). The fracture is visualized on T2-weighted images as a region of increased signal intensity and on T1-weighted images as an often linear region of decreased signal intensity with variable distraction of the fragment from the remainder of the glenoid. Plain films and computed tomography also show the fracture well (Fig. 22). If the fracture is displaced, it is often repaired with the bone abnormality by internal fixation methods. The MRI appearance is varied and depends on the age of the lesion. Acutely, a hemorrhagic effusion is usually present and the labrum and capsule are lifted away from the underlying glenoid. The labrum may be discreetly torn (Fig. 23) but is often fragmented and markedly inhomogeneous and predominately of increased signal intensity on axial MR images (Fig. 24). In the chronic case, the Bankart lesion may be partially healed and fibrosed down to the glenoid, making its detection more difficult by MRI, especially when there is a paucity of joint fluid present. In these cases, arthrography may be necessary to demonstrate the lesion by lifting the torn labrum up and

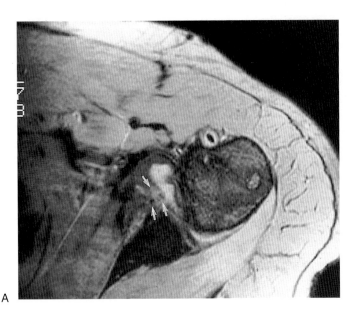

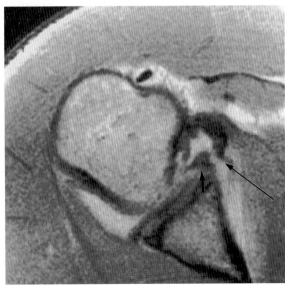

A   B

FIG. 20. Bankart lesion. **A:** Gradient echo axial image to the inferior portion of the joint demonstrates marked irregularity of the inferior glenohumeral labral ligamentous insertion site *(arrows)* in this patient who is status post anterior dislocation of the shoulder. The findings are consistent with visualization of a Bankart lesion. **B:** Axial proton density image demonstrates detachment of the anteroinferior labrum *(short arrow)* and a tear of the inferior glenohumeral ligament *(long arrow)* in another patient.

away from the glenoid to allow its detection (Fig. 25). As described previously, imaging in ABER may demonstrate an otherwise occult Bankart lesion by placing stress on the inferior glenohumeral ligament attachment site and partially disrupting a healed (or partially healed) labral tear, thus allowing its detection. Occasionally, the ABER position may demonstrate subluxation or dislocation (Fig. 26).

Bankart Variations

With the Bankart lesion, the scapular periosteum ruptures as the labral ligamentous attachment is avulsed from the glenoid. With Bankart variant lesions, the scapular periosteum remains attached to the labral ligamentous complex. If the labral ligamentous complex is displaced medially and

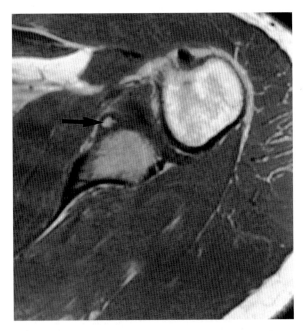

FIG. 21. Osseous bankart: Axial T1-weighted image demonstrates a small bony fragment *(arrow)* in a patient with a surgically proven Bankart lesion.

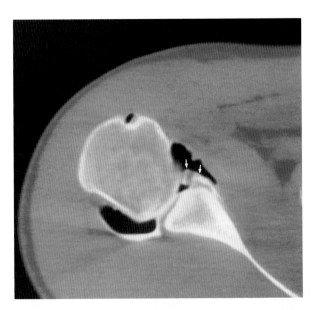

FIG. 22. Bankart lesion with fracture. Single axial image from a CT arthrogram demonstrates a fracture of the anteroinferior glenoid with an attached segment of the glenoid labrum *(arrows)*. (Courtesy M. Percy, Somerset West, South Africa.)

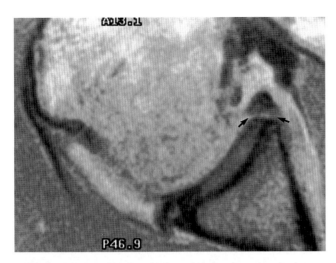

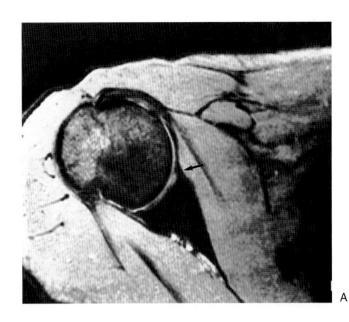

FIG. 23. Discreet Bankart lesion. Axial proton density image through the anterior inferior portion of the joint demonstrates a discreet tear through the anterior labrum *(arrows)* in a patient after a recent dislocation.

A

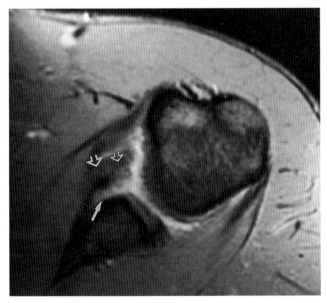

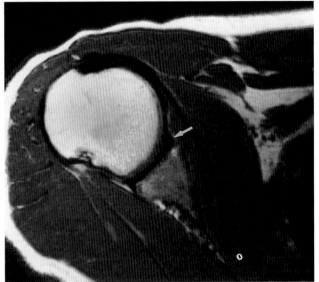

B

FIG. 24. Bankart lesion. Gradient echo axial image to the anteroinferior portion of the joint demonstrates avulsion of the inferior glenohumeral labral ligamentous complex *(open arrows)*. A cleft of fluid can be seen extending beneath the torn ligamentous attachment *(large arrow)*. It is not possible to determine whether the lesion represents a typical Bankart lesion or whether the periosteum is attached, making this a Perthes lesion. Nonetheless, the degree of irregularity of the labral ligamentous structures is consistent with complete avulsion and a Bankart lesion.

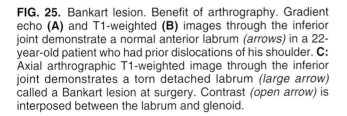

FIG. 25. Bankart lesion. Benefit of arthrography. Gradient echo **(A)** and T1-weighted **(B)** images through the inferior joint demonstrate a normal anterior labrum *(arrows)* in a 22-year-old patient who had prior dislocations of his shoulder. **C:** Axial arthrographic T1-weighted image through the inferior joint demonstrates a torn detached labrum *(large arrow)* called a Bankart lesion at surgery. Contrast *(open arrow)* is interposed between the labrum and glenoid.

C

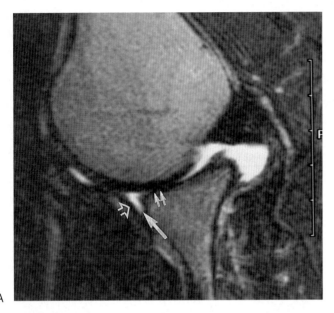

A

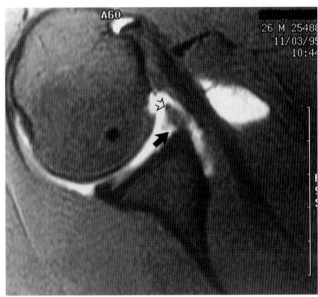

B

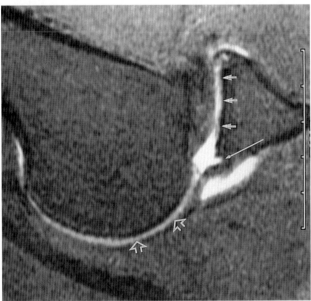

C

FIG. 26. **A:** Abduction and external rotation (ABER) image demonstrating slight anterior subluxation in chronic dislocator. T2-weighted image obtained in ABER demonstrates a cleft of fluid *(thick arrow)* between the glenoid and the detached and anteriorly displaced glenoid labrum *(open arrow)*. Note the anteriorly located contact site between the humerus and underlying glenoid *(small arrows)* indicating subluxation. **B:** Severe subluxation demonstrated on ABER view. Axial arthrographic image demonstrates a large cleft beneath the anterior labrum at its insertion onto the glenoid *(closed arrow)*, mimicking a meniscoid labrum variant. The labrum *(open arrow)* appears in appropriate position. **C:** Image obtained in the ABER position demonstrates essentially dislocation of the humeral head *(open arrows)* from the glenoid *(short arrows)*. The labrum is partially detached *(long arrow)* in this chronic subluxer.

shifted inferiorly (see Fig. 19E,F), rolling up on itself like one rolls a long shirt sleeve on a hot day, the lesion is referred to as an ALPSA lesion (9). ALPSA is an acronym that stands for *a*nterior *l*abroligamentous *p*eriosteal *s*leeve *a*vulsion (9). In the acute case, there is not usually a diagnostic dilemma for the arthroscopist. A problem arises in the chronic setting (9) after some attempt at healing occurs as most patients are treated conservatively after the first dislocation. If an ALPSA lesion is present, the labrum is not located in its original position and heals in its medially displaced position (9) (Fig. 27). Thus, there is a high likelihood that the patient will redislocate. With the chronic ALPSA lesion, fibrous tissue is deposited upon the medially displaced labral ligamentous complex and then the entire lesion resynovializes along the articular surface (9). To help visualize this lesion, the glenoid surface and glenoid labrum can

arthroscopically be thought of as a "made bed." The synovium (quilt) extends over the glenoid face and up and over the glenoid labrum (pillow). It can be difficult for the surgeon to make the distinction between whether the heaped up region covered by synovium is labrum or synovial-lined fibrous tissue deposited on a medially displaced labrum (9). Thus, it has been postulated that some of these lesions have been missed arthroscopically in the chronic setting (9). MRI offers an advantage in the chronic situation in that subtle ALPSA lesions may be discovered as the displaced labrum can be identified as being displaced, especially when an effusion or contrast is present in the joint (Fig. 28). Also, subtle ALPSA lesions may be diagnosed in the ABER position (Fig. 29), in which the medial displacement can be visualized at the insertion point of the inferior glenohumeral ligament onto the underlying glenoid. Usually, the mid portion

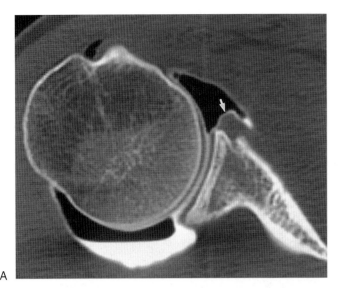
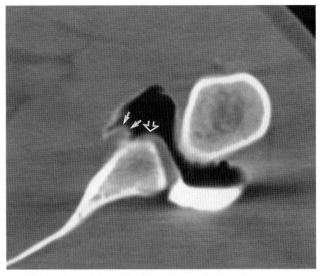

A   B

FIG. 27. ALPSA lesion. **A:** CT arthrographic axial image through the mid inferior joint demonstrates medial displacement of the labral ligamentous attachment *(arrow)*. This is consistent with and characteristic of an ALPSA lesion. **B:** Single CT arthrographic axial image through the joint demonstrates medial displacement of the labral ligamentous complex *(closed arrows)* from the expected location of the labrum and ligament attachment *(open arrow)*. The findings are characteristic of an ALPSA lesion. (Courtesy M. Percy, Somerset West, South Africa.)

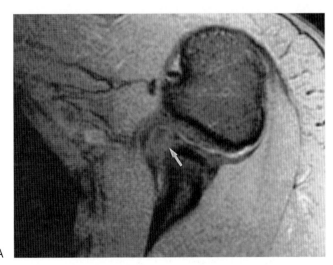
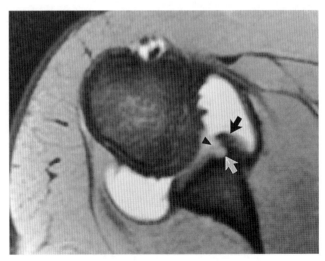

A   B

FIG. 28. Chronic ALPSA lesion. **A:** Patient with surgically proven chronic ALPSA lesion. Axial gradient echo image to the anteroinferior portion of the joint demonstrates diffuse increased signal intensity and indistinctness to the anteroinferior glenoid labrum *(arrow)*. This is not unlike many normal patients exhibiting the magic angle phenomenon. **B:** Different patient with same history. Axial saline arthrographic gradient echo image demonstrates medial displacement of the labrum *(black arrow)* from the glenoid, indicating an ALPSA lesion. The cleft between the labral ligamentous attachment and the residual labrum is seen *(white arrow)*. Note the medium signal intensity tissue within the cleft *(arrowhead)*, indicating resynovialization. The surgeon sees only the small crevice filled in with the contrast material, making it difficult to identify at arthroscopy. (Courtesy A. Stauffer, Mission Viejo, CA.)

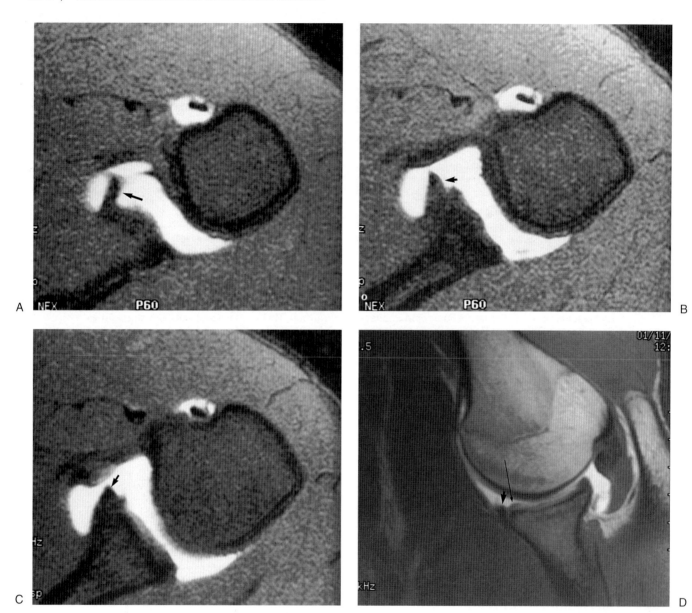

FIG. 29. ALPSA lesion. **A:** Axial arthrographic image of the inferior portion of the joint demonstrates the anterior band of the inferior glenohumeral ligament *(arrow)* coursing up to its insertion point. **B:** Axial image 4 mm more superior than **(A)** demonstrates the labral ligamentous insertion region *(arrow).* **C:** Axial image 4 mm superior to **(B)** demonstrates the anterior glenoid labrum *(arrow).* The inferior glenohumeral ligament has already inserted onto it. **D:** Image in abduction and external rotation (ABER) demonstrates medial displacement of the anterior labrum ligamentous complex *(short arrow)* with respect to the glenoid *(long thin arrow).* The medial displacement is better appreciated on the ABER view than the axial images. (Courtesy A. Glowchesky, Longview, TX.)

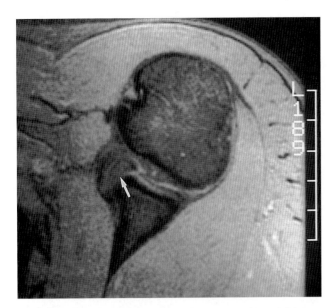

FIG. 30. Chronic ALPSA lesion. Gradient echo axial image of the anteroinferior portion of the joint demonstrates diffuse increased signal intensity within the anterior labral ligamentous attachment site *(arrow)*. A diagnosis of abnormality could not be made with confidence with this image alone. The labrum turned out to be a fibrous resynovialized, medially displaced, mass in a patient who was a multiple dislocator.

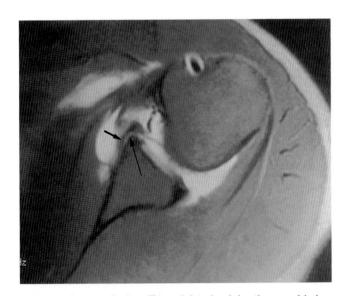

FIG. 31. Perthes lesion. T1-weighted axial arthrographic image with fat saturation demonstrates contrast *(long thin arrow)* material extending beneath a minimally detached anterior labrum. Note the still attached scapular periosteum *(small thick arrow)*. The patient was a multiple dislocator.

FIG. 32. Perthes lesion. **A:** Axial gradient echo arthrographic image demonstrates a somewhat flattened but attached anteroinferior labrum *(arrow)*. **B:** Image obtained 4 mm more superior than **(A)** demonstrates subtle increased signal intensity *(arrow)* at the base of the labrum. We were uncertain whether this represented a tear. **C:** Oblique axial image obtained in the abducted and externally rotated position demonstrates avulsion of the inferior glenohumeral labral ligamentous complex from the glenoid *(arrow)*. The patient was a chronic dislocator.

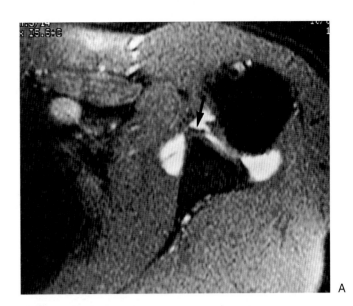

A

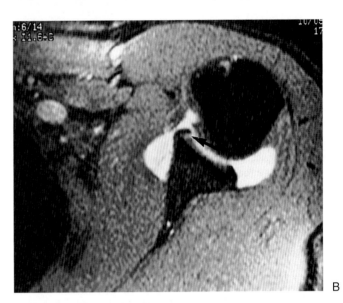

B

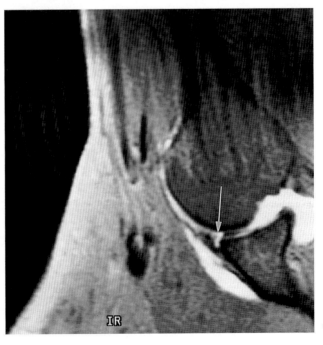

C

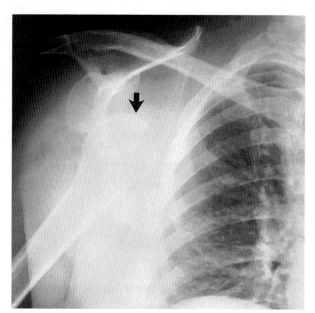
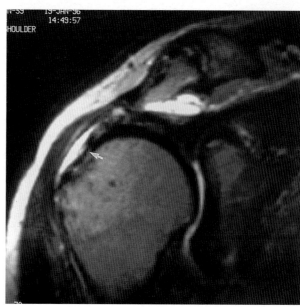

A   B

FIG. 33. A: Plain film demonstrates an anterior glenohumeral dislocation *(arrow)*. **B:** Rotator cuff tear in 55-year-old patient after anterior dislocation. Coronal T2-weighted image demonstrates a tear of the distal supraspinatus *(arrow)* in this patient after initial anterior dislocation.

of the anterior labrum is abnormal along with the inferior portion in the chronic ALPSA lesion, allowing the radiologist to make the diagnosis of an abnormality. If the mid anterior labrum is not visualized as being abnormal on MRI (in my experience, this is not an uncommon appearance), then the chronic ALPSA lesion can be difficult to diagnose with conventional MRI technique. The fibrous, medialized, resynovialized mass can appear strikingly normal on MR images in a patient with a paucity of joint fluid and magic angle artifact (Fig. 30).

Another type of variation in Bankart lesion has been termed the *Perthes lesion* after the German physician who initially described it at the turn of the century (44). If the labral ligamentous avulsion occurs with an intact scapular periosteum and if the periosteum is stripped medially, becoming redundant, the lesion is referred to as a Perthes lesion (Fig. 31). It is distinguished from the ALPSA lesion by redundant periosteum versus the rolled up medially displaced periosteum labral mass, which is medially displaced. With the Perthes lesion, the humeral head may repeatedly sublux into a "pseudojoint" in a severely unstable patient or the labrum may lay back down onto the glenoid in a remarkably normal position. It can then become resynovialized with the redundant but intact periosteum ballooning out medially (see Fig. 19*G,H*). A patient with a Perthes lesion in which the labrum reapproximates its normal position and becomes resynovialized looks normal at arthroscopy and can look normal at MRI. This type of lesion can be the most difficult to diagnose, and it is uncertain how commonly it occurs. Imaging with the ABER sequence may help visualize these lesions (Fig. 32). In one case, a patient with a remote history of dislocation was given the diagnosis by an orthopedist of

primary impingement as the cause for shoulder pain. The patient was a relatively poor historian and did not relate or emphasize the fact that the dislocation had occurred during adolescence (the patient was now in his early 60s). An MR arthrogram including ABER disclosed a large Perthes lesion (see Fig. 4). The patient received an acromioplasty after a negative diagnostic arthroscopy. A partial rotator cuff tear was present. Careful evaluation of the arthroscopic videotape revealed that the anteroinferior labral ligamentous attachment site appeared normal—probably because resynovialization had occurred, and stress was not placed on the ligament by probing during arthroscopy; therefore, the lesion was not appreciated. Reevaluation of the arthroscopic videotape in concert with the MR arthrogram led the surgeon to conclude that a Perthes lesion was probably present.

Older Patient (Mid-30s and Older)

Because of age-related collagen degeneration, the weak link in shoulder stabilizers shifts from the labral ligamentous attachment in a younger patient to other structures in the older patient (45). A cadaveric study performed by Bigliani et al. (45) demonstrated that, if dislocating forces were placed across the shoulder joint, the labral ligamentous complex would tear in various places. As the cadavers were predominantly older, it was common for the tear of the ligamentous complex to occur at the humeral interface or in the mid ligament. A study by Neviaser et al. (6,7) demonstrated that surgical evaluation after anterior dislocation in patients older than age 40 revealed a paucity of Bankart lesions and Bankart variants.

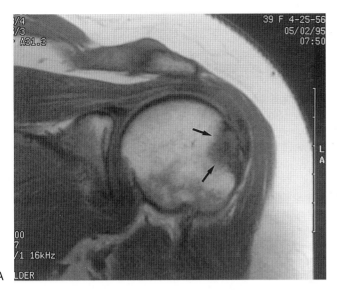
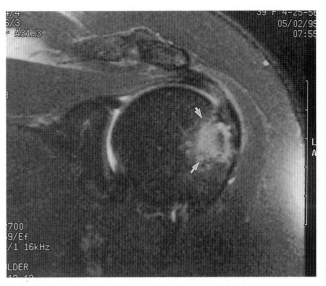

FIG. 34. Nondisplaced greater tuberosity fracture after anterior dislocation. Thirty-nine–year-old woman after anterior dislocation with continued pain. **A:** T1-weighted oblique coronal image demonstrates bone trabecular injury representing essentially a nondisplaced greater tuberosity fracture *(arrows)*. **B:** T2-weighted image demonstrates the high signal intensity indicating edema *(arrows)*. The plain films were normal.

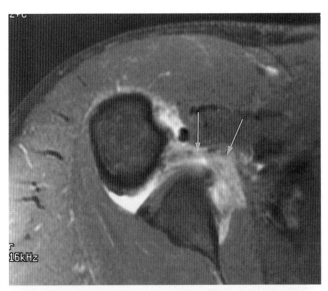
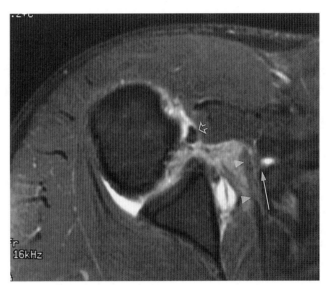

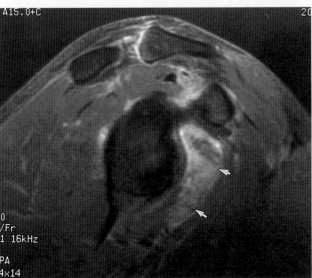

FIG. 35. Subscapularis avulsion from the humerus following anterior dislocation. **A:** Thirty-five year old who sustained a fall while mountain climbing dislocating the shoulder anteriorly. Axial arthrographic image demonstrating the inferior portion of the joint shows a disrupted subscapularis tendon *(arrows)*. **B:** Image 4 mm superior to **(A)** demonstrates the torn subscapularis *(arrowheads)* displaced anteriorly and oriented in a more anterior direction than usual (direction of arrow). Note the dislocated long head of the biceps tendon *(open arrow)*. **C:** Sagittal T1-weighted arthrographic image demonstrates abnormal signal intensity within the subscapularis muscle *(arrows)* indicating edema.

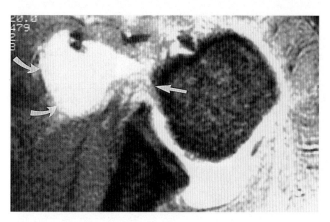

FIG. 36. Humeral avulsion of the glenohumeral ligament lesion. Axial saline arthrographic image through the inferior portion of the joint demonstrates a rent in the anterior capsule at its interface with the humerus *(arrows)*, allowing contrast material to extravasate anteriorly to form a puddle in front of the joint *(curved arrows)*. At surgery, the subscapularis tendon was intact and the defect was seen in the anterior capsule only.

The lesions resulting from initial anterior dislocation of the shoulder in a patient older than mid-30s can be conveniently grouped into three categories, some of which are surgical candidates and others of which are candidates for conservative therapy.

One third of the patients suffering an initial anterior dislocation of the shoulder after the age of 40 tear the supraspinatus tendon (6,7) (Fig. 33). Another one third of the patients suffer a fracture of the greater tuberosity. This is thought to, in effect, represent an avulsion of the rotator cuff or an extensive Hill-Sachs fracture (6,7) (Fig. 34). These fractures are often nondisplaced, occult at plain film evaluation, and should be treated conservatively. The other one third of patients older than age 40 who suffer an initial anterior dislocation of the shoulder suffer an avulsion of the subscapularis and capsule from the lesser tuberosity (6,7) (Fig. 35). In many cases, chronic recurrent instability develops in these patients and they are considered surgical candidates. Clinically, distinguishing between these three possibilities can be difficult (6,7). This is coupled with the difficulty in determining whether an anterior dislocation or severe subluxation in actuality even occurred. Older patients often do not realize that they actually dislocated their shoulder because the dislocation reduces quickly. The patients are only aware of the fact that they suffered a severe injury. Careful questioning as to the mechanism of injury is often required to determine what actually happened. Conventional MRI often suffices in the diagnosis of the injuries resulting from a fall on an outstretched arm in a patient older than 40. MRI is an effective tool for the diagnosis of the abnormalities in this setting and routine use of MR arthrography is probably not necessary.

With respect to MRI, the diagnosis of a rotator cuff tear is the same as is discussed in Chapter 6. The important aspect of this diagnosis to the radiologist is considering it as a possibility after obtaining the history.

Greater tuberosity fractures, when they are nondisplaced and occult at plain film, often appear as an inhomogeneous region of predominantly decreased signal intensity on T1-weighted sequences, which become bright on T2-weighted sequences. I prefer fast spin-echo with fat saturation or multiplanar inversion recovery as a diagnostic sequence of choice. With a distracted fragment, the fragment and rotator cuff are pulled away from the remainder of the humerus, and this is best diagnosed with plain films. The integrity of the rotator cuff, however, is best assessed with MRI.

Patients suffering an avulsion of the subscapularis from the lesser tuberosity also avulse the glenohumeral capsule from the humerus in association (see Fig. 35). Often times, the long head of the biceps tendon dislocates from the bicipital groove as a result of the loss of the transverse bicipital ligament, which is, in part, formed by fibers of the subscapularis tendon. Sometimes, the capsule itself is avulsed from the humerus without an accompanying tear of the subscapularis (Fig. 36). This lesion is referred to as the HAGL (*h*umeral *a*vulsion of the *g*lenohumeral *l*igament) (46,47). It has not been shown that this lesion has an age predilection (47).

Other Associated Abnormalities

With anterior dislocation of the humeral head, the posterosuperior margin of the proximal humerus impacts against the anteroinferior glenoid as it dislocates out (Fig.

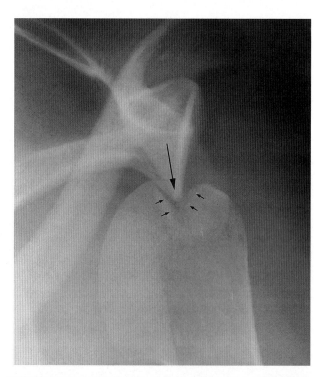

FIG. 37. Anterior dislocation. Note the anterior-inferiorly dislocated humeral head with a large Hill-Sachs deformity *(small arrows)* impacted against the anteroinferior glenoid *(long arrow)*.

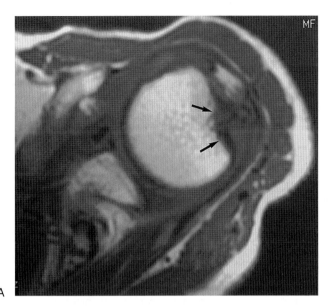

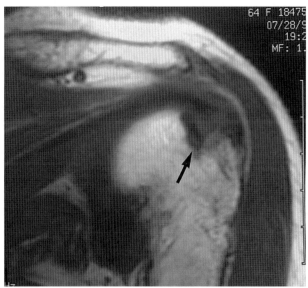

FIG. 38. Hill-Sachs deformity. **A:** Axial T1-weighted image demonstrates a large impaction fracture of the posterosuperior humeral head *(arrows)* in a patient who had a dislocation consistent with the Hill-Sachs fracture. **B:** Oblique coronal T1-weighted image demonstrates the Hill-Sachs fracture from a different perspective *(arrow)*.

37). This impaction fracture is called the *Hill-Sachs fracture* (Fig. 38) and is commonly seen in the acute situation as an area of edema on T2-weighted sequences in association with irregularity of the posterosuperior humeral head. In the chronic situation, the indentation resulting from the impaction may be visualized as irregularity of the posterosuperior humeral head, or, if the lesion is purely chondral, the Hill-Sachs may not be seen at all.

It is important to distinguish the Hill-Sachs deformity from the "bare area" that exists in this region, which often looks irregular on MRI. Typically, this irregularity at the in-

sertion of the infraspinatus tendon has a subarticular cystic appearance (Fig. 39). The easiest way to distinguish between the two is by history. A patient who has never dislocated a shoulder does not have a Hill-Sachs fracture.

POSTERIOR INSTABILITY

The position of risk for a posterior dislocation of the shoulder is that of adduction internal rotation (48,49) (Fig. 40). With internal rotation, the posterior capsule and labrum

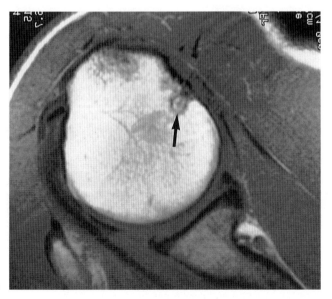

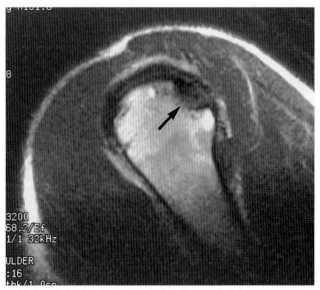

FIG. 39. Irregularity of posterior superior humeral head mimicking a Hill-Sachs lesion. Note the cystic irregularity of the posterior superior humeral head *(arrow)* commonly seen. The patient did not have a dislocation history. **B:** Note the irregularity in this young baseball pitcher, probably owing to posterosuperior impingement. The patient was not a dislocator.

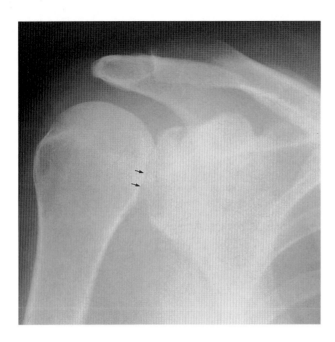

FIG. 40. Posterior dislocation. Anteroposterior radiograph demonstrates a strikingly normal appearing right shoulder. The shoulder was locked in internal rotation and a small trough *(arrows)* can be seen along the medial margin. The shoulder was in fact posteriorly dislocated and locked.

becomes taut. By adducting the humerus, further stress is put on the posterior capsule. Therefore, a force impacting on the anterior portion of the joint in this position forces the humerus posteriorly against an already stressed capsule and a subluxation or dislocation results in injury to those already stressed structures. Typically, what occurs is a labral capsular disruption posteriorly known as a *reverse Bankart* (Fig. 41) and injury to the humeral head anteriorly (impaction injury on the posterior glenoid) known as a *reverse Hill-Sachs* (Fig. 42). The anterior injury may be an impaction fracture

or an avulsion, depending on the status of the subscapularis tendon during the dislocation. During a clonic-tonic seizure, which often places the patient in decerebrate posturing (adduction internal rotation of the shoulder), with a fall to the ground, the patient often dislocates posteriorly, avulsing the lesser tuberosity. This is, in part, due to the fact that the subscapularis is in spasm, thus avulsing the lesser tuberosity. Other times, the lesser tuberosity may be purely impacted. A posterior dislocation can result in tear of the subscapularis, often just a partial tear of the articular surface.

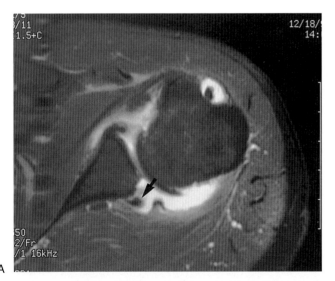

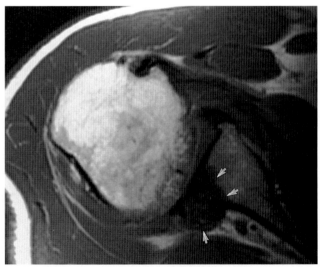

A   B

FIG. 41. A: Reverse Bankart. T1-weighted axial arthrographic image with fat saturation demonstrates displacement of the posterior bony glenoid and labrum *(arrow)* posteromedially as a result of a posterior dislocation of the shoulder. **B:** Chronic reverse Bankart: T1-weighted axial image through the mid joint demonstrates marked irregularity and slight expansion of the posterior portion of the bony glenoid *(arrows)*. This patient had a history of remote posterior dislocation and the findings were thought to represent healing changes.

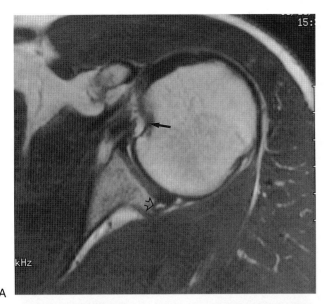

A

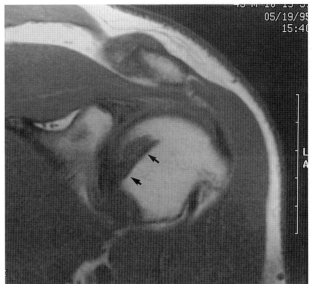

B

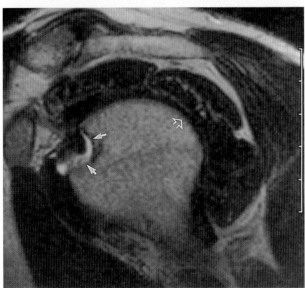

C

FIG. 42. Reverse Hill-Sachs lesion in a patient who suffered a posterior dislocation. **A:** Axial fast spin-echo T2 image without fat saturation demonstrates an impaction fracture of the anterior medial portion of the humeral head *(arrow)*. A small paralabral cyst indicative of a posterior labral tear is seen posteriorly *(open arrow)*. Note that the posterosuperior humeral head is intact. **B:** Oblique coronal T1-weighted image demonstrates a trough-like reverse Hill-Sachs lesion *(arrows)*. This appearance led to the description of the trough sign on plain films. **C:** Oblique sagittal T2-weighted image demonstrates a reverse Hill-Sachs fracture *(arrows)* anterosuperiorly. Note that the posterosuperior humeral head *(open arrow)* is within normal limits.

FIG. 43. Reverse Bankart labral tear and capsular disruption. Single T1-weighted arthrographic image with fat saturation to the mid joint demonstrates a partial detachment of the posterior labrum with contrast extending beneath the labrum *(arrow)* indicative of a tear. A torn portion of the capsule *(small dark arrow)* can be seen floating within the contrast. Both lesions were proved surgically.

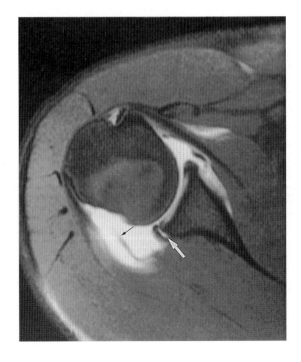

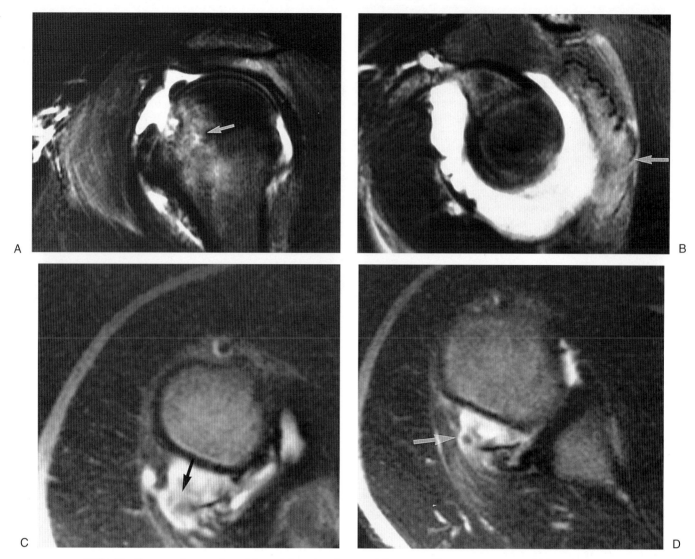

FIG. 44. Reverse humeral avulsion of the glenohumeral ligament. Twenty-two–year-old bicycle messenger after posterior dislocation. **A:** Oblique sagittal coronal turbo spin-echo T2 image with fat saturation demonstrates a reverse Hill-Sachs fracture and resulting edema *(arrow).* **B:** Oblique sagittal coronal turbo spin-echo T2 image with fat saturation demonstrates edema within the teres minor muscle *(arrow).* **C** and **D:** Axial T2-weighted images demonstrate the avulsion of the posterior inferior capsule

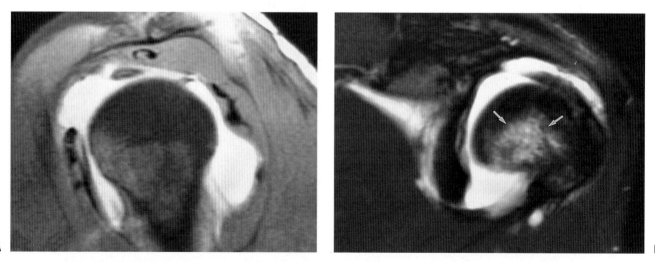

FIG. 45. Multidirectional instability after suspected dislocation in a 35-year-old woman after injury (uncertain mechanism). Sagittal T1-weighted arthrographic image demonstrates no osseous abnormality. Note the capacious capsule, which is a subjective and often unreliable determination with imaging. **B:** Oblique coronal T2-weighted fast spin-echo with fat saturation image demonstrates the anterior bone trabecular injury *(arrows)* suggesting a probable posterior subluxation.

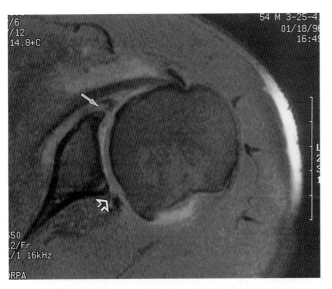

FIG. 46. Multidirectional instability. Axial arthrographic T1-weighted image demonstrates a tear of both the anterior *(arrow)* and posterior *(open arrow)* labrum in a patient with clinical multidirectional instability.

The lesions resulting from posterior dislocation can be extremely subtle with MRI and the radiologist needs to have a high index of suspicion by knowing the mechanism of injury before evaluating. Again, if partial healing and resynovialization has occurred, the lesions can be quite subtle and perhaps best detected with MR arthrography if a defect persists where the tear is located (Fig. 43). Additionally, my colleagues and I have seen four cases of humeral avulsion of the posterior portion of the inferior glenohumeral ligament as the result of a posterior dislocation, which could be termed the *reverse HAGL lesion* (Fig. 44).

MULTIDIRECTIONAL INSTABILITY

Imaging is often not used in cases of multidirectional instability, except when the diagnosis is in question or the multidirectional instability is a cause of shoulder pain but is not suspected (Fig. 45). The spectrum of abnormalities is wide and varied, but often times degenerative changes of the glenohumeral joint are found in association with labral degeneration and tearing.

OTHER CONSIDERATIONS

In the chronic, recurrent instability patient, posttraumatic degenerative changes may develop (Fig. 46). These changes are typical of those occurring in other joints and consist of articular cartilage defects (chondromalacia), subarticular cyst formation and sclerosis, joint space narrowing, and, often times, proliferative synovitis. One interesting entity that can develop in the shoulder as a result of trauma or degeneration is the glenoid labral cyst (50–52). These cysts are analogous to those that form about other joints and, in particular, the knee where a tear of the meniscus can lead to a paraarticular meniscal cyst (51). With a frank tear of the labrum or capsule, joint fluid can be extruded into the paraarticular soft tissues (Fig. 47). If the tear does not immediately heal, a cyst can form at the site of the tear, and a ball-valve mechanism

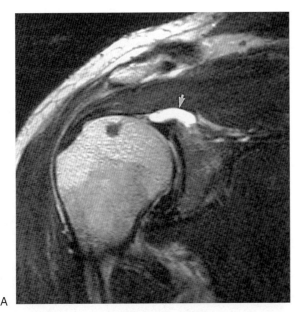

A

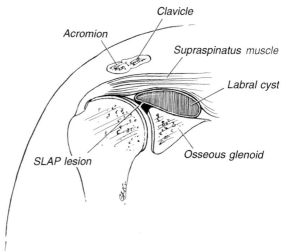

B

FIG. 47. Paralabral cyst. **A:** Oblique coronal T2-weighted image in a patient with a surgically proven SLAP lesion demonstrates a paralabral cyst *(arrow)*. The labral tear is not shown on this T2-weighted image. **B:** Diagram showing the relationship between the cyst and tear. **C:** Anterior paralabral cyst *(arrow)*. This would be difficult to distinguish from a sublabral hole and fluid within the subscapularis recess. Arthroscopic photograph **(D)** and diagram **(E)** of the cyst seen on image **(C)**. *(Continued on next page.)*

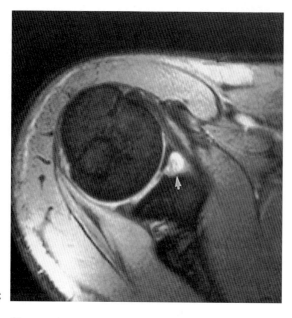

C

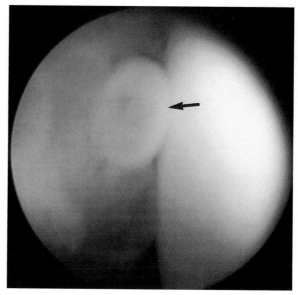

D

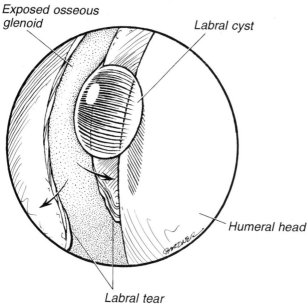

Exposed osseous glenoid

Labral cyst

Humeral head

Labral tear

E

FIG. 47. Continued.

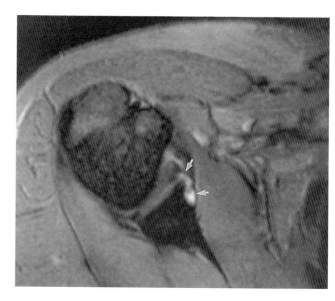

A

FIG. 48. Paralabral cyst formation in a patient who suffered remote anterior dislocation. **A:** Axial gradient echo image demonstrates a labral cyst beneath the scapular periosteum (arrows) anteroinferiorly. (Continued on next page.)

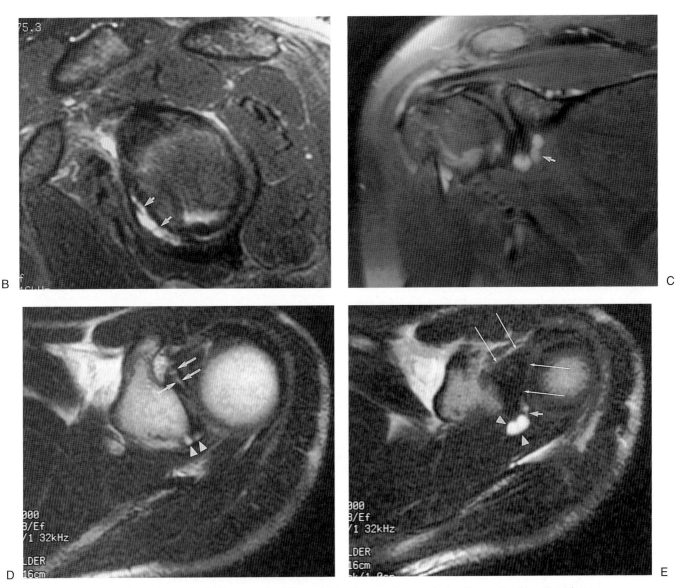

FIG. 48. *Continued.* **B:** Oblique sagittal T2-weighted image demonstrates the cyst adjacent to the anteroinferior glenoid *(arrows).* **C:** Oblique coronal fast spin-echo (FSE) T2-weighted image demonstrates the multiloculated cyst *(arrow).* **D:** SLAP lesion with paralabral cyst. Axial fast spin-echo T2-weighted image at the top of the joint demonstrates two small rounded fluid collections adjacent to the posterosuperior labrum *(arrowheads).* Note anteriorly the irregular increased signal intensity extending to the anterosuperior labrum *(arrows).* Anteriorly this could represent a sublabral hole. At arthroscopy, a SLAP lesion was found. **E:** Axial FSE T2-weighted image 4 mm more superior than **(D)** demonstrates the bean-shaped paralabral cyst *(arrowheads)* connecting to the labrum via a small stalk, indicating a labral tear *(small arrow).* Note the delta shaped insertion of the biceps tendon *(long thin arrows).*

may develop, allowing the cyst to grow. Alternatively, degeneration may lead to a disruption in the integrity of the labrum or capsule, allowing a cyst to form, typically near the labrum or the labrum may become somewhat dehiscent, allowing joint fluid to extrude beneath the dehiscent portion, forming a paraarticular cyst. Nonetheless, the cysts vary in size and are almost universally positioned immediately adja-

cent to the joint or close to it, thus lending credence to the theory of an articular origin as opposed to arising de novo in the soft tissues (Fig. 48). The clinical presentation of a patient with a labral cyst varies and depends on the status of the labrum and the proximity of the cyst to nerves that may be impinged upon. If the patient has a patent labral tear, the overwhelming clinical presentation may be that of glenohumeral instability. If the patient has dissection of the cyst through the paraarticular soft tissues to compress a nerve, denervation phenomenon may be the clinical presentation (50,51). If the suprascapular nerve is compressed either in the suprascapular notch or in the spinoglenoid notch, denervation of the supraspinatus or infraspinatus may occur. The nerve also provides pain fibers to the joint (50,51). The patient has weakness of those rotator cuff muscles and pain.

REFERENCES

1. Crues JV, Ryu RK. The shoulder. In: Stark D, Bradley WG, eds. *Magnetic resonance imaging.* St Louis: Mosby, 1991:2424–2458.
2. Freiberger RH, Kaye JJ. *Arthrography.* New York: Appleton-Century-Crofts, 1979.
3. Silliman J, Hawkins R. Current concepts and recent advances in the athlete's shoulder. *Clin Sports Med* 1991; 10:693-705.
4. Silliman J, Hawkins R. Classification and physical diagnosis of instability of the shoulder. *Clin Orthop Rel Res* 1993;291:7–19.
5. Lippitt S, Harryman D. Diagnosis and management of AMBRI syndrome. *Techniques Orthop* 1991;6:61–73.
6. Neviaser RJ, Neviaser TJ, Neviaser JS. Concurrent rupture of the rotator cuff and anterior dislocation of the shoulder in the older patient. *J Bone Joint Surg [Am]* 1988;70 (9):1308–1311.
7. Neviaser RJ, Neviaser TJ, Neviaser JS. Anterior dislocation of the shoulder and rotator cuff rupture. *Clin Orthop Rel Res* 1993;291:103–106.
8. O'Brien SJ, Warren RF, Schwartz E. Anterior shoulder instability. *Orthop Clin North Am* 1987;18:395–408.
9. Neviaser TJ. The anterior labroligamentous periosteal sleeve avulsion lesion: a cause of anterior instability of the shoulder. *Arthroscopy* 1993;9 (1):17–21.
10. Bankart ASB. The pathology and treatment of recurrent dislocation of the shoulder joint. *Br J Surg* 1938;26:23–29.
11. Arciero RA, St PP. Acute shoulder dislocation. Indications and techniques for operative management. *Clin Sports Med* 1995;14 (4):937–953.
12. Hintermann B, Gachter A. Arthroscopic findings after shoulder dislocation. *Am J Sports Med* 1995;23 (5):545–551.
13. McGlynn FJ, Caspari RB. Arthroscopic findings in the subluxating shoulder. *Clin Orthop* 1984;183:173–178.
14. Peterfy CG. Magic angle phenomenon as a cause of increased signal in the glenoid labrum. 1994, *personal communication.*
15. Erickson SJ, Cox IH, Hyde JS, Carrera GF, Strandt JA, Estkowski LD. Effect of tendon orientation on MR imaging signal intensity: a manifestation of the "magic angle" phenomenon. *Radiology* 1991;181 (2):389–392.
16. Cvitanic O, Tirman PFJ, Feller JF, Stauffer AE, Carroll K. Can abduction and external rotation of the shoulder increase the sensitivity of MR arthrography in detecting anterior glenoid labral tears? *Am J Roentgenol* 1997;169:837–844.
17. Protzman RR. Anterior instability of the shoulder. *J Bone Joint Surg* 1980;62-A (6):909–918.
18. Zarins B, Rowe CR. Current Concepts in the diagnosis and treatment of shoulder instability in athletes. *Med Sci Sports Exerc* 1984;16:444–448.
19. Turkel SJ, Panio MW, Marshall JL, Girgis FG. Stabilizing mechanisms preventing anterior dislocation of the glenohumeral joint. *J Bone Joint Surg [Am]* 1981;63A:1208–1217.
20. Lippitt S, Matsen F. Mechanisms of glenohumeral joint stability. *Clin Orthop Rel Res* 1993;291:20–27.
21. Zlatkin MB, Bjorkengren AG, Gylys MV, Resnick D, Sartoris DJ. Cross-sectional imaging of the capsular mechanism of the glenohumeral joint. *Am J Roentgenol* 1988;150 (1):151–158.
22. O'Brien SJ, Neves MC, Arnoczky SP, et al. The anatomy and histology of the inferior glenohumeral ligament complex of the shoulder. *Am J Sports Med* 1990;18 (5):449–456.
23. Detrisac DA, Johnson LL. *Arthroscopic shoulder anatomy: pathologic and surgical implications.* Thorofare, NJ: SLACK, 1987.
24. Rockwood CA, Matsen FAI. *The shoulder,* 1st ed. Philadelphia: WB Saunders, 1990:622.
25. Warner JJP. The gross anatomy of the joint surfaces, ligaments, labrum, and capsule. In: Matsen FA, Fu FH, Hawkins RJ, ed. *The shoulder: a balance of mobility and stability.* Rosemont, IL: American Academy of Orthopedic Surgeons, 1992:7–27.
26. Kumar VP, Balasubramaniam P. The role of atmospheric pressure in stabilising the shoulder. An experimental study. *J Bone Joint Surg [Br]* 1985;67 (5):719–721.
27. Kumar VP, Satku K, Balasubramaniam P. The role of the long head of biceps brachii in the stabilization of the head of the humerus. *Clin Orthop* 1989;244:172–175.
28. Goss TP. Anterior glenohumeral instability. *Orthopedics* 1988;11 (1):87–95.
29. Pappas AM, Goss TP, Kleinman PK. Symptomatic shoulder instability due to lesions of the glenoid labrum. *Am J Sports Med* 1983;11 (5):279–288.
30. McAuliffe TB, Dowd GS. Avulsion of the subscapularis tendon. A case report. *J Bone Joint Surg [Am]* 1987;69 (9):1454–1455.
31. McNiesh LM, Callaghan JJ. CT Arthrography of the shoulder: variations of the glenoid labrum. *Am J Radiol* 1987;149:963–966.
32. Neuman CH, Petersen SA, Jahnke AH, et al. MRI in the evaluation of patients with suspected instability of the shoulder joint including a comparison with CT-arthrography. *Fortschr Röntgenstr* 1991;154 (6):593–600.
33. DePalma AF, Callery G, Bennett GA. *Shoulder joint: variational anatomy and degenerative lesions of the shoulder.* Presented at AAOS Instructional Course Lectures, 1949;255–281.
34. Williams MM, Synder SJ, Buford D. The Buford complex—the cord like middle glenohumeral ligament and absent anterosuperior labrum complex: a normal anatomic capsulolabral variant. *Arthroscopy* 1994;10 (3):241–247.
35. Tirman P, Feller J, Palmer W, Carroll K, Steinbach L, Cox I. The Buford complex—a variation of normal shoulder anatomy: MR arthrographic imaging features. *Am J Roentgenol* 1996;166:869–873.
36. Snyder SJ. Diagnostic arthroscopy: normal anatomy and variations. In: Snyder SJ, ed. *Shoulder arthroscopy.* New York: McGraw-Hill, 1994:179–214.
37. Moseley HJ, Overgaard B. The anterior capsular mechanism in recurrent dislocation of the shoulder: morphological and clinical studies with special reference to the glenoid labrum and glenohumeral ligaments. *J Bone Joint Surg [Br]* 1962;44B:913–927.
38. Tirman PFJ, Stauffer AE, Crues JV, Turner RM, Schobert WE, Nottage WM. Saline MR arthrography in the evaluation of glenohumeral instability. *Arthroscopy* 1993;9 (5):550–569.
39. Palmer WE, Caslowitz PL. Anterior shoulder instability: diagnostic criteria determined from prospective analysis of 121 MR arthrograms. *Radiology* 1995;197 (3):819–825.
40. Neumann CH, Petersen SA, Jahnke AH. MR imaging of the labral-capsular complex: normal variations. *Am J Roentgenol* 1991;157 (5):1015–1021.
41. Snyder SJ. Arthroscopic evaluation and treatment of shoulder instability. In: Snyder SJ, ed. *Shoulder arthroscopy.* New York: McGraw-Hill, 1994:179–214.
42. Neviaser TJ. The GLAD lesion: another cause of anterior shoulder pain. *Arthroscopy* 1993;9 (1):22–23.
43. Bankart ASB. Recurrent of habitual dislocation of the shoulder joint. *BMJ* 1923;2:1132.
44. Perthes G. Uber operationen bei habitaller schulterluxationen. *Deutsch Z Chir* 1906;85:199–227.
45. Bigliani LU, Pollock RG, Soslowsky LJ, Flatow EL, Pawluk RJ, Mow VC. Tensile properties of the inferior glenohumeral ligament. *J Orthop Res* 1992;10:187–197.
46. Wolf E. *Arthroscopic management of shoulder instability.* Presented at Arthroscopy Association of North America Annual Meeting, Instructional Course No. 201, Boston, MA, 1992.
47. Wolf EM, Cheng JC, Dickson K. Humeral avulsion of glenohumeral ligaments as a cause of anterior shoulder instability. *Arthroscopy* 1995;11:600–607.
48. Hawkins RJ, Koppert G, Johnston G. Recurrent posterior instability (subluxation) of the shoulder. *J Bone Joint Surg* 1984;66A:169–174.

49. Wirth MA, Rockwood CAJ. Traumatic glenohumeral instability: pathology and pathogenesis. In: Matsen FAI, Fu FH, Hawkins RJ, eds. *The shoulder: a balance of mobility and stability.* Rosemont, IL: American Academy of Orthopedic Surgeons, 1993:279–304.

50. Fritz RC, Helms CA, Steinbach LS, Genant HK. Suprascapular nerve entrapment: evaluation with MR imaging. *Radiology* 1992;182 (2):437–444.

51. Tirman P, Feller J, Janzen D, Peterfy C, Bergman A. Association of glenoid labral cysts with labral tears and glenohumeral instability: radiologic findings and clinical significance. *Radiology* 1994;190 (3):653–658.

52. Catalano JB, Fenlin JM. Ganglion cysts about the shoulder girdle in the absence of suprascapular nerve involvement. *J Shoulder Elbow Surg* 1994;3 (1):34–41.

Shoulder Magnetic Resonance Imaging,
edited by Lynne S. Steinbach, et al.
Lippincott–Raven Publishers, Philadelphia © 1998.

CHAPTER 8

Long Bicipital Tendon Including SLAP Lesions

Lynne S. Steinbach

Anatomic Review	**Partial and Full-Thickness Tears**
Magic Angle Phenomenon	**Subluxation and Dislocation**
Tenosynovitis	**SLAP Lesions**
Tendinosis	**Miscellaneous**

ANATOMIC REVIEW

The long head of the biceps functions as a flexor and medial rotator of the shoulder. It is active in abduction and external rotation (ABER) of the shoulder, assisting in limiting external rotation of the glenohumeral joint (1) and in preventing proximal migration of the humeral head (2,3). The tendon arises from the long head of the biceps muscle within the upper one third of the arm and courses superiorly through the intertubercular sulcus (bicipital groove) of the humerus, arcing over the humeral head as it passes as an intracapsular but extrasynovial structure inferior to the supraspinatus tendon, inserting on the supraglenoid tubercle and/or the glenoid labrum (4,5) (Fig. 1). It attaches on or near the superior and posterior glenoid labrum. Portions of the long head fibers also support and form the anterior labrum. As a result of the close relationship to the glenoid labrum, this tendon contributes to superior and anterior glenohumeral joint stability (1,6).

The biceps tendon is covered by several anatomic structures as it courses in the intertubercular sulcus (Fig. 2). The pectoralis major tendon covers the intertubercular sulcus inferiorly, blending with the capsular ligament. More cranially, the biceps tendon is held in the bicipital groove by the transverse humeral ligament, an extension of the subscapularis tendon that covers the bicipital groove. Further cranial, when it becomes intraarticular, the biceps tendon is covered anteriorly by the coracohumeral ligament, superior glenohumeral ligament, and the supraspinatus and subscapularis

tendons, which thicken the capsule and act as the chief stabilizers of the tendon.

The sheath for the long head of the biceps tendon communicates with the glenohumeral joint. The presence of small amounts of fluid or contrast in the tendon sheath is common in asymptomatic volunteers (7). As a corollary, contrast and fluid normally flow into the biceps tendon sheath during an magnetic resonance (MR) arthrogram (Fig. 3).

MAGIC ANGLE PHENOMENON

A short segment of the long bicipital tendon located proximal to the intertubercular groove lies 55 degrees to MR imagers with a vertical static magnetic field. Therefore, this region can exhibit higher signal intensity on short TE images related to structural anisotropy of the collagen, which is susceptible to the "magic angle" phenomenon (8) (see Fig. 1). This elevated signal intensity can mimic a rotator cuff or biceps tendon lesion on short TE images; however, this signal should decrease in the normal tendon on longer TE images.

TENOSYNOVITIS

A large amount of fluid in the biceps tendon sheath without associated increase in glenohumeral joint fluid is suggestive of biceps tenosynovitis (7,9), but this accepted concept requires further study.

An abnormal amount of fluid in the tendon sheath, biceps tenosynovitis, is usually caused by degeneration or trauma, including impingement. It can also be related to a synovitis from an inflammatory arthropathy such as rheumatoid arthritis. The Yergason test, which stresses the biceps tendon, aids in diagnosing this condition. Pain is produced in the biceps

L. S. Steinbach: Department of Radiology, University of California, San Francisco, San Francisco, California 94143

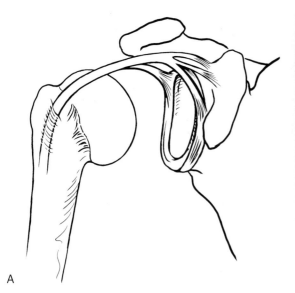

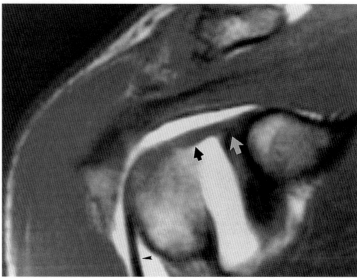

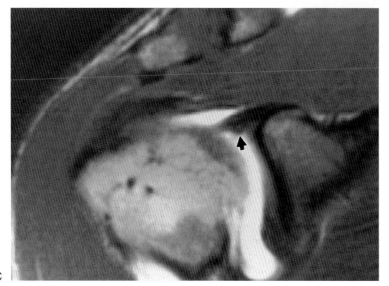

FIG. 1. A: The long head of the biceps tendon travels up the intertubercular groove to insert on the supraglenoid tubercle with a variable insertion on the superior labrum. This drawing demonstrates a bifid insertion. **B:** A corresponding oblique coronal gadolinium MR arthrogram (T1-weighted with fat saturation) delineates the intertubercular *(arrowhead)* and intraarticular *(black arrow)* portions of the tendon before it inserts on the superior labrum *(white arrow)*. **C:** The normal superior labrum is seen as a low signal intensity triangular structure on an image obtained more posterior to **(B)** *(arrow)*.

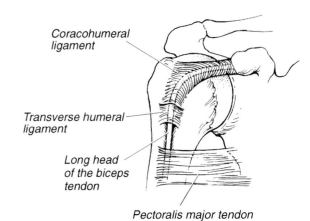

FIG. 2. The biceps tendon is held in place in the intertubercular sulcus by the pectoralis major tendon, transverse humeral ligament (an extension of the subscapularis tendon), and the coracohumeral ligament from cranial to caudal.

Coracohumeral ligament

Transverse humeral ligament

Long head of the biceps tendon

Pectoralis major tendon

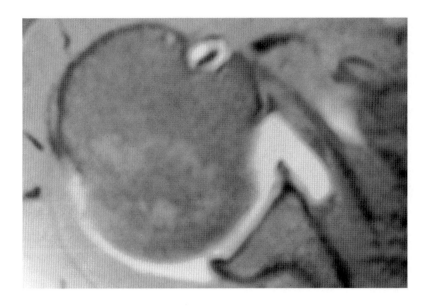

FIG. 3. A normal axial image from a gadolinium MR arthrogram (T1-weighted with fat saturation) demonstrates high signal intensity contrast in the glenohumeral joint and in the biceps tendon sheath. The biceps tendon sheath normally communicates with the glenohumeral joint.

groove when the arm is placed in forced supination. This test does not stress the rotator cuff tendons, which allows for distinction from rotator cuff impingement.

MR studies usually demonstrate an abnormal amount of fluid in the tendon sheath (10,11) (Fig. 4). The fluid should completely surround the tendon to comfortably make this diagnosis. The vessels in the intertubercular groove should not be mistaken for abnormal fluid (9). Occasionally, a stenosing tenosynovitis in the sheath with internal adhesions is seen. This is best detected with MR arthrography in which there is a lack of passage of contrast beyond a certain region of the tendon sheath.

Biceps tenosynovitis can be treated conservatively or with aspiration and injection of medications such as anesthetizing agents and steroids. Tenodesis is performed when pain persists.

TENDINOSIS

Inflammation and degeneration of the tendon results in tendinosis. This is a condition that can be seen in all age groups. Patients complain of pain over the anterior aspect of the shoulder. It may be localized to the intertubercular groove or radiate caudal or cephalad to it. The pain is usually gradual in onset. The long head of the biceps tendon may be impinged when it courses in the region of the critical zone under the supraspinatus tendon. This can result in tenosynovitis and tendinosis. Chronic tendinosis can lead to rupture of the tendon. A history of acute trauma or overuse of the shoulder is less common.

Microscopically, the tendon may demonstrate increased vascularity, hypercellularity, and fibrosis. The severity of tendinosis is related to its duration and the age of the patient (12). Tendinosis can lead to adhesive capsulitis and tendon rupture.

Intrinsic high signal intensity within the tendon on T1-

and T2-weighted MR images or enlargement of the tendon may be related to inflammation or degeneration (Fig. 5). If the abnormal signal is diffuse, it is termed tendinosis. As previously discussed, the magic angle phenomenon may affect the biceps tendon as it goes from the intraarticular region into the bicipital groove, a region that may lie approximately 55 degrees to the static magnetic field on short TE images. This appearance can simulate a mild tendinosis. This is also a common location for impingement. Because this location is a frequent site of magic angle phenomenon and if there is

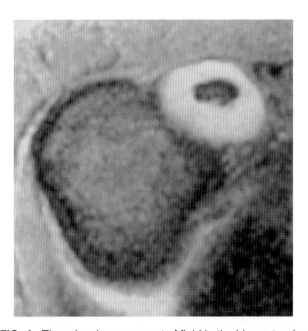

FIG. 4. There is a large amount of fluid in the biceps tendon sheath on this axial gradient echo T2*-weighted MR image. The fluid completely surrounds the tendon and is out of proportion to that seen in the glenohumeral joint, consistent with tenosynovitis.

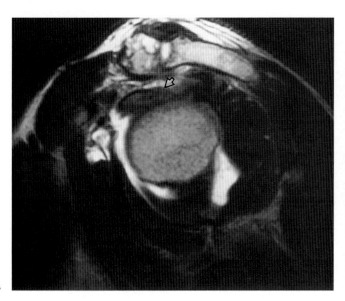
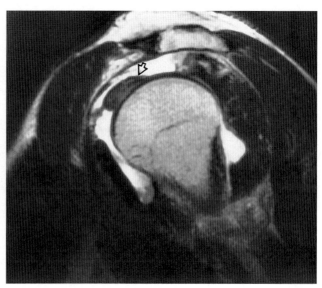

FIG. 5. A and **B:** The biceps tendon is enlarged with diffuse intermediate to high signal intensity on these consecutive oblique sagittal T2-weighted MR images *(arrows).* The findings were consistent with tendinosis. Incidentally noted is degenerative change of the acromioclavicular joint, characterized by hypertrophy and abnormal high signal intensity in **(A).**

a lack of increased signal intensity on T2-weighted MR images, the clinician may put the magic angle phenomenon as the top possibility when describing this appearance.

PARTIAL AND FULL-THICKNESS TEARS

Most tears of the long head of the biceps tendon occur at the proximal portion of the bicipital groove, usually in patients older than age 40 years as a result of impingement. Musculotendinous ruptures are infrequent and are usually associated with significant trauma.

Neer (13) has stated that biceps tendon ruptures are extremely uncommon without coexisting rotator cuff abnormalities and has classified full-thickness tears of the long head of the biceps tendon into three types. Type 1 is a tear without retraction; type 2 is a tear with partial retraction; Type 3 is a self-attaching tear without retraction. This latter type of tear can be difficult to diagnose clinically and magnetic resonance imaging (MRI) can be of help in this situation. Some clinicians have found it difficult to distinguish fibrous tissue in the bicipital groove from the bicipital tendon itself.

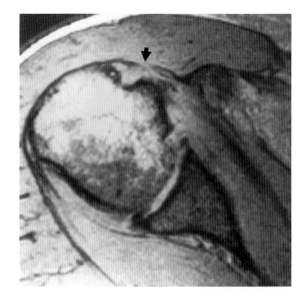

FIG. 6. An axial gradient echo MR image shows an empty bicipital groove. The biceps tendon is absent because of a full-thickness tear of the tendon with distal retraction. There was also a tear of the transverse humeral ligament *(arrow)* and avulsion of the subscapularis tendon from the lesser tuberosity of the humerus.

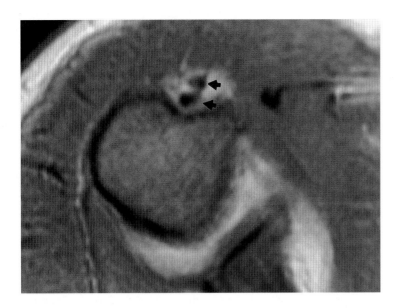

FIG. 7. There is a longitudinal split of the biceps tendon in the intertubercular sulcus *(arrows)*, well demonstrated on this axial gadolinium MR arthrogram obtained with T1 weighting and fat saturation. This could potentially be confused with a bifid biceps tendon (congenital variant) and a loose body (see Fig. 30).

When there is distal retraction of the muscle, there is absence of the tendon in all or a portion of the bicipital groove (Fig. 6). The tendon may also be split longitudinally (Fig. 7). This is most common superiorly. A bifid biceps tendon can be mistaken for a longitudinal split of the biceps tendon. The distinction from a tear can be difficult, but is more likely if the bifid tendon is seen on all axial MR images and extends into the glenohumeral joint toward the attachment on the supraglenoid tubercle. The labral attachment should also appear intact to distinguish from a SLAP lesion associated with a longitudinal biceps tendon tear. A full-thickness rupture is usually treated conservatively rather than surgically.

Partial thickness tears may present as thinning, irregularity, fragmentation, or increased signal intensity on MR images (Fig. 8).

SUBLUXATION AND DISLOCATION

Medial subluxation or dislocation of the biceps tendon may present as an isolated lesion, but it is usually seen in association with large rotator cuff tears.

The clinical presentation of biceps tendon dislocation and rotator cuff tear can be similar and accurate diagnosis is important. The patient may experience snapping of the tendon and there are several provocative tests that have been used to diagnose this disorder (14,15).

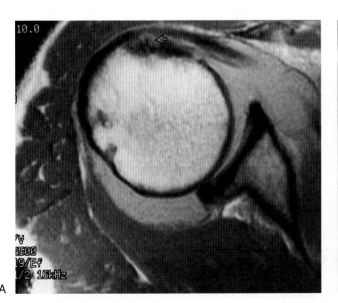
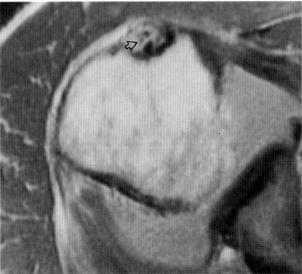

FIG. 8. This patient had a partial thickness tear of the long head of the biceps tendon. **A:** The tendon is attenuated and irregular on a more cranial T1-weighted axial MR image *(arrow)*. **B:** There is fragmentation of the tendon on a T1-weighted axial MR image obtained more caudally *(arrow)*.

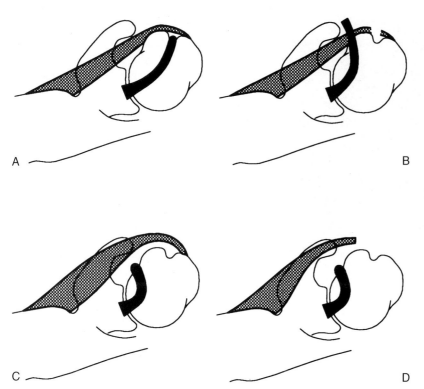

A   B

C   D

FIG. 9. A: Normal relationship of the long head of the biceps to the intertubercular sulcus, subscapularis tendon (hatched region), and glenohumeral joint. **B:** When the transverse humeral ligament is torn but the subscapularis tendon is intact, the biceps can sublux or dislocate medially superficial to the subscapularis tendon. When the subscapularis tendon avulses off of the lesser tuberosity but is otherwise intact **(C)** or is completely torn **(D)**, the biceps tendon can slip medially beneath the subscapularis tendon and can lie anterior to or inside the glenohumeral articulation. The biceps tendon can lie within the substance of a partially torn subscapularis tendon (not shown, see Fig. 11).

Biceps tendon subluxations and dislocations are usually seen in the setting of a disruption of the overlying stabilizing structures including the subscapularis tendon (Figs. 9C,D and 10), the transverse humeral ligament (Figs. 9B and D), and/or the coracohumeral ligament. Experimental transverse humeral ligament disruption infrequently results in tendon dislocation. The coracohumeral ligament is believed to be the major stabilizer and disruption of this structure (which is frequently associated with a subscapularis tendon tear) often results in dislocation of the bicipital tendon (16).

The long bicipital tendon subluxes superficially to an intact subscapularis tendon if the transverse humeral ligament (Figs. 9B) or coracohumeral ligament is torn (17,18). The subscapularis tendon may avulse from the lesser tuberosity but still be continuous with the transverse humeral ligament, allowing the biceps tendon to slip medially under the subscapularis (see Fig. 9C). A partial subscapularis tendon tear may result in the tendon dislocating medially into the substance of the torn subscapularis tendon (Fig. 11). A shallow bicipital groove, flattening of the lesser tuberosity, and a supratubercular ridge can also predispose to subluxation and dislocation (19–22) (Fig. 12).

Biceps tendon subluxations and dislocations can be identified by ultrasound (23), computed tomography (CT),

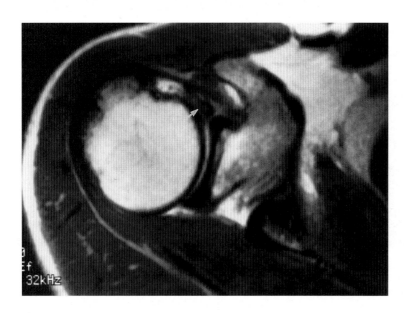

FIG. 10. The biceps tendon lies medial to the intertubercular sulcus and anterior to the superior glenohumeral joint *(arrow)* on an axial fast spin-echo T2-weighted MR image. This patient has an avulsed subscapularis tendon (analogous to Fig. 9D).

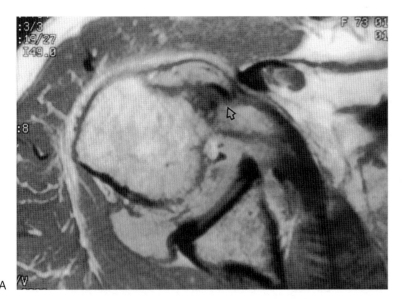
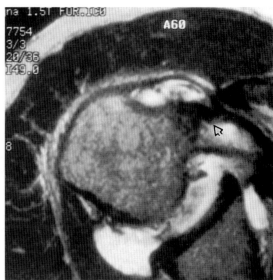

FIG. 11. The biceps tendon dislocated medially into the substance of a partially torn subscapularis tendon *(arrow)* on axial T1- **(A)** and T2-weighted **(B)** MR images.

arthrography, and MRI. This can be seen in all imaging planes on MRI but is easiest to identify on axial images (10,11,17,18). Axial MR images obtained with internal and external rotation may bring out subtle subluxation and dislocation, but most are readily apparent on routine axial MR images. The dislocated tendon is located medial to the bicipital groove (Figs. 10–13). If the subscapularis tendon is completely torn or if it is detached from the lesser tuberosity, the long head of the biceps tendon lies deep to the subscapularis tendon and may relocate anterior to or within the gleno-

humeral joint (17) (see Fig. 8-9D and Fig. 14). This appearance can mimic a labral tear or a loose body, but interpretation is clear once it is seen that the biceps tendon is missing from the intertubercular groove.

SLAP LESIONS

The long head of the biceps tendon originates through and is continuous with the superior labrum (see Fig. 1). A superior quadrant labral tear with anterior and posterior compo-

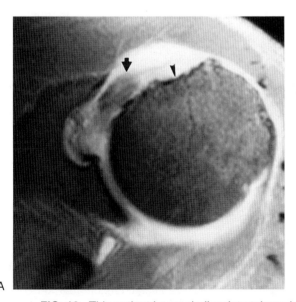
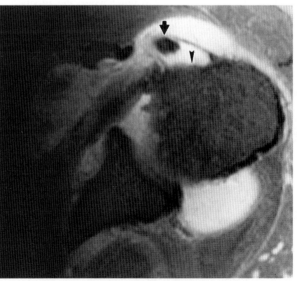

FIG. 12. This patient has a shallow intertubercular sulcus (bicipital groove) *(arrowhead)*, which predisposes him to subluxation and dislocation. **A:** Note that the tendon is medially dislocated *(arrow)* on a more cranial axial image from a gadolinium arthrogram (T1-weighted with fat saturation). **B:** The tendon is just subluxed on a more caudal image *(arrow).*

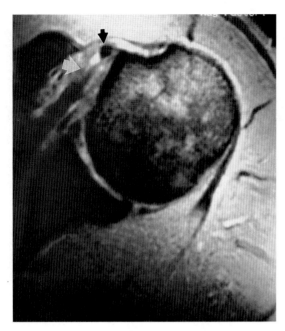

FIG. 13. There is a full-thickness tear of the subscapularis tendon *(white arrow)*, allowing the biceps tendon to dislocate medial to the intertubercular sulcus *(black arrow)*. This is well seen on an axial gradient echo T2*-weighted MR image.

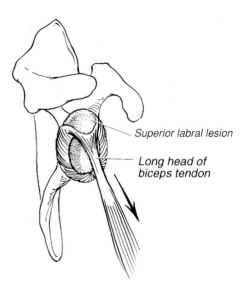

FIG. 15. Overloading of the long head of the biceps tendon can result in a superior labral (SLAP) tear.

nents of the tear is called a SLAP lesion (*superior labrum* from *anterior* to *posterior* relative to the biceps tendon insertion on the supraglenoid tubercle) (24,25). This usually results when the long head of the biceps tendon is overloaded, resulting in a tear or avulsion of the superior labrum from the glenoid (Fig. 15). There may be involvement of the biceps tendon and associated rotator cuff tears. SLAP lesions are seen in the following situations: (a) during the follow-through phase of pitching and throwing when the biceps

muscle contracts with deceleration; (b) following a fall on an outstretched abducted arm with associated superior glenohumeral compression and a proximal subluxation force; and (c) upon catching a heavy falling object. Repetitive stress on the biceps tendon and glenohumeral instability can also produce a SLAP lesion.

A lesion of the superior labrum can contribute to anterior shoulder instability because the long head of the biceps tendon and superior glenoid labrum play a role in glenohumeral joint stability (1). A retained biceps tendon stump at the superior glenoid from a tear can cause glenoid and humeral head chondromalacia via a "windshield wiper"

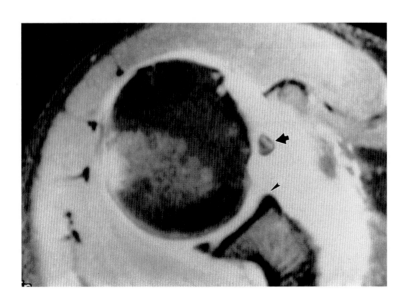

FIG. 14. The biceps tendon has dislocated far medially and lies near the anterior aspect of the glenohumeral joint *(arrow)* in association with a full-thickness subscapularis tendon tear on this axial gadolinium MR arthrogram. The patient also had an anterior labral tear *(arrowhead)* accompanied by humeral avulsion of the inferior glenohumeral ligament (a HAGL lesion).

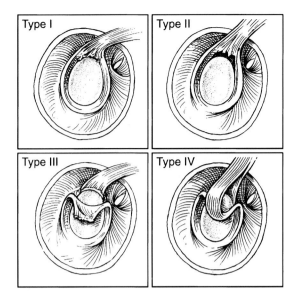

FIG. 16. The original four types of SLAP lesion. Type I—degenerative fraying of the superior labrum; type II—type I lesion with detachment of the biceps tendon and superior labrum from the glenoid; type III—tear of the central portion of the superior labrum without involvement of the biceps tendon; type IV—type III lesion with extension of the tear into the proximal portion of the biceps tendon.

mechanism and it is important to remove it before this occurs (26).

Clinical diagnosis of SLAP lesions can be difficult. Patients with this disorder frequently present with a painful locking, pseudosubluxation, or snapping sensation. This can be difficult to distinguish from instability, biceps tendinosis, and impingement.

Identification and classification of SLAP lesions by CT and MRI can be challenging. SLAP lesions can be seen by CT arthrography (27), but they are best seen on MRI wherein there is routine multiplanar imaging and improved soft tissue contrast (28).

Four types of SLAP lesion were originally described (Fig. 16). *Type I* lesions consist of degenerative fraying that primarily involves the superior glenoid labrum (29). The biceps

tendon is intact. These lesions show labral irregularity and slight increase in signal intensity on MRI, and are the most difficult to identify with MRI. Type I SLAP lesions were seen in 11% of patients in a retrospective series by Cartland et al. (28). These lesions are treated with arthroscopic debridement of the degenerative labrum. *Type II* lesions are the most common (seen in 41% of the series by Cartland and coworkers) and have similar superior labral fraying with detachment of the superior labrum and long head of the biceps tendon from the osseous glenoid, resulting in instability. The labral appearance is similar to type I lesions on MRI, with an additional globular region of high signal intensity between the superior glenoid and the labrum, representing the biceps anchor tear. Treatment of the Type II SLAP lesion involves debridement of the labrum and reattachment of the detached biceps anchor to the

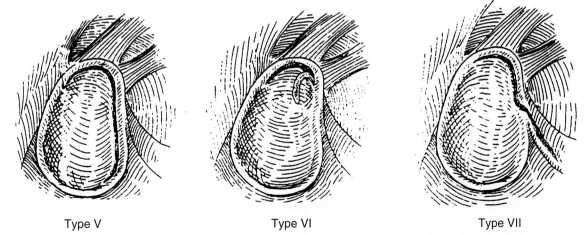

Type V   Type VI   Type VII

FIG. 17. Further classification of SLAP lesions with three additional types. Type V—anteroinferior Bankart lesion that extends superiorly to a torn biceps tendon; type VI—unstable radial or flap tears associated with separation of the biceps anchor; type VII—anterior extension of the superior labral tear beneath the middle glenohumeral ligament. (From ref. 30, with permission.)

superior glenoid. A *type III* SLAP lesion is seen in about one third of SLAP lesions and presents as a crescentic vertical tear that involves the central portion of the superior labrum with displacement or buckling of the labrum into the joint (similar to a bucket handle tear). The biceps tendon is normal. The treatment of this type of tear is variable. The labrum may be debrided, reattached, or resected. A *type IV* SLAP lesion is a type III tear of the superior labrum with extension of the tear into the proximal long head of the biceps tendon. It presents on MRI as a diffuse high signal intensity lesion in the superior portion of the labrum and proximal portion of the biceps tendon. These patients have functional instability. Fifteen percent of SLAP lesions in the series by Cartland et al. were Type IV. Treatment of the type IV SLAP lesion may involve resection of the torn labrum or suture repair of bucket handle tears. If the biceps tear involves more than half of the tendon, and the patient has symptoms referable to the tendon, biceps tenodesis may also be performed. A complex SLAP lesion may consist of a combination of two or more types, usually types II and IV.

Three more types of SLAP lesions have been described recently by Maffet et al. (30) (Fig. 17). *Type V* lesions represent an anteroinferior Bankart lesion that extends superiorly to a torn biceps tendon. *Type VI* lesions are unstable radial or flap tears associated with separation of the biceps anchor. *Type VII* lesions involve anterior extension of the superior labral tear beneath the middle glenohumeral ligament.

Various mechanisms of injury lead to certain types of SLAP lesions (31). Traction injuries often produce a type II SLAP lesion. Patients who fall on an outstretched hand more commonly have a type III, IV, or V lesion. Athletes who use overhead shoulder motion and patients with atraumatic instability tend to get type I or II SLAP lesions, whereas patients who have traumatic instability are prone to type V or VII lesions.

The superior labrum and biceps tendon can be evaluated in all three planes, with the tear most easily characterized in the oblique coronal and axial planes. SLAP lesions are best demonstrated on MRI with the shoulder in external rotation, which provides traction on the long head of the biceps, enhancing the detection of imbibition of contrast, posterior and superior extent of the tear, and separation at the site of the tear.

It is difficult sometimes to completely characterize the lesions according to the various subtypes using MRI. The main function of the MRI is to identify the lesions of the superior labrum and biceps tendon (Figs. 18–27). SLAP lesions are best evaluated when there is fluid or contrast in the joint. SLAP lesions should also be sought when imaging in the ABER position (see Fig. 24D). This provocative position may enhance evaluation of the SLAP lesion by causing fluid to be further pushed into the superior labrum.

SLAP lesions can also be associated with paralabral cysts (Figs. 25 and 26). At times, these cysts may be the red flag that alerts the radiologist of the underlying labral tear. They often lie medial to the tear in the suprascapular notch and can produce entrapment of the suprascapular nerve, which courses through this region. Associated denervation changes may be identified in the supraspinatus and infraspinatus muscles.

Fifteen to twenty-five percent of SLAP lesions are associated with a full- or partial thickness tear of the rotator cuff (Figs. 21, 27) anterior instability (Fig. 19), humeral head fracture, chondromalacia of the humeral head, and acromioclavicular joint arthritis (29) (Fig. 27). It is especially important to carefully scrutinize the superior labrum and biceps tendon in these situations.

Labral fraying and irregularity can be seen in asymptomatic shoulders, often in patients of older age. This appearance can simulate a type I or II SLAP lesion (32). It is crucial to keep this in mind and to correlate symptoms with the appearance on MRI.

Care must be taken to distinguish a SLAP lesion from normal variants involving the anterosuperior labrum. These normal variants include the sublabral recess and Buford complex

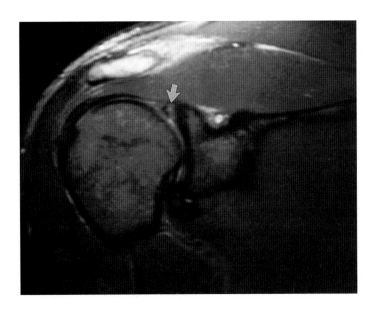

FIG. 18. A type III SLAP lesion is seen on this oblique-coronal fat-saturated fast spin-echo T2-weighted image *(arrow)*. The high signal intensity extends up to the superior portion of the labrum. The overlying biceps tendon was intact.

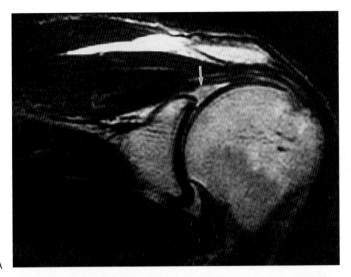

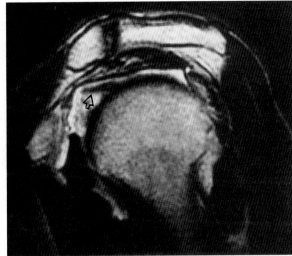

A

B

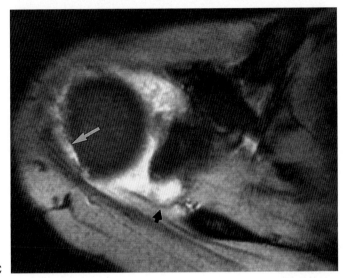

C

FIG. 19. SLAP lesion in a patient with anterior instability. **A:** There is a tear of the posterosuperior labrum *(arrow)* manifest as high signal intensity and irregularity on an oblique coronal T2-weighted MR image. **B:** There is also a tear of the long head of the biceps tendon, which is thinned and flattened on this T2-weighted oblique sagittal MR image *(arrow)*. The tendon was totally avulsed from the superior glenoid. **C:** There is a Hill-Sachs lesion *(white arrow)* associated with the anterior instability, as well as a posterosuperior paralabral cyst *(black arrow)* extending from the superior labral tear.

(32–34) discussed in Chapter 7 of this book. A type II SLAP lesion may simulate a sublabral recess, which is located at the glenoid margin of some superior labra, inferior to the biceps tendon insertion of the superior glenoid tubercle, and has been seen in 19 of 26 (73%) cadaver shoulders in one study (32). Contrast material or fluid accumulates in this area (Fig. 28). This normal variant is smoothly marginated, usually symmetric, and lacks imbibition of contrast into the superior labrum, helping to separate it from a SLAP lesion. The articular cartilage of the superior glenoid extends to the attachment of a sublabral recess, unlike most type II SLAP lesions in which there is often a gap between the glenoid articular cartilage and attachment of the superior labrum and biceps tendon. The sublabral recess is distinguishable from a type III SLAP lesion in which fluid signal intensity extends into the substance of the superior labrum, resembling a bucket-handle tear of the knee (Fig. 29). The sublabral foramen and the Buford complex are associated with a cordlike middle glenohumeral ligament, which should further distinguish them from SLAP lesions.

MISCELLANEOUS

The tendon sheath of the long head of the biceps may contain osteochondral loose bodies or may be involved by synovial chondrometaplasia. Occasionally, the loose body can mimic a split or bifid tendon (Fig. 30). Careful attention to the conventional radiograph excludes an ossified loose body.

Osteophytes extending from the bicipital groove can lead to tendinous disease and should be mentioned when seen by MRI. Friction on the tendon sheath may produce a tenosynovitis.

Calcific tendinitis can involve the proximal or distal portions of the tendon and may be overlooked on MRI unless the deposits produce morphologic distortion. The calcific deposits are particularly evident on gradient echo imaging because of magnetic susceptibility. The blooming effect makes the calcifications darker and larger. Surrounding edema and tenosynovitis is occasionally seen in association with calcific tendinitis.

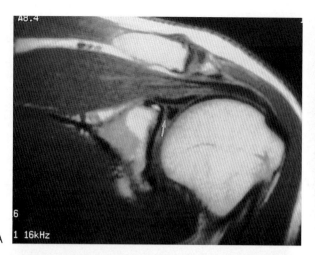

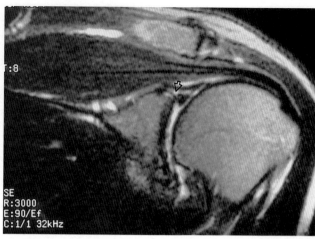

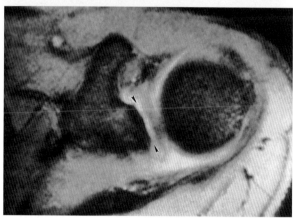

FIG. 20. Type IV SLAP lesion in a 58-year-old man. **A:** There is intermediate signal intensity extending between the base of the labrum in the superior aspect and underneath the biceps tendon on this oblique coronal T1-weighted MR image *(arrow)*. **B:** This region is high signal intensity on a T2-weighted oblique coronal MR image *(arrow)*. **C:** Fluid signal intensity tracks in the tear between the labrum and the glenoid from anterior to posterior on this axial gradient echo MR image *(arrowheads)*.

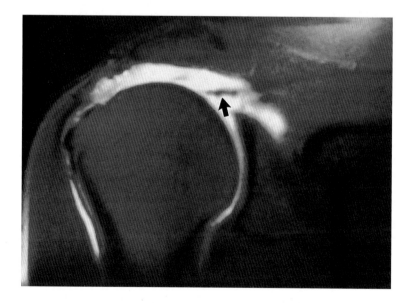

FIG. 21. Type IV SLAP lesion in a patient with a supraspinatus tendon tear. The superior labrum is absent and the long head of the biceps tendon is detached from the superior glenoid consistent with a type IV SLAP lesion. Gadolinium fills in the region of the torn supraspinatus tendon on this fat-saturated T1-weighted MR arthrogram.

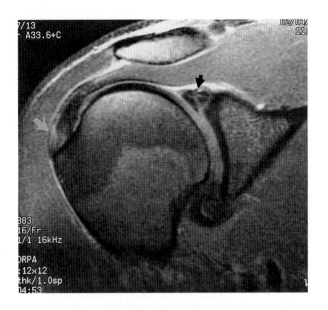

FIG. 22. This 18-year-old baseball pitcher has a complex superior labral tear that extends to the superior labral surface *(black arrow)* on an oblique coronal fat-saturated T1-weighted indirect intravenous gadolinium MR arthrogram. The supraspinatus tendon is thickened with diffuse high signal intensity from diffusion of intravenous gadolinium near its insertion on the greater tuberosity, consistent with tendinosis *(white arrow)*.

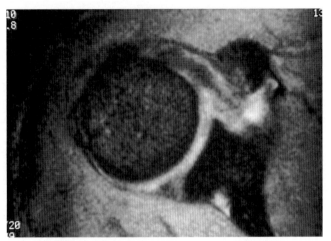

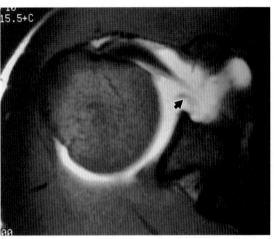

A   B

FIG. 23. A: This baseball player had a SLAP lesion that was not well seen on a routine, noncontrast axial gradient echo MR image. The anterosuperior labrum can be ghosted by the magic angle phenomenon. **B:** The patient came back for an intraarticular MR arthrogram. The torn avulsed labrum was easily identified surrounded by high signal intensity gadolinium on this fat saturated T1-weighted MR study *(arrow)*.

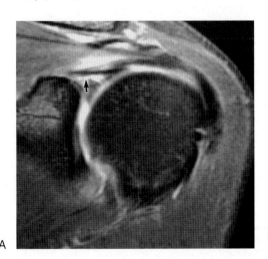

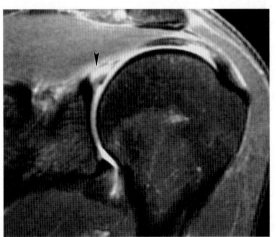

A   B

FIG. 24. A: There is high signal intensity gadolinium in the upper portion of the superior labrum on this oblique coronal fat-saturated MR arthrogram *(arrow)*. The overlying biceps tendon is intact. **B:** The gadolinium extends into the superior labrum posterior to the biceps tendon *(arrowhead)*. (*Continued on next page*.)

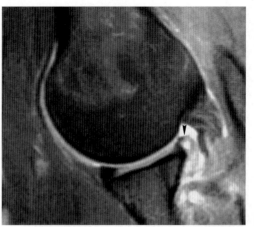

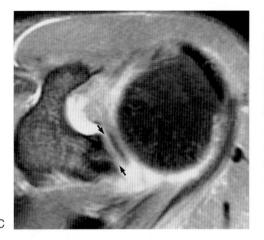

FIG. 24. *Continued.* **C:** The tear is seen extending between the labrum and the glenoid on this axial fat saturated T1-weighted MR image *(arrows).* **D:** The superior labral tear is also well seen on this fat-saturated T1-weighted MR image taken in the ABER position *(arrowhead).*

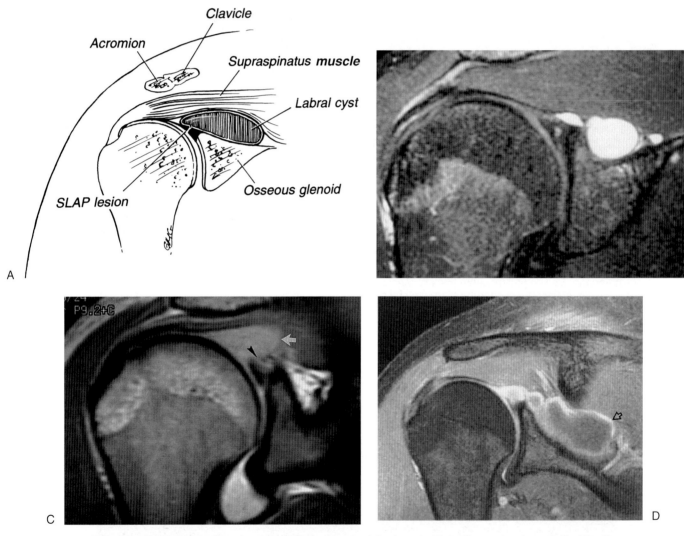

FIG. 25. SLAP lesions can be associated with paralabral cysts that often extend medially into the suprascapular notch. This is shown diagrammatically in **(A)**. **B:** Oblique coronal fat-saturated fast spin-echo T2-weighted MR image demonstrates a paralabral cyst adjacent to a superior labral tear. **C:** Oblique coronal fat-saturated T1-weighted MR arthrogram. The gadolinium within the glenohumeral joint is high signal intensity. The superior labral tear *(arrowhead)* and the cyst *(arrow)* do not take up the gadolinium and are of intermediate signal intensity. **D:** This patient had an intravenous gadolinium MR arthrogram. The high signal intensity gadolinium surrounds the paralabral cyst on this oblique coronal fat saturated T1-weighted MR image *(arrow).*

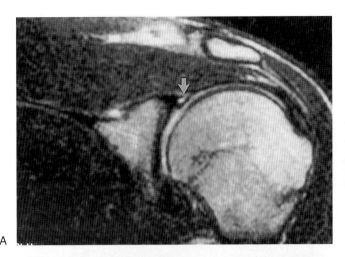

A

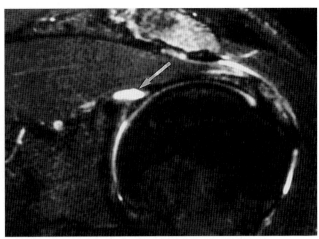

B

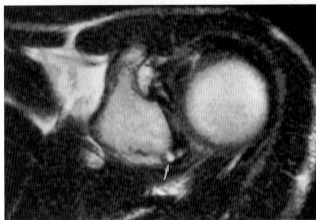

C

FIG. 26. This teen-aged swimmer and weightlifter developed a SLAP lesion with a paralabral cyst. **A:** The superior labral tear is well seen on this oblique coronal T2-weighted MR image *(arrow).* **B:** The paralabral cyst is shown filled with intravenous gadolinium on a fat-saturated oblique coronal posterior to the previous image *(arrow).* **C:** An axial T1-weighted MR image shows that the cyst extended posterior to the glenoid *(arrow).*

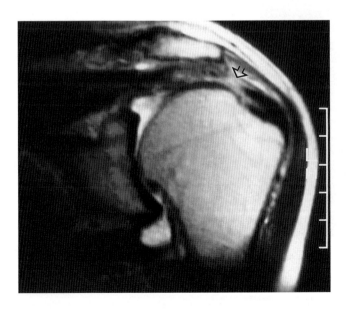

FIG. 27. SLAP lesion. This patient had complete absence of the superior labrum in association with a full-thickness supraspinatus tendon tear *(arrow)* seen on an oblique coronal T2-weighted MR image.

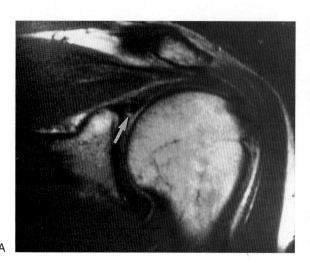

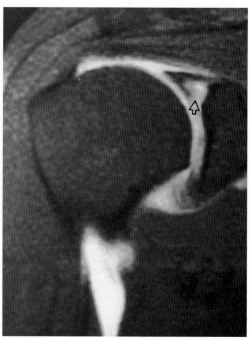

A

B

FIG. 28. Sublabral recess in different patients. **A:** This man has a small sublabral recess filled with fluid on a fast spin-echo oblique coronal MR image *(arrow)*. **B:** This is a much larger sublabral recess, distended with gadolinium on an oblique coronal MR image from a fat-saturated T1-weighted MR arthrogram *(arrow)*.

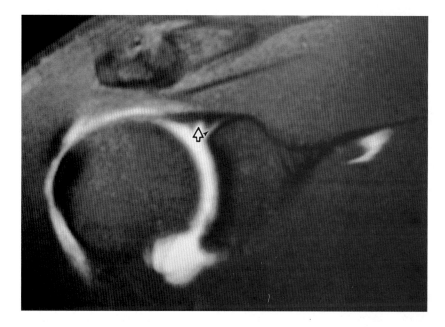

FIG. 29. There is a sublabral recess *(arrowhead)* and a superior labral tear *(arrow)* on this fat-saturated T1-weighted oblique coronal MR image taken from a gadolinium MR arthrogram.

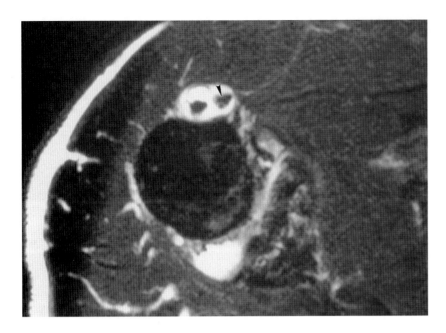

FIG. 30. There are two low signal intensity rounded structures in the distended biceps tendon sheath on this axial gradient echo MR image. One was the biceps tendon and the other was an osseous loose body (arrowhead).

REFERENCES

1. Rodosky MW, Harner CD, Fu FH. The role of the long head of the biceps muscle and superior glenoid labrum in anterior stability of the shoulder. *Am J Sports Med* 1994;22:121–130.
2. Neer CS. Impingement lesions. *Clin Orthop Rel Res* 1983;173:70.
3. Kumar VP, Satku K, Balasubramaniam P. The role of the long head of the biceps brachii in the stabilization of the head of the humerus. *Clin Orthop* 1989;244:172–175.
4. Detrisac DA, Johnson LL. *Arthroscopic shoulder anatomy: pathologic and surgical implications.* Thorofare, NJ: SLACK, 1987.
5. Vangness CT, Jorgenson SS, Watson T, Johnson DL. The origin of the long head of the biceps from the scapula and glenoid labrum. *J Bone Joint Surg* 1994;76-B:951–954.
6. Warner JJP, McMahon PJ. The role of the long head of the biceps brachii in superior stability of the glenohumeral joint. *J Bone Joint Surg* 1995:336.
7. Needell SD, Zlatkin MB, Sher JS, Murphy BJ, Uribe JW. MR imaging of the rotator cuff: peritendinous and bone abnormalities in an asymptomatic population. *Am J Roentgenol* 1996;166:863–867.
8. Erickson SJ, Prost RW, Timins ME. The "magic angle" effect: background physics and clinical relevance. *Radiology* 1993;188:23–25.
9. Kaplan PA, Bryans KC, Davick JP, Otte M, Stinson WW, Dussault RG. MR imaging of the normal shoulder: variants and pitfalls. *Radiology* 1992;184:519–524.
10. Erickson SJ, Fitzgerald SW, Quinn SF, Carrera GF, Black KP, Lawson TL. Long bicipital tendon of the shoulder: normal anatomy and pathologic findings on MR imaging. *Am J Roentgenol* 1992;158:1091–1096.
11. Tuckman GA. Abnormalities of the long head of the biceps tendon of the shoulder: MR imaging findings. *Am J Roentgenol* 1994;163:1183–1188.
12. DePalma AF, Callery GE. Bicipital tenosynovitis. *Clin Orthop* 1954;3:69.
13. Neer CS. *Shoulder reconstruction.* Philadelphia: WB Saunders, 1990.
14. Slatis P, Aalto K. Medial dislocation of the tendon of the long head of the biceps brachii. *Acta Orthop Scand* 1979;50:73.
15. Burkhead WZ Jr. The shoulder. In: Rockwood CA Jr., III MF, eds. Philadelphia: WB Saunders, 1990.
16. Petersson CJ. Spontaneous medial dislocation of the tendon of the long head of the biceps brachii: an anatomic study of prevalence and pathomechanics. *Clin Orthop* 1986;211:224–227.
17. Cervilla V, Schweitzer ME, Ho C, Mott A, Kerr R, Resnick D. Medial dislocation of the biceps brachii tendon: appearance at MR imaging. *Radiology* 1991;180:523–526.
18. Chan TW, Dalinka MK, Kneeland BJ, Chevrot A. Biceps tendon dislocation: evaluation with MR imaging. *Radiology* 1991;179:649–652.
19. Meyer AW. Spontaneous dislocation of the long head of the biceps brachii. *Arch Surg* 1926;13:109–119.
20. O'Donoghue DH. Subluxating biceps tendon in the athlete. *Clin Orthop* 1982;164:26–29.
21. Nevaiser RJ. Lesions of the biceps and tendinitis of the shoulder. *Orthop Clin North Am* 1980;11:343–348.
22. Levinsohn EM, Santelli ED. Bicipital groove dysplasia and medial dislocation of the biceps brachii tendon. *Skeletal Radiol* 1991;20:419–423.
23. Farin PU, Jaroma H, Harju A, et al. Medial displacement of the biceps brachii tendon: evaluation with dynamic sonography during maximal external shoulder rotation. *Radiology* 1995;195:845.
24. Snyder SJ, Karzel RP, Del Pizzo W, Ferkel RD, Friedman MJ. SLAP lesions of the shoulder. *Arthroscopy* 1990;6:274–279.
25. Andrews JR, Carson WG, McLeod WD. Glenoid labrum tears related to the long head of the biceps. *Am J Sports Med* 1985;13:337–341.
26. Burkhart SS, Fox DL. SLAP lesions in association with complete tears of the long head of the biceps tendon: a report of two cases. *Arthroscopy* 1992;8:31–35.
27. Hunter JC, Blatz DJ, Escobedo EM. SLAP lesions of the glenoid labrum: CT arthrographic and arthroscopic correlation. *Radiology* 1992;184:513–518.
28. Cartland JP, Crues JV III, Stauffer A, Nottage W, Ryu RKN. MR imaging in the evaluation of SLAP injuries of the shoulder: findings in 10 patients. *Am J Roentgenol* 1992;159:787–792.
29. Rames RD, Karzel RP. Injuries to the glenoid labrum, including SLAP lesions. *Orthop Clin North Am* 1993;24:45–53.
30. Maffet, Gartsman GM, Moseley B. Superior labrum-biceps tendon complex lesions of the shoulder. *Am J Sports Med* 1995;23:93.
31. Urban WP Jr, Caborn DNM. Management of superior labral anterior to posterior lesions. *Oper Techniq Orthop* 1995;5:223.
32. Smith DK, Chopp TM, Aufdemorte TB, et al. Sublabral recess of the superior glenoid labrum: study of cadavers with conventional nonenhanced MR imaging, MR arthrography, anatomic dissection, and limited histologic examination. *Radiology* 1996;201:251–256.
33. Tuite MJ, Orwin JF. Anterosuperior labral variants of the shoulder: appearance on gradient-recalled-echo and fast spin-echo MR images. *Radiology* 1996;199:537–540.
34. Tirman PFJ, Feller JF, Palmer WE, Carroll KW, Steinbach LS, Cox I. The Buford Complex—a variation of normal shoulder anatomy. MR arthrographic imaging features. *Am J Roentgenol* 1996;166:869–873.

Shoulder Magnetic Resonance Imaging,
edited by Lynne S. Steinbach, et al.
Lippincott–Raven Publishers, Philadelphia © 1998.

CHAPTER 9

MR Imaging of the Postoperative Shoulder

John F. Feller, Tom D. Howey, and Brad R. Plaga

Even though most patients who undergo shoulder surgery have a satisfactory outcome, persistent or recurrent symptoms related to the postoperative shoulder are a common and difficult clinical problem. For the radiologist, interpretation of magnetic resonance imaging (MRI) findings in the postoperative shoulder can be equally challenging. There are significant anatomic changes as a result of the surgery as well as the frequent presence of ferromagnetic artifact, which can

compromise image quality. This difficulty is compounded by the fact that there is a paucity of scientific work published to date on MRI of the shoulder following surgery. As a result, the practicing radiologist may find himself or herself resisting the desire to sneak a postoperative shoulder MRI case into the stack of films being read by another radiologist in their group.

Difficult problems are best approached by gaining a thorough understanding of their more basic components. This chapter first reviews the technique for postoperative shoulder imaging. The common surgical procedures used for the treatment of impingement, rotator cuff tears, instability, and SLAP lesions (superior quadrant labral tear with anterior and posterior components of the tear) are then discussed, including their potential for complications. Finally, normal and ab-

---

J. F. Feller: Department of Radiology, Stanford University School of Medicine, Stanford, California 94305; and Desert Medical Imaging, Indian Wells, California 92210

T. D. Howey and B. R. Plaga: Department of Surgery, University of South Dakota; and Orthopaedic Associates, LTD., Sioux Falls, South Dakota 57005

normal postoperative MRI findings are reviewed. Abnormal postoperative MRI findings are categorized as follows: (a) residual or recurrent findings related to the original condition for which surgery was performed, (b) a complication of surgery, or (c) findings completely unrelated to either the original condition or the surgery (1).

MAGNETIC RESONANCE TECHNIQUE

A good clinical and surgical history is helpful when creating optimal protocol for the MRI scan. Correlative conventional radiographs of the shoulder are also helpful for accurate MRI interpretation, especially in the postoperative setting. Even though various field strength MRI systems are used for shoulder imaging, the following general protocol is appropriate for use on a high field strength 1.5 Tesla MRI unit. In general, MRI of the postoperative shoulder is performed using the same protocol used for routine shoulder MRI.

The patient is scanned in a supine position, using a commercially available dedicated shoulder coil. The arm is positioned at the patient's side in external rotation, and the coil is centered on the lesser tuberosity. Three orthogonal planes are essential for adequate anatomic assessment including axial, oblique sagittal, and oblique coronal imaging planes. Imaging should extend from the acromioclavicular joint through the lateral aspect of the humeral head and from the inferior aspect of the acromion through the glenohumeral joint. A slice thickness of 3 to 4 mm is used with a 0.5- to 1-mm interslice gap, in combination with an imaging matrix of 256×192 and a 12- to 16-cm field of view.

An example of a routine pulse sequence protocol includes the following: (a) T2*-weighted axial gradient recalled echo imaging, (b) intermediate-weighted axial fast spin-echo imaging with frequency-selective fat suppression, (c) T1-weighted oblique coronal spin-echo imaging, (d) T2-weighted fast spin-echo oblique coronal imaging with frequency selective fat suppression, and (e) T2-weighted fast spin-echo oblique sagittal imaging obtained without frequency-selective fat suppression. With routine shoulder imaging, there is occasionally incomplete fat suppression when using the frequency-selective fat saturation in conjunction with a fast spin-echo sequence because of bulk susceptibility artifact/magnetic field inhomogeneity related to the curved external surface of the shoulder. Incomplete fat suppression is a more common problem when imaging the postoperative shoulder because of the presence of magnetic susceptibility effects and ferromagnetic artifact related to the prior surgery. If this occurs, then a fast inversion recovery sequence is obtained, which is not as dependent on field homogeneity for reliable suppression of fat signal intensity.

The indications for MR arthrography of the postoperative shoulder are the following: (a) to confirm a humeral surface partial thickness tear, (b) to distinguish a subtle full-thickness rotator cuff tear from a partial thickness tear, (c) to evaluate the glenoid labrum, capsule, and glenohumeral ligaments in the context of instability, and (d) to distinguish SLAP lesions from normal variants of the glenoid labrum (2). Direct MR arthrography is performed by intraarticular injection of dilute gadolinium contrast agent using fluoroscopic guidance. T1-weighted spin-echo images are then obtained in all three routine planes using frequency-selective fat suppression. A T2-weighted fast spin-echo sequence is also obtained in the oblique coronal plane in conjunction with frequency-selective fat suppression to evaluate the bone marrow and extraarticular soft tissues. If the initial pulse sequence obtained demonstrates incomplete fat suppression because of the presence of ferromagnetic artifact from prior surgery, then the T1-weighted sequences are obtained without frequency-selective fat suppression and the T2-weighted fast spin-echo sequence is replaced with a fast inversion recovery sequence.

IMPINGEMENT

Primary impingement frequently is associated with certain osseous configurations or pathologic changes involving the coracoacromial arch or less likely the acromioclavicular joint. In particular, the anteriorly hooked acromion or inferiorly directed subacromial osteophyte has a high association with the clinical syndrome of impingement (3). Proliferation of the soft tissues of the acromioclavicular joint and osteophyte formation involving the acromioclavicular joint may also cause primary impingement. Secondary impingement syndrome may be caused by a variety of shoulder disorders, the most important of which is glenohumeral instability.

Conservative Treatment

Whether the impingement syndrome is primary or secondary, conservative nonoperative treatment is the mainstay of treatment for this disease process. Most patients respond to well-controlled activity modification and a physical therapy program (4,5,6,7). If symptoms continue, a corticosteroid injection can be considered, but the physician and patient must understand the potential consequences of repeated steroid injections, which include possible rupture of the rotator cuff.

Total Acromionectomy

Many techniques have been described for the surgical decompression of the shoulder for the treatment of impingement syndrome. Currently, there continues to be an evolution of the most appropriate method for the surgical treatment of impingement syndrome. Earlier authors advised complete excision of the acromion (8,9,10). This is done through an anterior approach to the shoulder and the entire

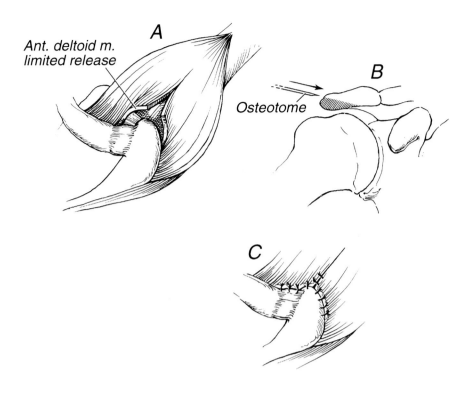

Ant. deltoid m. limited release

Osteotome

FIG. 1. Open anterior acromioplasty. **A:** Limited surgical release of the anterior deltoid muscle. **B:** Bony resection of the anterior inferior portion of the acromion with an osteotome. **C:** Reattachment of the anterior deltoid to the anterior acromion.

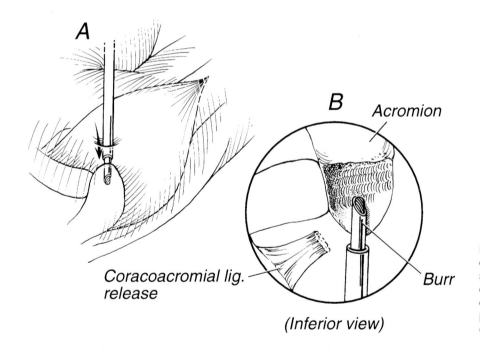

Coracoacromial lig. release

Acromion

Burr

(Inferior view)

FIG. 2. Arthroscopic subacromial decompression. **A:** Insertion of an arthroscope into the subacromial space. **B:** A cautery is used to release the coracoacromial ligament and an acromioplasty burr is used to remove the undersurface of the acromion.

acromion is excised. This technique is not currently recommended, because it leads to significant weakness of the anterior deltoid, which causes significant patient morbidity (11).

Anterior Acromioplasty

The current recommended surgical approach is that described by Neer (6), the anterior and inferior partial resection of the acromion (Fig. 1). Through an anterior open incision, the anterior and inferior portion of the acromion is resected. With osseous resection, it is also important to release the coracoacromial ligament. Upon closure of the wound, the anterior deltoid is firmly reattached to the anterior acromion, usually through drill holes and large sutures. Adequate removal of the anterior acromion and the undersurface of the acromion is readily seen through this approach. The rotator cuff is also easily inspected so that a repair can be performed if needed. If the acromioclavicular joint is also found to be arthritic, the distal end of the clavicle can also be resected (*Mumford procedure*) (12,13). Some surgeons do this routinely whereas others reserve distal clavicle resection pending intraoperative and preoperative findings. Failure of complete subacromial resection, incomplete coracoacromial ligament release, rupture of the deltoid repair, scar formation, and acromial fracture are all potential causes of failure with this technique.

Arthroscopic Decompression

The expansion of arthroscopic capabilities has led to the development of arthroscopic subacromial decompression (Fig. 2). The results of this technique have been as favorable in some studies as the traditional open technique; however, other studies have shown a less favorable result using the arthroscopic technique (14,15). In all studies, there is thought to be a significant learning curve with the arthroscopic approach. Arthroscopic techniques involve the insertion of an arthroscope into the subacromial space and the use of a burr to remove the undersurface of the acromion. A cautery is also used to release the coracoacromial ligament. The advantages are a shorter recovery time, less pain, performance in an outpatient setting, and no need to release the anterior deltoid muscle. Arthroscopic decompression can be a difficult procedure because the view afforded in the subacromial space is somewhat limited. Because of this limited view, there is a significant learning curve with this procedure, which may be the reason for a higher failure rate in most studies. A common error is insufficient excision of the acromion and consequently failure to relieve the patient's pain. One advantage of the arthroscopic technique is that the glenohumeral joint is easily inspected for possible concomitant disease. If a rotator cuff tear is found during arthroscopy, arthroscopic repair may be used, but such technique is still in development and many surgeons convert to an open repair if a tear is found. The distal clavicle can also be resected using a burr. Some surgeons prefer to use the arthroscopic technique for the younger athlete whereas others use it for all patients.

Complications

The incidence of failure ranges from 3% to 11% (6,12, 14,15). As discussed, arthroscopic decompressions may carry a higher rate of recurrence. Causes for failure include incomplete decompression, postoperative scar formation, infection, acromion fracture, large irreparable cuff defects,

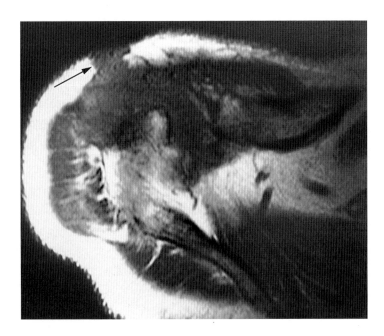

FIG. 3. Postoperative scar tissue. T1-weighted axial image demonstrates a low signal intensity band in the anterior subcutaneous fat following open acromioplasty *(arrow).*

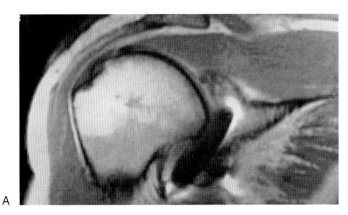
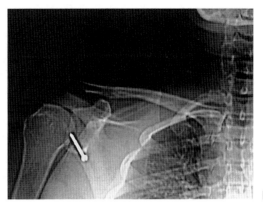

FIG. 4. Ferromagnetic artifact. **A:** T1-weighted coronal image shows ferromagnetic artifact at the anteroinferior glenoid. **B:** Computed tomography localizer scan demonstrates a fixation screw in the anteroinferior glenoid as part of a prior Bristow procedure.

anterior deltoid weakness secondary to large acromial defects or failure of the deltoid repair, rehabilitation failure, and incorrect diagnosis such as an unrecognized unstable os acromiale (16). Many of these complications can be documented with MRI.

Summary of Acromial Decompression Techniques

1. Partial or total acromionectomy—rarely used
2. Open anterior acromioplasty—commonly used
3. Arthroscopic decompression—commonly used

Postoperative Magnetic Resonance Imaging Findings

MRI following shoulder surgery demonstrates general surgical findings such as scar formation and ferromagnetic artifact (1). Scar tissue formation is best identified on MRI by a band of decreased signal intensity in the subcutaneous fat on all pulse sequences. It is usually most conspicuous on the T1-weighted images because it is surrounded by high signal intensity subcutaneous fat (Fig. 3). Scar tissue in the deep soft tissues of the shoulder may efface normally identifiable soft tissue planes and distort anatomy. Ferromagnetic artifact is due to two sources: (a) metallic orthopedic devices deliberately placed in the shoulder (e.g., staples, screws, suture anchors) (Fig. 4) and (b) microscopic, clinically insignificant pieces of metal that are left behind by metallic orthopedic tools (e.g., motorized burr, bone saw, sucker). The latter appear as small round or target-shaped foci of decreased signal intensity and are most conspicuous on gradient recalled echo images (blooming artifact) because of greater sensitivity to magnetic susceptibility effects (Fig. 5). The use of titanium surgical devices and fast spin-echo

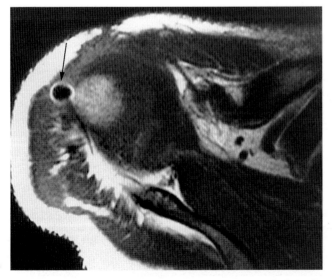
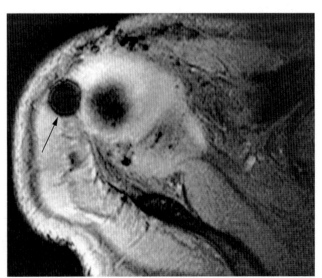

FIG. 5. Ferromagnetic artifact. **A:** T1-weighted axial image shows ferromagnetic artifact *(arrow)* resulting from prior open anterior acromioplasty. **B:** T2*-weighted axial gradient echo image demonstrates blooming of the artifact *(arrow)*, which appears larger and more conspicuous.

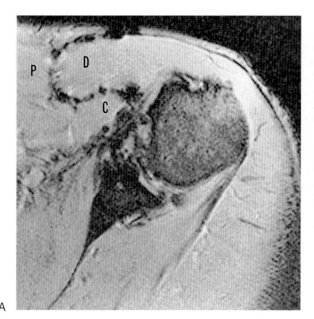
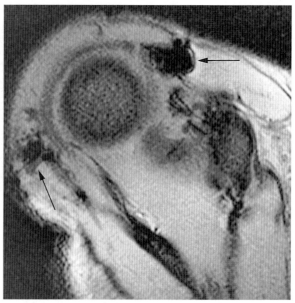

A B

FIG. 6. Open versus arthroscopic surgery patterns. **A:** T2*-weighted axial gradient echo image demonstrates a pattern of ferromagnetic artifact along the deltopectoral interval, lateral to the coracobrachialis muscle, and at the subscapularis insertion consistent with a prior open Bankart repair. D, deltoid muscle; P, pectoralis muscle; C, coracobrachialis muscle. **B:** T2*-weighted axial gradient echo image shows ferromagnetic artifact resulting from the anterior and posterior portals *(arrows)* of arthroscopic surgery.

imaging tends to minimize the problem of ferromagnetic artifact obscuring pertinent anatomy and pathology on MRI. Although the presence of postoperative scar tissue and ferromagnetic artifacts are nonspecific MR findings of prior surgery, the pattern of involvement can be specific with regard to the type of surgery that has been performed. It is usually possible to distinguish prior open surgery from prior arthroscopic surgery, for example (Fig. 6).

In addition to nonspecific postoperative changes, specific MRI findings indicative of a prior acromioplasty have been well described (17). First, osseous morphologic changes are

seen involving the acromion, dependent on the amount of bone resected including scalloping or flattening of the undersurface and/or nonvisualization of the anterior third of the acromion (Fig. 7). Second, there is a subtle decrease in signal intensity of the marrow of the remaining distal acromion on all pulse sequences. This may be due to postoperative fibrosis or sclerosis in the bone marrow (Fig. 8). Third, there is loss of the subacromial-subdeltoid fat plane (Fig. 9). Fourth, focal interruption of the coracoacromial ligament may be seen if this ligament was released (Fig. 10). Fifth, a cluster of ferromagnetic artifacts is identified at the anterior

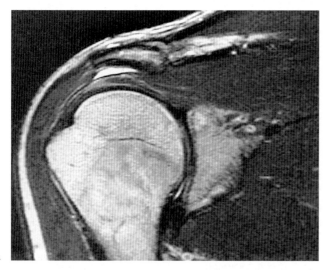
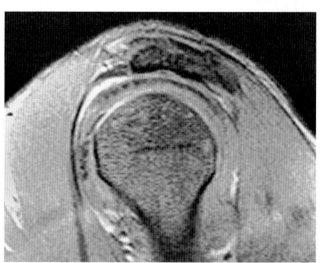

A B

FIG. 7. Acromioplasty. T2-weighted coronal image and T2*-weighted sagittal gradient echo image demonstrate scalloping of the undersurface of the acromion following acromioplasty.

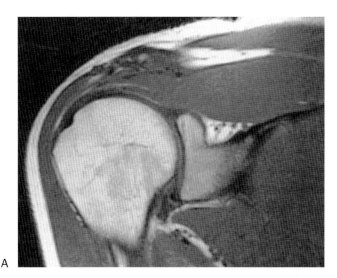
A

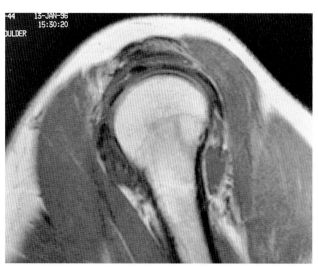
B

FIG. 8. Acromioplasty. T1-weighted coronal and sagittal images demonstrate decreased marrow signal intensity in the acromion following acromioplasty.

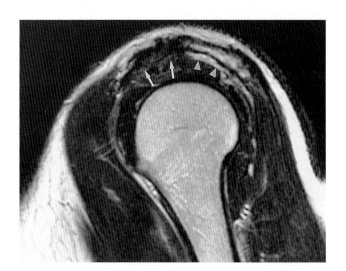

FIG. 9. Acromioplasty. T2 fast spin-echo sagittal image shows absence of the subacromial-subdeltoid fat plane anteriorly *(arrows)*. More posteriorly, this fat plane is intact *(arrowheads)*.

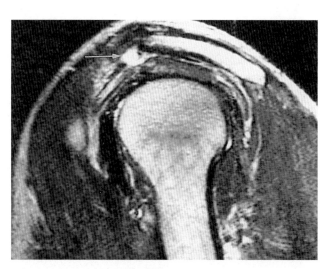

FIG. 10. Coracoacromial ligament release. T2-weighted sagittal image documents focal interruption of the coracoacromial ligament *(arrow)*, which was surgically released in conjunction with an acromioplasty.

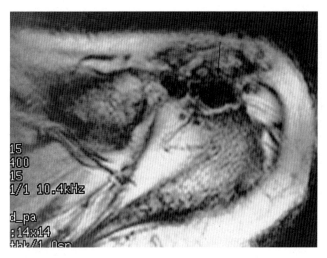

FIG. 11. Arthroscopic acromioplasty. T2*-weighted axial GRE image demonstrates ferromagnetic artifact *(arrow)* at the anteroinferior aspect of the acromion following acromioplasty.

margin of the acromion, presumably because of the motorized burring of the acromion (Fig. 11). Finally, some authors have noted diffuse intermediate signal intensity in the rotator cuff tendons and muscles on T2-weighted images (1). The etiology of this finding is uncertain, but may reflect postsurgical edema or preexisting degenerative change or tendonitis. In the setting of a concomitant Mumford procedure, there is also surgical absence of the distal clavicle and acromioclavicular joint (Fig. 12).

General postoperative complications following shoulder surgery are usually accurately diagnosed clinically. In the context of a diagnostic dilemma clinically, MRI reliably distinguishes between these entities, including hematoma formation, myositis ossificans (see Figure 3 in Chapter 11), wound infection, cellulitis, abscess formation, septic arthritis, osteomyelitis, reactive synovitis (Fig. 13), pseudoaneurysm, and denervation atrophy (Fig. 14). If there is clinical suspicion for infection or synovitis, then intravenous gadolinium contrast agent should be used as part of the MR examination. This allows reliable distinction between phleg-

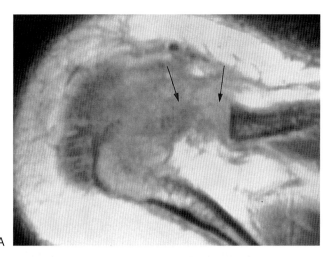

A

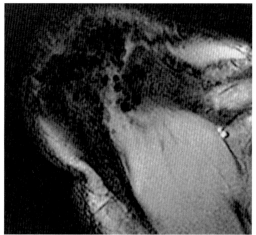

B

FIG. 12. Mumford procedure. **A:** T1-weighted axial image reveals surgical absence of the distal clavicle and acromioclavicular joint *(arrows)*. **B:** T2*-weighted axial gradient echo image shows ferromagnetic artifact at the site of surgical resection. **C:** Conventional radiograph (anteroposterior, external rotation) confirms excision of the acromioclavicular joint and distal clavicle.

C

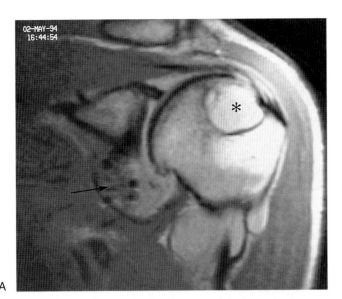
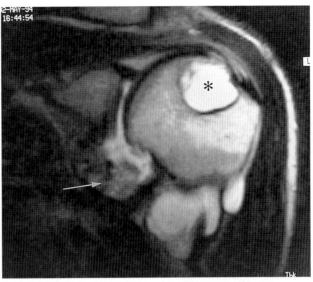

FIG. 13. Postoperative reactive synovitis. Intermediate and T2-weighted coronal images demonstrate a large glenohumeral joint effusion, cystic erosions *(*)*, and associated synovitis *(arrows)* 3 months after an open Bankart repair.

mon (inflammatory soft tissue mass) and abscess, and between joint effusion and underlying synovitis.

In the clinical setting of recurrent or residual impingement syndrome following an acromioplasty, MRI is helpful for determining the cause of surgical failure. Possible causes include an incompletely resected subacromial osteophyte or type III acromion (Fig. 15), an unstable, unfused os acromiale (16) (Fig. 16), significant acromioclavicular joint osteoarthritis (Fig. 17), rupture of the tendon for the long head of the biceps, and interval development of a rotator cuff tear.

Owen et al. (17) noted a 64% sensitivity, 82% specificity, and 74% accuracy predicting residual or recurrent impingement on the basis of a postoperative MRI study. Magee et al. (18) found a 84% sensitivity, 87% specificity, 95% positive predictive value, but only 50% negative predictive value in a similar study. This suggests that impingement syndrome, even in the postoperative setting, remains a clinical diagnosis. Postoperative MRI is helpful, however, for documenting anatomic or pathologic causes of recurrent shoulder pain in the appropriate clinical setting (Fig. 18).

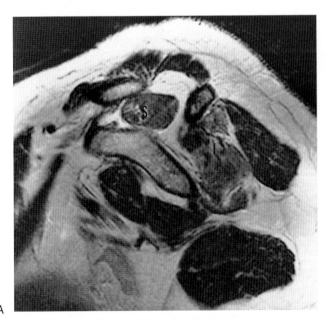
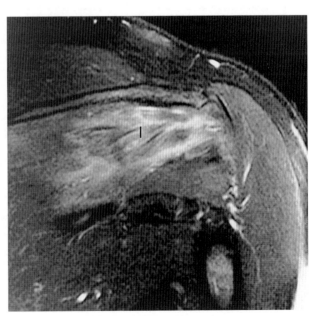

FIG. 14. Denervation atrophy. T2 fast spin-echo (FSE) sagittal image and T2 FSE fat-suppressed coronal image show denervation atrophy of the supraspinatus (S) and infraspinatus (I) muscles. This was due to neuropraxia involving the suprascapular nerve as a result of arthroscopic surgery.

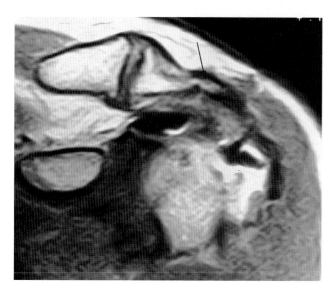

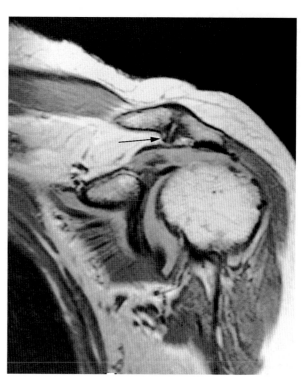

FIG. 15. Recurrent impingement syndrome. Intermediate-weighted coronal image demonstrates an incompletely resected or recurrent subacromial osteophyte *(arrow)* associated with a recurrent rotator cuff tear in a patient who had previously undergone an acromioplasty and rotator cuff repair.

FIG. 17. Acromioclavicular joint osteophytes. Intermediate-weighted coronal image shows inferiorly directed osteophytes *(arrow)* arising from the acromioclavicular joint which resulted in recurrent impingement syndrome and a rotator cuff tear following a remote acromioplasty.

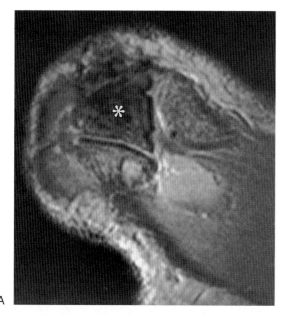

A

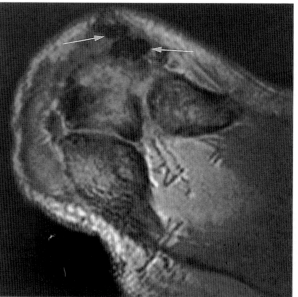

B

FIG. 16. Unstable os acromiale. T2*-weighted axial gradient echo images demonstrate an unfused os acromiale (*) in a 30-year-old man with recurrent impingement syndrome following an open acromioplasty. This diagnosis was missed at the time of the original surgery. Ferromagnetic artifact from the prior acromioplasty is also seen *(arrows)*.

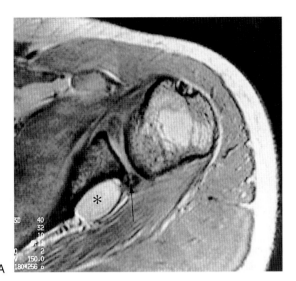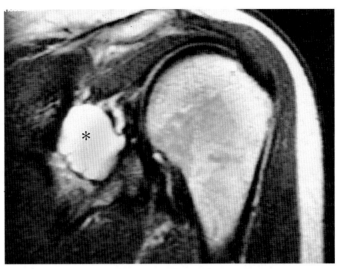

FIG. 18. Posterior labral tear and associated labral cyst. T2*-weighted axial gradient echo image and T2-weighted coronal image in a swimmer who had previously undergone sternoclavicular joint surgery, open acromioplasty, and arthroscopic surgery for unexplained shoulder pain. The subsequent MRI documents the presence of a posterior labral tear *(arrow)* and an associated labral cyst *(*)* extending into the spinoglenoid notch.

ROTATOR CUFF TEARS

For the surgeon, it is extremely important to have an understanding before surgery of the size of the rotator cuff tear, the thickness of the tear, and the condition of the rotator cuff musculature so that adequate preoperative planning can be done. The approach to treatment of these injuries varies greatly according to these factors.

Nonoperative Treatment

Nonoperative treatment includes rest, nonsteroidal antiinflammatory medications, physical therapy, avoidance of activities, and judicious use of subacromial steroid injections. Success of these modalities varies from 33% to 90% (19,20,21). Patients with acute extensions of a chronic tear, less than 1 year of symptoms, and no significant loss of active motion or strength tend to respond best to nonoperative treatment. Younger patients with higher activity levels and all patients with significant functional limitations do not respond as well to nonoperative treatment.

Operative Treatment

Surgical management until recently has required opening the shoulder and direct repair or supplementing the rotator cuff defect (12,22,23). Arthroscopic techniques have evolved that give the surgeon the option of repair using a "mini" incision or a totally arthroscopic repair (13). With large tears, various tendon "substitutions" are available. Surgical manage-

ment may also involve the debridement of the remaining cuff for pain relief. Each of these techniques is described below.

Open Rotator Cuff Repair

In almost all described techniques of rotator cuff repair, acromial decompression is performed. Most patients have a narrowed subacromial outlet so that adequate acromioplasty is required for pain relief (24,25,26). This is done through an anterosuperior approach over the acromion. A small portion of the anterior deltoid insertion on the acromioclavicular joint and the anterolateral acromion is released. The deltoid is then carefully split 3 to 4 cm distally. The distal clavicle is resected only if acromioclavicular arthritis is present or if further exposure of the supraspinatus tendon is needed. The rotator cuff tendons are mobilized and any thickened subacromial bursal material is removed. Significantly retracted tendons may require a release of the tendon with relaxing incisions. The edges of the cuff are freshened with a small area of resection. With most defects, the cuff is then reattached to a trough in the bone in the area of the greater tuberosity. This can be done using the traditional method of heavy nonabsorbable sutures through drill holes (Fig. 19) or with the advent of bone anchor devices the suture can be reattached to the bone using one of these devices (Fig. 20). The bone anchors are usually metallic materials; however, the newer devices are being manufactured using bioabsorbable materials. If a horizontal component is found, then a side-to-side tendon repair is used. The deltoid is then carefully reattached to the acromion through drill holes and to the deltotrapezius fascia.

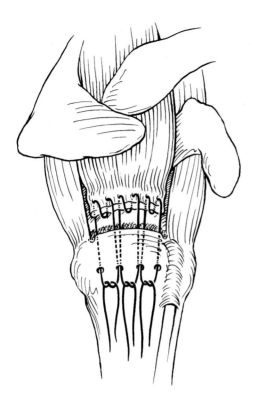

FIG. 19. Tendon-to-bone rotator cuff repair. A trough is formed in the humerus as close as possible to the anatomic insertion site of the torn tendon. The edge of the torn rotator cuff is sutured deep into the trough, using drilled holes and nonabsorbable sutures.

Arthroscopic "Mini" Open Technique

The arthroscopic "mini" open technique combines an arthroscopic and open approach and can be used for smaller cuff tears. Standard arthroscopic portals are used to perform a subacromial decompression and then a lateral incision is performed. Through this incision, the deltoid is not released but is split to expose the greater tuberosity. A trough is then produced in the bone, and the cuff is repaired using standard drill holes and sutures or with suture anchors. Early short-term results are comparable to results of open techniques (27,28).

Arthroscopic Rotator Cuff Repair

Similar to the limited open technique, a subacromial decompression is performed through arthroscopic portals. Using percutaneously placed suture anchors, two point fixation devices, staples, or tied sutures, the rotator cuff is reattached to the bone. This technique is in its early development and is technically demanding. Its use in large chronic tears is limited because of the inability to completely mobilize the cuff or transpose substitute tendons. Early results of smaller tears have been comparable to those of open techniques (27,28); however, long-term follow-up and the lack of ability to repair large tears has limited this technique and it should be used only after careful consideration.

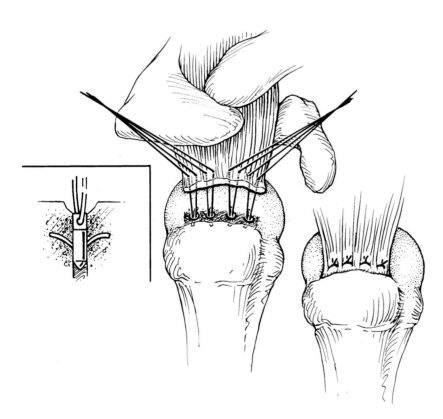

FIG. 20. Tendon-to-bone rotator cuff repair. Suture anchors can also be used to facilitate surgical reattachment of the torn rotator cuff to the humerus.

Surgical Treatment of Massive Cuff Tears

Treatment of large tears that are not amenable to direct repair include subacromial decompression with debridement of the rotator cuff remnants, autogenous or allograft tendon grafts, and local tendon transfers. Rockwood et al. (29) had satisfactory results in 85% of their patients who underwent acromial decompression and debridement of the nonviable rotator cuff tissue. For patients to do well with this technique, a strong deltoid muscle and intact biceps tendon is needed.

Tendon allografts have been tried with variable success (30). In this technique, the allograft is used to fill a large defect and to reattach the remaining cuff tendons to bone. Another option is to transfer a local tendon to fill the defect. Tendons used include the subscapularis, latissimus dorsi, and deltoid. Cofield described the transfer of the subscapularis tendon in defects involving the supraspinatus tendon (31). Latissimus dorsi transfer is used for large tears of the posterior portion of the cuff, teres minor, and infraspinatus (32). Finally, in Europe, the middle deltoid has been used as a transfer (33).

Complications

Review of failed rotator cuff surgeries revealed persistent subacromial impingement in 90% of patients and the presence of a large or massive tear at the index operation in 97% (34). A weak or detached deltoid is also a significant contributor to failure of rotator cuff surgery as it is in subacromial decompressions. Other contributors to failure include infection, denervation of the deltoid muscle (axillary nerve injury), surgical adhesions, denervation of the cuff muscles (suprascapular nerve injury), failure of the repair, subsequent tears in a new area of the cuff, failure of grafts or transfers to heal, and failed rehabilitation. Neurovascular complications resulting from arthroscopy portal placement are of particular concern during arthroscopic procedures (13).

Summary of Surgical Options for Rotator Cuff Tears

Direct suture of the tendon
Suture of the tendon to bone (direct suture versus suture anchors)
Mobilization of the tendons with direct, rotational, or transpositional flaps
Autograft, allograft
Free tendon grafts

Summary of Surgical Techniques for Rotator Cuff Tears

Open rotator cuff repair with subacromial decompression
"Mini" open arthroscopically assisted repair and subacromial decompression
Arthroscopic repair
Acromial decompression with debridement of the rotator cuff

Postoperative Magnetic Resonance Imaging Findings

The postoperative findings on MRI following rotator cuff repair usually include those findings associated with an acromioplasty because this procedure is commonly performed in conjunction with the rotator cuff repair. Additional findings depend on the precise type of cuff repair performed (1,17,18,35). For a tendon-to-tendon or tendon-to-bone rotator cuff repair, intermediate signal intensity is frequently identified within the repaired tendon on T2-weighted images (Fig. 21). This may be due to postoperative granulation tissue, or sutures and can be indistinguishable from tendonitis or a partial thickness rotator cuff tear. There is also frequent loss of the subacromial-subdeltoid fat plane (Fig. 22). Fluid may also be present in the subacromial-subdeltoid bursa. Patients with tendon-to-bone repairs also demonstrate a surgical trough at the site of tenodesis in the humeral head superolaterally (Fig. 23). Ferromagnetic artifact may also be seen at the site of the tendon-to-bone repair (Fig. 24).

The MR findings of general postoperative complications following rotator cuff repair are the same as those following acromioplasty described above. Additional potential complications more specifically related to attempted rotator cuff repair include detachment of the deltoid from the anterolateral acromion, and residual or recurrent rotator cuff tear. Deltoid

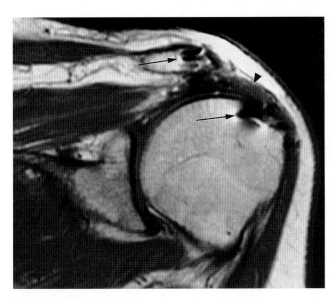

FIG. 21. Intact rotator cuff repair. T2-weighted coronal image demonstrates ferromagnetic artifact *(arrows)* resulting from prior rotator cuff repair and acromioplasty. Intermediate signal intensity is seen in the repaired supraspinatus tendon *(arrowhead)*.

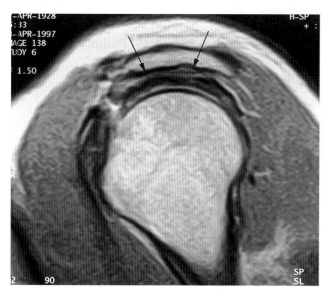

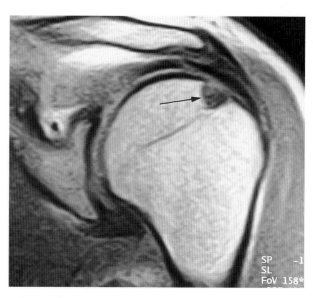

FIG. 22. Intact rotator cuff repair. T2 fast spin-echo sagittal image shows loss of the subacromial-subdeltoid fat plane *(arrows)* following rotator cuff repair, acromioplasty, and coracoacromial ligament release.

FIG. 23. Intact tendon-to-bone rotator cuff repair. Intermediate-weighted coronal image demonstrates a surgical trough *(arrow)* in the humeral head following tendon-to-bone rotator cuff repair.

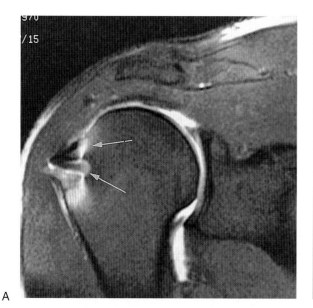

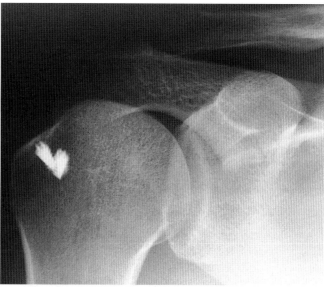

A

B

FIG. 24. Intact suture anchor rotator cuff repair. **A:** T1-weighted fat-suppressed coronal image from a dilute gadolinium arthrogram reveals an intact rotator cuff repair. Ferromagnetic artifact *(arrows)* is caused by metallic suture anchors. **B:** Conventional radiograph (anteroposterior, external rotation) confirms the presence of the metallic suture anchors.

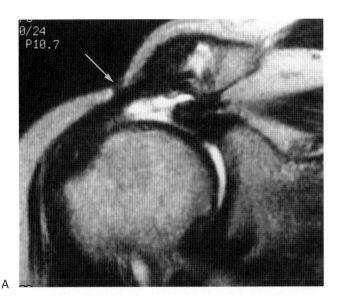

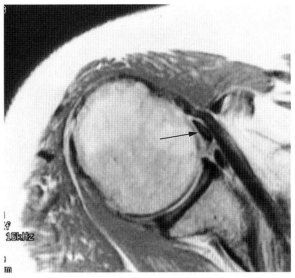

FIG. 25. Recurrent rotator cuff tear with biceps dislocation. **A:** T2 fast spin-echo (FSE) coronal image shows a large recurrent rotator cuff tear with associated retraction. Ferromagnetic artifact is seen *(arrow)*. **B:** Intermediate-weighted axial FSE image demonstrates an associated medial dislocation of the biceps tendon *(arrow)*.

detachments are reliably diagnosed with MRI with an accuracy approaching 100%. If this diagnosis is missed, the deltoid retracts and atrophy becomes irreparable, resulting in considerable disability. Avascular necrosis of the humeral head and rupture or dislocation of the biceps tendon have also been described following rotator cuff repair and are also reliably diagnosed with MRI (36) (Fig. 25).

Owen et al. (17) demonstrated an 86% sensitivity, 92% specificity, and a 90% accuracy for the MR diagnosis of a residual or recurrent full-thickness rotator cuff tear follow-

ing repair of the rotator cuff. Magee et al. (18) reported similar results with an 84% sensitivity and 91% specificity. Diagnostic MR criteria include focal full-thickness fluid signal intensity in the tendon or complete nonvisualization of a portion of the cuff on T2-weighted images (Figs. 26 and 27). Care must be taken not to confuse ferromagnetic artifact in a repaired tendon for a recurrent rotator cuff tear (Fig. 28). Useful secondary signs include the presence of retraction or atrophy of the involved muscle belly (35) (Fig. 29). Obscuration of the subacromial-subdeltoid fat plane and the pres-

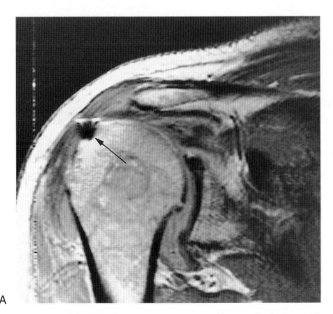

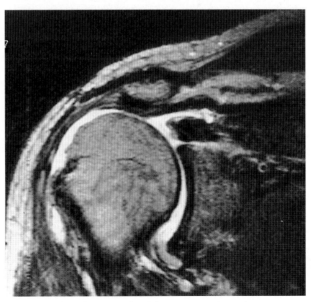

FIG. 26. Recurrent rotator cuff tear. **A:** Intermediate-weighted coronal image demonstrates ferromagnetic artifact *(arrow)* from a prior tendon-to-tendon rotator cuff repair. **B:** T2-weighted coronal image confirms the presence of a large recurrent rotator cuff tear with associated retraction.

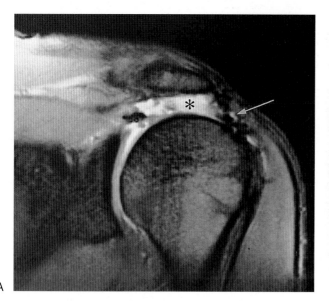
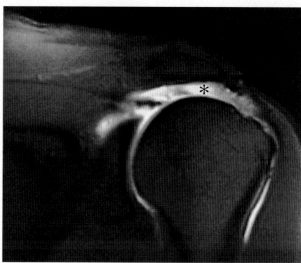

A   B

FIG. 27. Recurrent rotator cuff tear. Spoiled gradient echo coronal image and T1-weighted fat-suppressed coronal image from a dilute gadolinium arthrogram reveal ferromagnetic artifact from a prior tendon-to-tendon rotator cuff repair *(arrow)* and a large recurrent tear of the supraspinatus tendon, which is filled with contrast *(*)*.

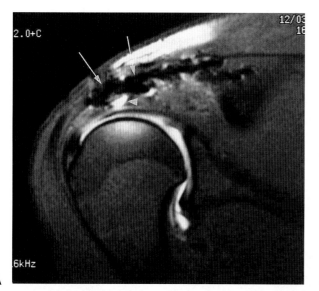
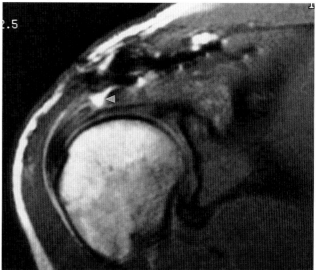

A   B

FIG. 28. Pseudo-tear of the rotator cuff resulting from ferromagnetic artifact. **A:** T1-weighted fat-suppressed coronal image from a dilute gadolinium arthrogram shows ferromagnetic artifact from a prior acromioplasty *(arrows)* and focal contrast signal intensity in the supraspinatus tendon *(arrowhead)* simulating a partial thickness rotator cuff tear. **B:** T1-weighted coronal image without contrast 1 week later confirms that this finding represents ferromagnetic artifact *(arrowhead)*. The rotator cuff is intact.

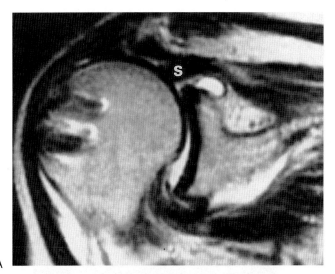

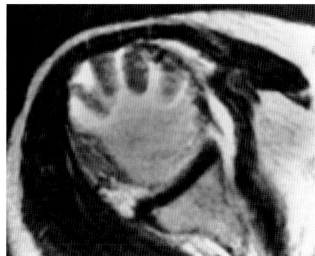

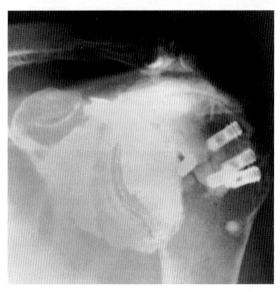

FIG. 29. Recurrent rotator cuff tear following suture anchor repair. **A** and **B:** T2-weighted coronal and axial images from a saline arthrogram demonstrate ferromagnetic artifacts in the humeral head from multiple metallic suture anchors. A large recurrent full-thickness tear of the supraspinatus tendon (S) is seen on the coronal image. **C:** A spot view from a conventional arthrogram confirms the presence of metallic suture anchors.

ence of fluid in the subacromial-subdeltoid bursa are of little usefulness in the assessment of the rotator cuff following surgery (17). MRI also does not reliably distinguish between expected postoperative changes following rotator cuff repair and residual or recurrent partial thickness tears of the rotator cuff. Magee et al. (18) found a sensitivity and specificity of 83% for the diagnosis of a partial thickness tear following rotator cuff repair; however, the positive predictive value was only 56%. The negative predictive value was 95%.

It is important to note that MR arthrography may reveal communication between the glenohumeral joint and the subacromial-subdeltoid bursa in the context of a clinically adequate rotator cuff repair (Fig. 30). In other words, a repaired rotator cuff need not be watertight to be functional (17). This may be due to interruption of the rotator interval (between the supraspinatus and subscapularis tendons) at surgery. Conversely, postoperative adhesions and granulation tissue may prevent the leakage of contrast material from the glenohumeral joint across a rotator cuff tear into the subacromial-subdeltoid bursa (17).

INSTABILITY

Classification

Glenohumeral instability can be classified on the basis of direction (anterior, posterior, inferior, or multidirectional), etiology (macrotrauma, repetitive microtrauma, or atraumatic), and degree of instability (dislocation or subluxation).

Anterior instability of the glenohumeral joint is the most common direction of shoulder instability and represents approximately 95% of cases (37). Rowe (38) reported on a series of 500 shoulder dislocations, of which 96% were the result of a major traumatic event and 98% occurred in the anterior direction. The incidence of posterior dislocations is estimated to be 2% to 3% and these dislocations are frequently locked with the humeral head trapped behind the glenoid. Posterior dislocations are usually the result of vehicular trauma, seizures, electroshock therapy, or prior shoulder surgery. Superior and inferior dislocations of the humeral head are quite uncommon and the result of severe

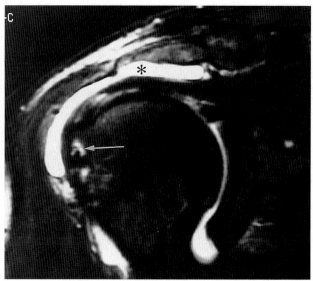

FIG. 30. Intact, but not watertight, rotator cuff repair. T1-weighted fat-suppressed coronal image from a dilute gadolinium arthrogram and T2 fast spin-echo fat-suppressed coronal image reveal ferromagnetic artifact from a prior rotator cuff repair *(arrows)*. Dilute gadolinium is identified in the subacromial-sub-deltoid bursa *(*)* despite the presence of an intact rotator cuff at repeat surgery.

trauma. Patients with multidirectional instability (MDI) have symptomatic inferior as well as anterior and/or posterior instability. Most patients with MDI demonstrate generalized ligamentous laxity and frequently have bilateral shoulder complaints and a history of trivial or no trauma.

Treatment of Recurrent Anterior Instability

Nonoperative

Conservative treatment of an acute instability episode (dislocation or subluxation) begins with a period of extremity rest and pain control with nonsteroidal antiinflammatory drugs. A

rehabilitation program that emphasizes regaining full range of motion and strengthening the dynamic stabilizers (rotator cuff and periscapular muscles) is then prescribed. Rockwood (39) has reported that 80% of patients with atraumatic anterior instability and 90% of those with posterior instability have successfully responded to such a nonoperative rehabilitation program. However, only 12% of patients with traumatic anterior instability had successful nonoperative treatment.

Operative Treatment (Open Procedures)

Surgical stabilization of the glenohumeral joint is reserved for those patients who, after an adequate trial of conservative treatment, continue to experience instability, pain, apprehen-

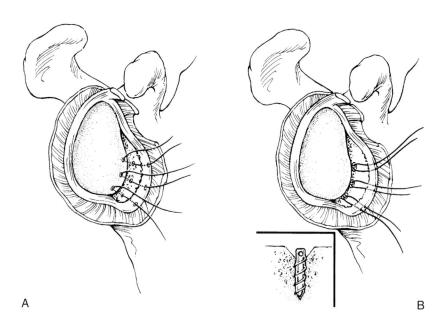

FIG. 31. A: Bankart repair with transglenoid drilling. The anterior labrum and joint capsule are reattached securely to the glenoid rim with sutures passed through drilled holes in the osseous glenoid. **B.** Suture anchor Bankart repair. Suturing is accomplished through approximately three suture anchors placed in the osseous glenoid.

sion, or loss of shoulder function. More than 30 open surgical procedures have been described for the treatment of anterior shoulder instability; however, many are of historical interest only. Open procedures can be grouped as capsulolabral repairs, subscapularis muscle procedures, coracoid transfers, and bone block procedures.

Capsular Repairs

Although Bankart is widely credited as the first to repair a torn anterior labrum back to the glenoid rim in 1923 (40), Perthes in 1906 actually recommended repair of the torn labrum to the glenoid. In any case, it has become accepted that tearing of the anterior labrum and the loss of the labral anchor for insertion of the inferior glenohumeral ligament complex is responsible for chronic anterior instability (37,41). The classical description of a *Bankart repair* is to repair the torn capsule back to the glenoid rim through drill holes in the margin of the glenoid (Fig. 31*A*). Recently, suture anchors have simplified the procedure by obviating the need for drill holes (see Fig. 31*B*). Instead, the anchors are placed along the articular margin of the glenoid (usually at the 3-, 4-, and 5-'o clock positions) and the capsule is tied down to these anchors. In addition to repairing the torn labrum, many surgeons also perform a capsulorrhaphy of the stretched out and redundant capsule, which is often seen in cases of recurrent anterior instability (Fig. 32). The Bankart

procedure with or without a capsulorrhaphy remains the gold standard operative procedure for anterior glenohumeral instability. Recurrent instability rates are 0% to 5% following a well-done Bankart procedure (42).

In 1956, *DuToit* described reattachment of the capsule back to the glenoid using metallic staples (43). In effect, this is similar to the original Bankart repair; however, loosening, migration, or penetration of cartilage by the staples can lead to severe arthritic complications.

Subscapularis Procedures

The *Putti-Platt procedure* involves the division of the subscapularis tendon approximately 1 inch medial to its humeral insertion. The lateral tendon stump is then sutured to the anterior glenoid rim and the medial subscapularis tendon and muscle are double breasted over the lateral stump. Thus, considerable shortening of the subscapularis and underlying capsule is achieved. This procedure results in significant loss of external rotation. Recurrence rates of 2% to 10% are reported, and early degenerative arthritic change has also been observed.

Transfer of the subscapularis tendon laterally from its lesser tuberosity insertion to the greater tuberosity was first described by *Magnuson and Stack* in 1940. The rationale for the procedure was to enhance the dynamic stabilizing force of the subscapularis on the humeral head. Instability recur-

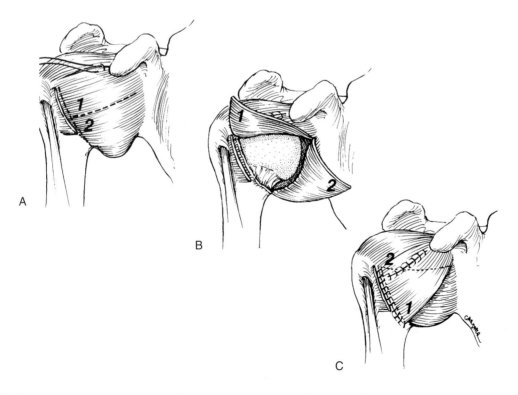

FIG. 32. Anterior capsulorrhaphy (capsular shift procedure). **A:** A T-shaped incision is placed in the anterior capsule. **B** and **C:** The superior and inferior flaps are overlapped and reattached, tightening and reinforcing the anterior capsule.

rence rates are low; however, the procedure has been associated with a loss of external rotation and with iatrogenic posterior subluxation and even dislocation of the humeral head from over tightening.

Coracoid Transfer

Osteotomy of the tip of the coracoid process and transfer to the anteroinferior glenoid margin where it is reattached with a screw is called the *Bristow procedure*. Various modifications to the original procedure have been described; however, the basics of the procedure are unchanged. It is believed that stability is achieved by a bone block effect as well as static and dynamic reinforcement of the anterior capsule. Instability rates following this procedure range from 5% to 13%. Non-union of the coracoid process to the glenoid rim, screw breakage, and migration are frequent problems with this procedure.

Bone Block

In the *Eden-Hybbinette procedure*, a block of iliac crest bone is transferred and secured to the anterior glenoid in an attempt to extend or deepen the glenoid cavity. This procedure is no longer routinely used unless there is a significant loss of anterior glenoid bone. A high rate of degenerative arthritic change caused by the nonphysiologic contact between the humeral head and bone block has been observed.

Arthroscopic Procedures

Johnson first performed arthroscopic staple capsulorrhaphy in the early 1980s and since then there has been tremendous interest and research in advancing arthroscopic shoulder procedures. Arthroscopically assisted stabilization procedures are less invasive, cause less perioperative pain, and can be performed in an outpatient setting. Unfortunately, the risk of recurrent instability following arthroscopic stabilization is higher than after an open procedure in most reports (44,45). Recurrence rates of 5% to 35% following arthroscopic procedures are reported. Recurrence rates have been particularly high for collision athletes such as football players. However, arthroscopic stabilization shows great promise in the treatment of throwing athletes such as baseball pitchers, by preserving a greater degree of shoulder motion, which is necessary in order to return to pitching.

At present, three arthroscopic techniques are used to manage anterior instability with capsular detachment: transglenoid suture technique, suture anchors, and a biodegradable tac made of polyglyconate.

Transglenoid Suture Technique

In the transglenoid suture technique, the torn labrum or capsule is reapplied to the anterior glenoid rim using horizontal mattress sutures, which are drilled from anterior to posterior through the scapula. A separate incision is then made posteriorly to tie the sutures over the infraspinatus fascia. Potential pitfalls of this technique are (a) failure to adequately decorticate the anterior glenoid rim and neck down to bleeding bone so the repaired capsule will heal to the bone, (b) repair of the torn labrum too medial on the scapular neck rather than at the articular margin, and (c) possible entrapment of the suprascapular nerve when tying the sutures over the infraspinatus muscle.

Suture Anchors

Over the past 5 years, there has been an explosion of interest in suture anchor devices for both open and arthroscopic surgery (see Fig. 31*B*). The first of these was the Mitek suture anchor (Mitek, Norwood, MA) (13). There are now several devices available that are similar in concept—the metallic anchor is buried in the bone with a suture attached to an eyelet on the anchor. The suture can then be used to tie down the torn soft tissue to the underlying bone. Thus, the arthroscopic application of these anchors in the case of a Bankart lesion is quite similar to the use of these anchors in an open repair. The difference being the anchors are placed through arthroscopic cannulas. The BioTak suture anchor (Concept, Inc., Largo, FL) is constructed of a long-lasting polylactide polymer that maintains its strength for 6 months and is resorbable.

Bioabsorbable Tac

To simplify the technical difficulties of transglenoid drilling and the arthroscopic placement and suture tying of suture anchors, a biodegradable tac made of polyglyconate has been developed (Acufex Microsurgical Inc., Mansfield, MA) (Fig. 33). In this technique, the torn capsulolabral tissue is advanced to the glenoid articular margin and tacked in place with two or three of these absorbable devices. The tacs are degraded over the next 4 to 6 weeks as capsular healing is completed.

Capsular Plication

In addition to the arthroscopic repair of Bankart lesions, several arthroscopic surgeons are also devising techniques to perform arthroscopic capsulorrhaphy using absorbable sutures as well as holium lasers. The long-term results of these procedures are presently unknown.

Complications

Any surgical procedure, arthroscopic or open, carries with it potential risks. The more common complications associated with surgical repairs for anterior shoulder instability in-

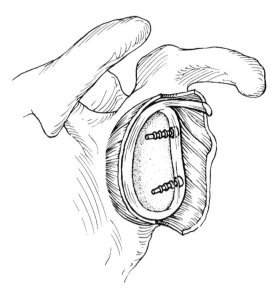

FIG. 33. Bankart repair with bioabsorbable tacs. The anterior labrum and capsular structures are reattached to the glenoid with two or three bioabsorbable tacs.

clude postoperative infection (less than 1%); recurrent anterior instability ranging from redislocation to subtle degrees of subluxation; neurovascular injury (the axillary and musculocutaneous nerves are at particular risk); metallic hardware complications including loosening, breakage, migration, and impingement; and the loss of glenohumeral motion (especially external rotation with the Magnuson-Stack, Putti-Platt, and Bristow procedures). Snyder states that no aspect of shoulder arthroscopy is more apt to result in complications than the surgical procedures for shoulder instability.

Summary of Anterior Glenohumeral Stabilization Procedures

Open techniques
  Extraarticular
    Bristow—coracoid transfer to anterior glenoid rim
    Putti-Platt—imbrication of subscapularis and capsule

Magnuson-Stack—lateral transfer of subscapularis tendon
    Eden-Hybbinette—bone block transfer to anterior glenoid rim
  Intraarticular
    Bankart—anatomic repair of labrum and capsule to glenoid
    Capsular shift—imbrication of the anterior capsule
    DuToit—repair of labrum and capsule with metal staple
Arthroscopic techniques
    Bankart repair—transglenoid sutures, suture anchors, absorbable tac
    Capsular plication—sutures, holium laser

Treatment of Recurrent Posterior Instability

Nonoperative

Patients with recurrent posterior instability must be carefully evaluated for evidence of generalized ligamentous laxity, connective tissue disorders such as Ehlers-Danlos syndrome, and MDI of the shoulder. Patients with voluntary instability need psychological evaluation. All patients with posterior instability should first undergo an aggressive shoulder strengthening program because a high percentage of patients with posterior instability respond to nonoperative treatment (39).

Operative Treatment (Open Procedures) for Posterior Instability

Posterior T-Plasty Capsulorrhaphy

Whereas the posterior capsule is not nearly as robust as the anterior glenohumeral capsule, particularly in the upper half of the capsule, the lower portion, which is reinforced by the posterior band of the inferior glenohumeral ligament, is usually quite substantial. A reefing of the posterior capsule has been described by Bowen and colleagues (46) with satisfactory results (Fig. 34). In addition to the capsular tightening,

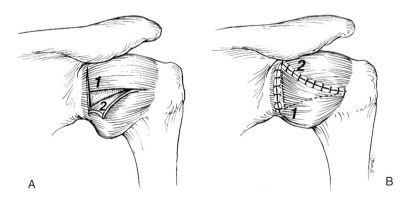

A   B

FIG. 34. Posterior capsulorrhaphy. A posterior capsule imbrication is performed consisting of a T-plasty capsulorrhaphy analogous to the anterior capsular shift procedure.

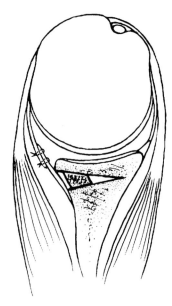

FIG. 35. Glenoid osteotomy. A wedge osteotomy with bone grafting is performed, improving glenoid version.

the joint is inspected for a reverse Bankart lesion of the posterior labrum, which, if present, is repaired in a manner analogous to the Bankart procedure for anterior labral tears. Rockwood (12) has also described a posterior capsular shift procedure that imbricates the posterior capsule with excellent results.

Posterior Glenoid Osteotomy

Version of the glenoid articular surface averages 6 degrees of retroversion (47). When glenoid version of greater than 25 to 30 degrees of retroversion exists in a patient with posterior instability, then consideration of osteotomizing the glenoid and bone grafting to correct the excessive retroversion can be entertained (Fig. 35). This osteotomy can be performed in conjunction with a posterior capsular procedure.

Posterior Bone Block

Rather than an opening wedge osteotomy of the glenoid, a posterior block of bone (analogous to the Eden-Hybbinette procedure) can be internally fixed to the posterior glenoid margin to help contain the humeral head in cases of severe posterior glenoid deficiency (Fig. 36).

Arthroscopic Treatment

The arthroscopic treatment of posterior instability continues to evolve with improved techniques and materials. The treatment of reverse Bankart lesions with absorbable tacs and suture anchors has recently been used; however, the results are very short term. Arthroscopic posterior capsular plication with sutures and the holium laser has also been reported.

Complications

The principal complication following a posterior shoulder procedure is recurrent posterior instability. As the patient regains postoperative motion, the posterior soft tissues stretch out and, unless good dynamic (muscular) stability is regained, dependence on the posterior capsule continues and it may ultimately fail, leading to recurrent instability. Rarely, the opposite can occur, for example, a very tight posterior reconstruction can cause the humeral head to be pushed out anteriorly.

Posterior glenoid osteotomy is technically a demanding procedure, and cracking or fracture of the articular surface can occur, giving rise to postoperative osteoarthritic changes. Excessive anteverting of the glenoid surface can cause anterior instability. Posterior bone blocks placed in too prominent a position can lead to severe degenerative joint changes. The axillary nerve is at risk as it exits the quadrangular space, and the suprascapular nerve can be injured in the spinoglenoid notch.

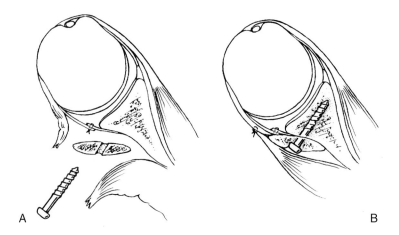

A   B

FIG. 36. Posterior bone block. A bone graft harvested from the iliac crest is internally fixed to the posterior glenoid.

Summary of Posterior Glenohumeral Stabilization Procedures

Open techniques

> Reverse Bankart repair—anatomic repair of torn posterior labrum
>
> T-Plasty capsulorrhaphy—imbrication of posterior capsule
>
> Glenoid osteotomy—opening wedge osteotomy of glenoid to decrease retroversion
>
> Bone block—internal fixation of iliac crest bone graft to posterior glenoid rim

Arthroscopic

> Reverse Bankart repair—suture anchors or absorbable tac
>
> Posterior capsular plication—sutures or laser

Treatment of Multidirectional Instability (MDI)

Patients with MDI of the shoulder have, by definition, inferior instability as well as anterior and/or posterior instability. Many of these patients (50% or more) exhibit generalized ligamentous laxity. Most have no history of a major traumatic event; however, some have either a history of repetitive microtrauma or minor trauma. All of these patients should first be treated with an aggressive rehabilitation program designed to strengthen the internal and external rotator muscles. Failure to respond to such a program after 6 to 8 months leads to consideration of surgery.

Operative Treatment

The operative approach chosen depends on the direction of greatest instability. In other words, if the clinical diagnosis reveals primarily anteroinferior instability, then a capsular shift procedure that plicates the anterior and inferior glenohumeral capsule is performed. Alternatively, if the direction of instability is posteroinferior, then the posterior capsule is approached. Rarely, both anterior and posterior procedures are necessary. Most authorities advocate open capsulorrhaphy for patients with MDI; however, some arthroscopists are performing anterior and posterior arthroscopic capsular plications by either a suture or laser technique.

Postoperative Magnetic Resonance Imaging Findings

There is a paucity of published scientific work dealing with the issue of MRI of the glenohumeral joint following

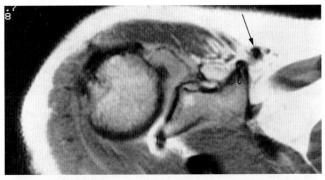
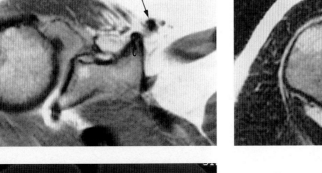
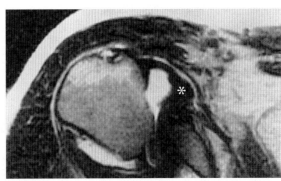
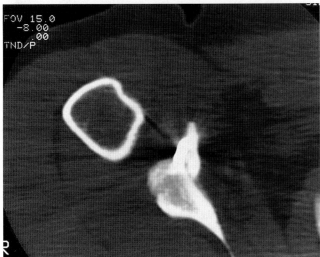

FIG. 37. Bristow procedure. **A:** Intermediate-weighted fast spin-echo (FSE) axial image from a saline arthrogram demonstrates a truncated coracoid process (C) with ferromagnetic artifact *(arrow)* near the coracoid tip. **B:** T2 FSE axial image demonstrates low signal intensity at the site of the coracoid transfer *(*)* to the anteroinferior glenoid. **C:** Axial computed tomography image confirms screw fixation of the coracoid transfer.

surgery for instability. In fact, there are currently no scientifically valid published studies addressing MRI of the shoulder in this patient population. The following discussion is, therefore, anecdotal.

There are MRI findings that suggest a prior history of specific glenohumeral stabilization surgeries. A shortened coracoid process with associated ferromagnetic artifact at the anteroinferior glenoid suggests a history of a prior Bristow procedure (see Fig. 4 and Fig. 37). Shortening and thickening of the subscapularis tendon suggests a previous Putti-Platt procedure or Magnuson-Stack procedure. The presence of grafted bone and ferromagnetic artifact at the anterior glenoid suggests a prior Eden-Hybbinette procedure. If there is ferromagnetic artifact within the anteroinferior osseous

glenoid, this suggests a history of either a DuToit procedure or a Bankart repair using metallic suture anchors (Figs. 38 and 39). If a transglenoid suture technique was used for a Bankart repair, then the drill hole tracts may be visible on MRI. If bioabsorbable tacs were used, normal marrow signal ultimately refills the predrilled holes in the glenoid as the tac is bioabsorbed (Fig. 40). Similar findings can be seen associated with the corresponding posterior stabilization surgeries (Fig. 41). In all cases, correlation with conventional radiograph findings and detailed surgical history is recommended.

Based on the growing body of evidence supporting the use of MR arthrography for the evaluation of glenohumeral instability before surgical intervention (2), this technique is

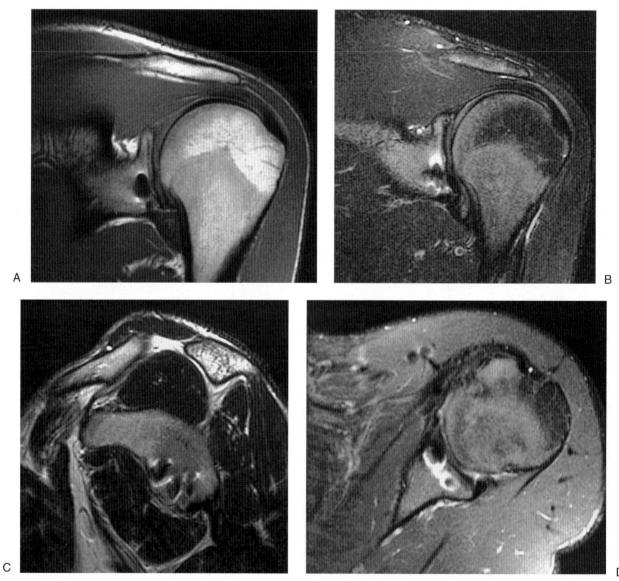

FIG. 38. Intact open Bankart repair with metallic suture anchors. T1-weighted coronal image, T2 fast spin-echo (FSE) fat-suppressed coronal image, T2 FSE sagittal image, and intermediate-weighted FSE axial image show multiple ferromagnetic artifacts involving the anteroinferior quadrant of the glenoid resulting from an open Bankart repair using three metallic suture anchors.

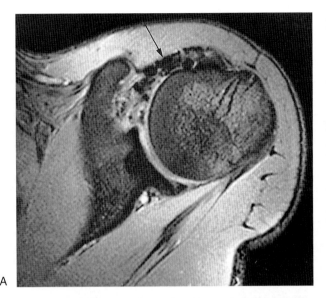

A

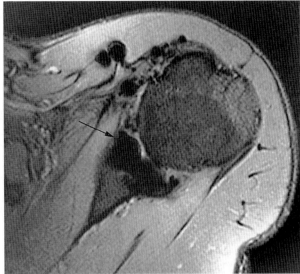

B

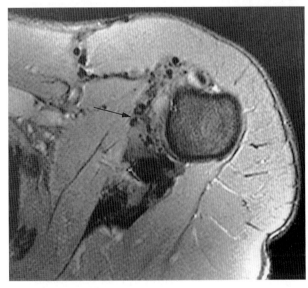

C

FIG. 39. Intact open Bankart repair and anterior capsulor-rhaphy. T2*-weighted gradient echo axial images demonstrate ferromagnetic artifact *(arrows)* along the anterior capsular structures and anteroinferior glenoid resulting from prior anterior capsular shift surgery in conjunction with an open Bankart repair.

also recommended for the postoperative assessment of patients who are seen with recurrent shoulder pain or instability following a surgical stabilization procedure. This is to facilitate evaluation of the dynamic stabilizers (i.e., the rotator cuff), which are extraarticular, as well as the static stabilizers (i.e., the glenohumeral ligaments and glenoid labrum), which are intraarticular (Fig. 42). In current practice, the orthopedic surgeon's decision to reoperate is usually based on the clinical history, physical examination, and conventional radiographs; however, MR arthrography is gaining more widespread use in this clinical setting.

In addition to the MR findings associated with general postoperative complications such as infection and hematoma formation, there are MR findings associated with more specific complications of prior surgical stabilization of the shoulder. Recurrent instability is one of the most common complications following a surgical stabilization procedure (12,13). Palmer et al. (48) have presented results of a study

assessing the MR arthrographic findings in recurrent shoulder instability following an anterior stabilization procedure. Twenty-three patients with a history of recurrent pain and instability following anterior stabilization surgery were imaged with MR arthrography as part of a larger study. The study was blinded and retrospective in design. All 23 patients underwent a second surgical procedure, the results of which served as the gold standard. At surgery, 20 of the patients (87%) demonstrated evidence of instability—seven were anterior in direction, eight were multidirectional, and five were posterior in direction. Other surgical findings included 15 failed surgical repairs (65%) and 14 posterior labral tears (61%). On MR arthrography, intraarticular contrast material extending through the inferior glenohumeral ligament labral complex at the site of a prior Bankart repair was the diagnostic criterion for a residual or recurrent Bankart lesion (Figs. 43 through 46). A similar finding involving the posterior labrum was the basis for diagnosing a

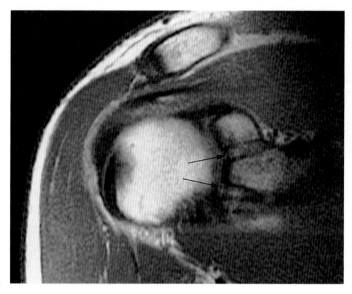
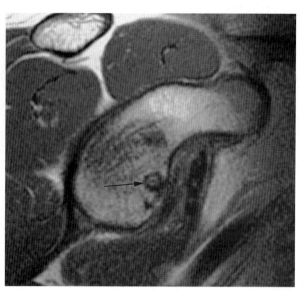

A   B

FIG. 40. Intact Bankart repair with bioabsorbable tacs. T1-weighted coronal and sagittal images reveal normal marrow signal within the tracts of bioabsorbable tacs *(arrows)* placed 1 year previously as part of a Bankart repair. The tacs have been resorbed, leaving only their original tracts, which are filled with normal-appearing bone marrow on magnetic resonance imaging.

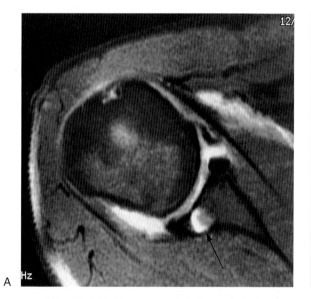
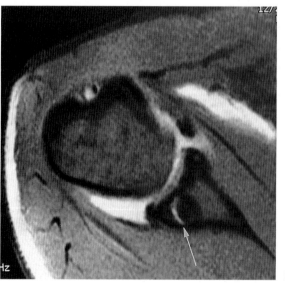

A   B

FIG. 41. Intact reverse Bankart repair. T1-weighted fat-suppressed axial images from a dilute gadolinium arthrogram show ferromagnetic artifact involving the posterior glenoid *(arrows)* resulting from a reverse Bankart repair. The repair appears intact.

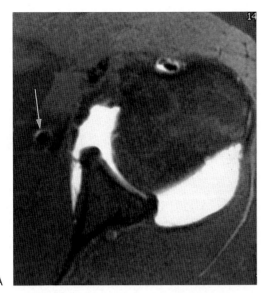
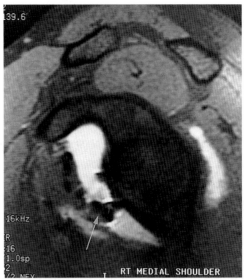

FIG. 42. Magnetic resonance arthrogram of an intact Bankart repair. T1-weighted fat-suppressed axial and sagittal images from a dilute gadolinium arthrogram demonstrate an intact anteroinferior labrum following a Bankart repair. Ferromagnetic artifact is seen in the anterior soft tissues *(arrow)*.

posterior labral tear (Fig. 47). MR arthrography demonstrated a 93% sensitivity and 88% specificity for the diagnosis of a failed repair, and an 86% sensitivity and 89% specificity for the diagnosis of a posterior labral tear. In summary, this study suggests that MR arthrography accurately assesses the symptomatic shoulder following anterior stabilization surgery and that both failed repairs and posterior labral tears account for residual or recurrent instability.

Other instability patterns are seen as a complication of prior shoulder stabilization surgery. If the subscapularis shortening is excessive, associated with a Putti-Platt, or associated with a Magnuson-Stack procedure, an overly tight anterior capsule may result in posterior subluxation of the humeral head. This can occur even in patients who did not have posterior instability preoperatively (42). Posterior glenoid osteotomy for posterior instability can result in anterior instability in an analogous fashion. This is usually due to excessive anteverting of the glenoid articular surface. Careful attention to the position of the humeral head relative to the glenoid is necessary on the axial MR images to avoid missing subtle glenohumeral subluxation (see Fig. 45A). MRI in provocative positions such as the abducted externally rotated position can also facilitate evaluation for subtle instability (2).

Because many of the shoulder stabilization surgical procedures involve the use of metal devices, loosening, breakage, or migration of the hardware into the intraarticular space can occur. These complications are readily diagnosed on conventional radiographs, but can be difficult to accurately assess on MRI because of associated ferromagnetic artifact.

Finally, secondary osteoarthritis is an important potential complication of these procedures. Possible causes include migration of orthopedic devices into the joint, altered joint

biomechanics, damage to the articular cartilage at the time of surgery, or loss of articular surface congruity as a result of the procedure.

MRI findings associated with this complication include focal or diffuse loss of articular cartilage, joint space narrowing, marginal osteophyte formation, and a spectrum of subchondral signal alteration representing edema, sclerosis, and cyst formation (Fig. 48). Osteochondral loose body formation can result.

SLAP LESIONS

The SLAP lesion as defined by Snyder et al. (13) consists of an injury to the superior labrum extending from anterior to posterior. The superior labrum is defined as the segment of labrum between the 10-o'clock and 2-o'clock positions of the glenoid. Usual mechanisms of injury include throwing and pitching, a fall onto an outstretched arm, or as a component of glenohumeral osteoarthritis. SLAP lesions are classified on the basis of the morphology of the injury and any associated injury of the biceps tendon anchor (13). The type I lesion consists of fraying and degeneration of the superior labrum with a normal biceps tendon anchor. The type II lesion demonstrates pathologic detachment of the superior labrum and biceps anchor from the superior glenoid with possible fraying of the superior labrum. The type III lesion presents with a vertical tear through a meniscoid-like superior labrum, producing a bucket-handle lesion that may displace into the glenohumeral joint. The biceps tendon anchor remains intact. Type IV lesions consist of a tear of the superior meniscoid-like labrum that extends into the biceps tendon. The biceps anchor and the remainder of the superior

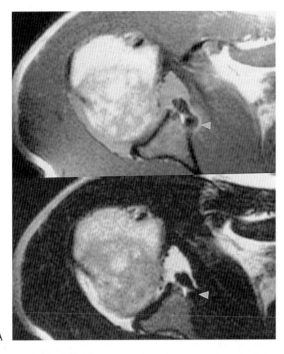

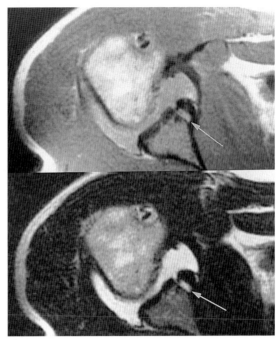

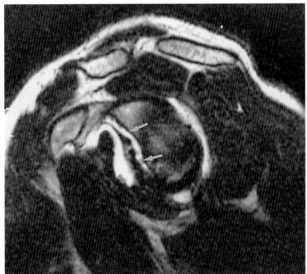

FIG. 43. Recurrent Bankart lesion. **A** and **B:** Paired intermediate and T2-weighted axial images from a saline arthrogram reveal ferromagnetic artifact involving the anteroinferior glenoid *(arrowheads)* resulting from a previous Bankart repair. A recurrent tear through the base of the anteroinferior labrum is well seen *(arrows)*. A longitudinal split of the biceps tendon is also seen on image **(B)**. **C:** T2-weighted sagittal image confirms the presence of a recurrent Bankart lesion *(arrows)*.

labrum remain well attached to the superior glenoid. Complex lesions include any combination of two or more other types of SLAP lesions. Most commonly this consists of a type II and a type IV lesion.

Operative Treatment

The treatment of SLAP lesions depends on the age of the patient, the clinical presentation, and the type of SLAP lesion present (13). For example, the presence of a type I SLAP lesion in an elderly patient may be seen as a component of osteoarthritis. When the superior labrum is frayed in a younger individual, however, it may be considered the primary disease and may be symptomatic. Treatment in this set-

ting consists of surgically shaving and debriding the degenerative tissue to remove any source of joint irritation or possible catching. The treatment of type II SLAP lesions is surgical reattachment of the labrum to the superior glenoid similar to the treatment of Bankart lesions in the context of instability. This may be accomplished with use of suture anchors, bioabsorbable tacs, and so on. Type III SLAP lesions occur only with a meniscoid-type labrum; therefore, it is adequate to simply debride the loose labral fragment with standard arthroscopic basket punches and mechanical shaving devices. The treatment of type IV lesions requires that both the biceps tendon and labrum be addressed. In a young patient, if the segment of damaged biceps tendon is small, the torn tissue is simply resected. If the torn segment is substantial (>30% of the thickness), then suture repair should be at-

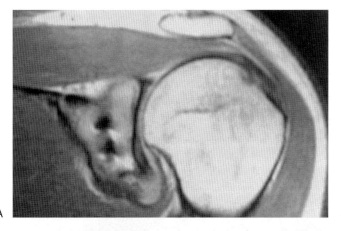

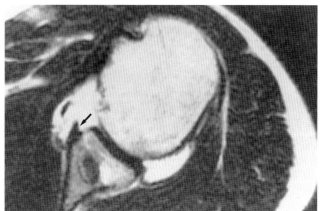

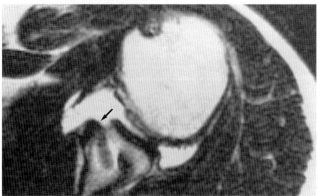

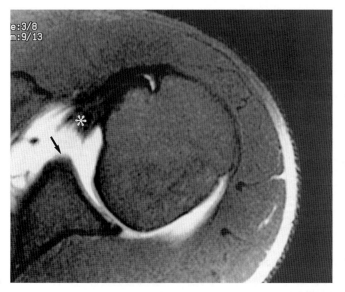

FIG. 44. Recurrent anterior labroligamentous periosteal sleeve avulsion (ALPSA) lesion. **A:** Intermediate-weighted coronal image from a saline arthrogram demonstrates ferromagnetic artifact from a Bankart repair using suture anchors. **B** and **C:** T2-weighted axial images also demonstrate a medially displaced recurrent ALPSA lesion *(arrows)*.

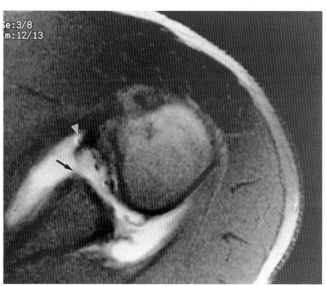

FIG. 45. Recurrent Bankart lesion and subscapularis tear. T1-weighted fat-suppressed axial images from a dilute gadolinium arthrogram show absence of the anteroinferior labrum *(arrows)* consistent with a recurrent Bankart lesion. There is also a full-thickness tear of the subscapularis tendon through which contrast extends *(*)*. Ferromagnetic artifact from a prior Bankart repair is also seen *(arrowhead)*.

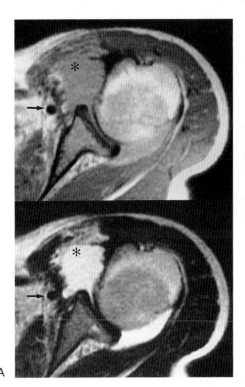

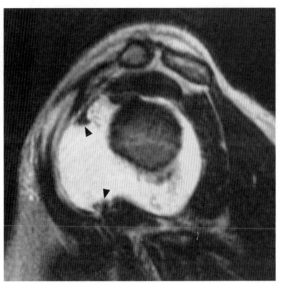

FIG. 46. Failed capsulorrhaphy. **A:** Paired intermediate and T2-weighted axial images from a saline arthrogram reveal ferromagnetic artifact from a prior anterior capsulorrhaphy *(arrows)*. Saline extends through the anterior capsular structures *(*)* because of traumatic failure of the capsulorrhaphy. **B:** T2-weighted sagittal image also demonstrates the margins of the disrupted anterior capsule *(arrowheads)*.

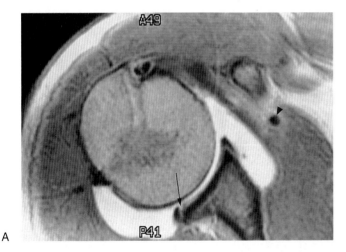

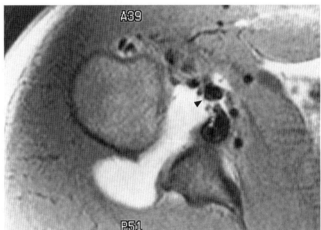

FIG. 47. Posterior labral tear associated with a prior Bankart repair. T1-weighted fat-suppressed axial images from a dilute gadolinium arthrogram demonstrate ferromagnetic artifact resulting from a previous Bankart repair *(arrowheads)*. Linear contrast extends through the base of the posterior labrum, reflecting a posterior labral tear *(arrow)*. A longitudinal split is also noted involving the tendon for the long head of the biceps within the bicipital groove.

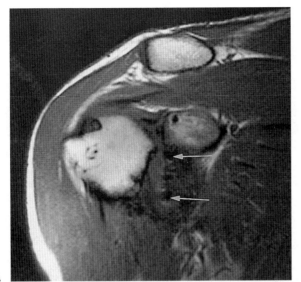

A

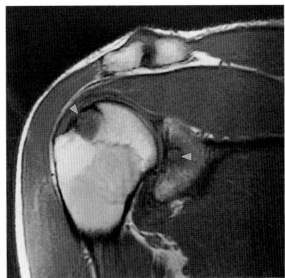

B

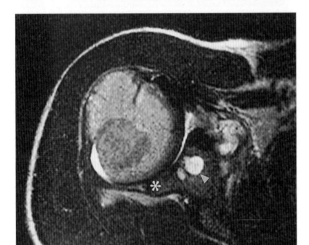

C

FIG. 48. Osteoarthritis following a Bankart repair. **A:** T1-weighted coronal image shows ferromagnetic artifact resulting from a previous Bankart repair *(arrows)*. **B and C:** T1-weighted coronal image and T2-weighted axial image demonstrate subchondral cyst (geode) formation *(arrowheads)* as well as remodeling and osteophyte formation involving the posterior glenoid as seen on the axial image *(*)*. The humeral head is also subtly subluxed posteriorly on the axial image.

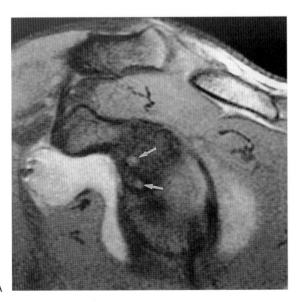

A

FIG. 49. Intact SLAP repair. **A:** T1-weighted fat-suppressed sagittal image from a dilute gadolinium arthrogram reveals two tracts in the anterosuperior quadrant of the glenoid *(arrows)* resulting from a previous SLAP lesion repair using two bioabsorbable suture anchors. *(Continued on next page.)*

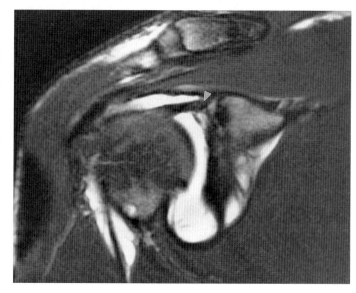

B   C

FIG. 49. *Continued.* **B** and **C**: T2 fast spin-echo fat-suppressed coronal images reveal an intact superior labrum *(arrow)* and an intact biceps anchor *(arrowhead).*

tempted. In an older patient with an intact rotator cuff, primary biceps tenodesis should be considered. Repair of type IV lesions also includes insertion of multiple sutures through the labrum and biceps stump in an attempt to reattach the detached segments.

Postoperative Magnetic Resonance Imaging Findings

The MRI findings following repair of SLAP lesions have not yet been reported. The most common indication for postoperative MRI following a SLAP lesion repair is recurrent

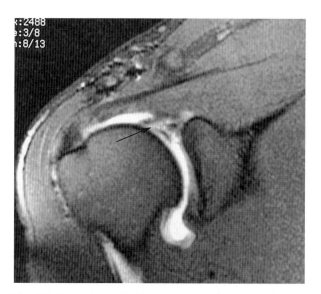

FIG. 50. Recurrent SLAP lesion. T1-weighted fat-suppressed coronal image from a dilute gadolinium arthrogram demonstrates linear contrast extending through the superior labrum *(arrow)* consistent with a recurrent SLAP lesion. The patient is a weight lifter who had undergone a previous SLAP lesion repair.

symptoms, suggesting the possibility of a recurrent SLAP lesion. Currently, dilute gadolinium MR arthrography is used for this evaluation. The criteria used for the MR arthrographic diagnosis of a recurrent SLAP lesion are similar to those used for diagnosing a recurrent labral tear following a Bankart repair (Figs. 49 and 50).

REFERENCES

1. Haygood TM, Oxner KG, Kneeland JB, Dalinka MK. Magnetic resonance imaging of the postoperative shoulder. *MRI Clin North Am* 1993;1:143–155.
2. Feller JF, Tirman PFJ, Steinbach LS, Zucconi F. Magnetic resonance imaging of the shoulder: review. *Semin Roentgenol* 1995;30:224.
3. Bigliani LU, Morrison D, April EW. The morphology of the acromion and its relationship to rotator cuff tears. *Orthop Trans* 1986;10:228.
4. Berry H, Fernandez L, Bloom B, et al. Clinical study comparing acupuncture, physiotherapy, injection and oral anti-inflammatory therapy in rotator cuff lesions. *Curr Med Res Opin* 1980;7 (2):121–126.
5. Neer CS II. Impingement lesions. *Clin Orthop* 1983;173:70–77.
6. Neer CS II. Anterior acromioplasty for the chronic impingement syndrome in the shoulder—a preliminary report. *J Bone Joint Surg* 1972;54A:41–50.
7. Rocks JA. Intrinsic shoulder pain syndrome. *Phys Ther* 1979;59 (2):153–159.
8. Armstrong JR. Excision of the acromion in treatment of the supraspinatus syndrome: report of 95 excisions. *J Bone Joint Surg* 1949; 31B:436–442.
9. Hammond G. Complete acromionectomy in the treatment of chronic tendonitis of the shoulder. *J Bone Joint Surg* 1962;44A:494–504.
10. Moseley HF. *Shoulder lesions,* 3rd ed. Edinburg: E and S Livingston, 1969.
11. Neer CS II, Marberry TA. On the disadvantages of radical acromionectomy. *J Bone Joint Surg* 1981;63A (3):416–419.
12. Rockwood CA Jr. *The shoulder.* Philadelphia: WB Saunders, 1990.
13. Snyder SJ. *Shoulder arthroscopy.* New York: McGraw-Hill, 1994.
14. Hurley JA, Anderson TE. Shoulder arthroscopy: its role in evaluating shoulder disorders in the athlete. *Am J Sports Med* 1990;18 (5):480–483.
15. Paulos LE, Franklin JL. Arthroscopic shoulder decompression development and application: a five year experience. *Am J Sports Med* 1990;18 (3):235–244.

16. Bigliani LU, Norris TR, Fischer J, et al. The relationship between the unfused acromial epiphysis and subacromial impingement lesions. *Orthop Trans* 1983;7 (1):138.

17. Owen RS, Iannotti JP, Kneeland JB, Dalinka MK, et al. Shoulder after surgery: MR imaging with surgical validation. *Radiology* 1993;186: 443–447.

18. Magee TH, Gaenslen ES, Seitz R, Hinson GA, Wetzel LH. MR imaging of the shoulder after surgery. *Am J Roentgenol* 1997;168:925–928.

19. Brown JT. Early assessment of supraspinatus tears and procaine infiltration as a guide to treatment. *J Bone Joint Surg* 1949;31B:423–425.

20. Itai E, Tabata S. Conservative treatment of rotator cuff tears. *Clin Orthop* 1992;275:165–173.

21. Wolfgang GL. Surgical repair of tears of the rotator cuff of the shoulder, factors influencing the result. *J Bone Joint Surg* 1974;56A:14–26.

22. Brems J. Rotator cuff tear: evaluation and treatment. *Orthopaedics* 1988;11:69.

23. McLaughlin HL. Lesions of the musculotendonous cuff of the shoulder. I. The exposure and treatment of tears with retraction. *J Bone Joint Surg* 1944;26:31–51.

24. Ogilvie-Harris DJ, Demazier A. Arthroscopic debridement versus open repair for rotator cuff tears. *J Bone Joint Surg* 1993;73B:416–420.

25. Parker NP, Calvert PT, Bayley TI, et al. Operative treatment of chronic ruptures of the rotator cuff of the shoulder. *J Bone Joint Surg* 1983;65B:171–175.

26. Rockwood CA Jr, Williams GR. The shoulder impingement syndrome: management of surgical treatment failures. *Orthop Trans* 1992;16: 739–740.

27. Paletta GA Jr, Warner JP, Altchek DW, et al. *Arthroscopic rotator cuff repair: evaluation of results and a comparison of techniques.* The 60th Annual Meeting of the American Academy of Orthopedic Surgeons, San Francisco, CA, 1993.

28. Weber SC, Shaefer RK. *Mini open versus traditional open technique in the management of tears of the rotator cuff.* The 60th Annual Meeting of the American Academy of Orthopedic Surgeons, San Francisco, CA, 1993.

29. Rockwood CA Jr, Williams GR, Burkhead WZ Jr. Debridement of irreparable degenerative lesions of the rotator cuff. *Orthop Trans* 1992;16:740.

30. Neviaser JS, Neviaser RJ, Neviaser TJ. The repair of chronic massive ruptures of the rotator cuff of the shoulder by use of a freeze-dried rotator cuff. *J Bone Joint Surg* 1978;60A:681–684.

31. Cofield RH. Subscapularis muscle transposition for repair of chronic rotator cuff tears. *Surg Gynecol Obstet* 1982;154:667–672.

32. Gerber C. Latissimus dorsi transfer for the treatment of irreparable tears of the rotator cuff. *Clin Orthop* 1993;275:152–160.

33. Augerean B. Rekonstruktion massiver rotator-enmanschettenrupturen mit einen deltoidlappen. *Orthopeide* 1991;20:315–319.

34. Bigliani LU, Cordaico FH, McIlveen ST, et al. Operative treatment of failed repairs of the rotator cuff. *J Bone Joint Surg* 1992; 74A:1505–1515.

35. Gusmer PB, Potter HG, Donovan WD, O' Brien SJ. MR imaging of the shoulder after rotator cuff repair. *Am J Roentgenol* 1997;168:559–563.

36. Sartoris DJ. Postoperative imaging of the shoulder. In: *Principles of shoulder imaging.* New York: McGraw-Hill, 1995.

37. Cain PR, Mutschler TA, Fu FH. Anterior stability of the glenohumeral joint: a dynamic model. *Am J Sports Med* 1987;15:144–48.

38. Rowe CA. Prognosis in dislocations of the shoulder. *J Bone Joint Surg* 1956;38A: 957–977.

39. Rockwood CA Jr, Burkhead WZ Jr, Brna J. *Subluxation of the glenohumeral joint; response to rehabilitative exercise in traumatic vs atraumatic instability.* American Shoulder and Elbow Surgeons 2nd Open Meeting, New Orleans, LA, 1986.

40. Bankart ASB. Recurrent or habitual dislocation of the shoulder joint. *BMJ* 1923;2:1132–1133.

41. Cooper DE, Arnoczky SP, O'Brien SJ, Warren RF, DiCarlo E, Allen AA. Anatomy, histology, and vascularity of the glenoid labrum. *J Bone Joint Surg* 1992;73A:46–52.

42. Rowe, CR, Patel D, Southmayd WW. The Bankart procedure: a long-term end-result study. *J Bone Joint Surg* 1978;60:1–16.

43. DuToit GT, Roux D. Recurrent dislocation of the shoulder. A 24 year study of the Johannesburg stapling operation. *J Bone Joint Surg* 1956;38A:1–12.

44. Hawkins RB. Arthroscopic stapling repair for shoulder instability: a retrospective study of 50 cases. *Arthroscopy* 1989;5:122–128.

45. Morgan CD, Bodenstab AB. Arthroscopic Bankart suture repair: technique and early results. *Arthroscopy* 1987;3 (2):111–122.

46. Bowen MK, Warren RF, Altchek DW, O'Brien SJ. Posterior subluxation of the glenohumeral joint treated by posterior stabilization. *Orthop Trans* 1991;15 (3):764.

47. Saha AK. Dynamic stability of the glenohumeral joint. *Acta Orthop Scand* 1971;42:491–505.

48. Palmer WE, Tung GA, Dupuy DE. *MR arthrographic findings in recurrent shoulder instability following anterior stabilization procedure.* Radiological Society of North America (RSNA) 81st Annual Meeting, Chicago, IL, 1995.

Shoulder Magnetic Resonance Imaging,
edited by Lynne S. Steinbach, et al.
Lippincott–Raven Publishers, Philadelphia © 1998.

CHAPTER 10

Evaluating Arthritic Changes in the Shoulder with MRI

Charles G. Peterfy, Van C. Mow, and Louis U. Bigliani

Over the past few years, there has been a growing interest in developing applications of magnetic resonance imaging (MRI) for arthritis. At the same time, it is becoming increasingly acknowledged that the shoulder is more frequently the target of arthritic disease than was previously appreciated. Imaging evaluation of the shoulder has traditionally focused on either rotator cuff disease or glenohumeral instability. It must be acknowledged, however, that this is an artificial dichotomy and that impingement syndrome and glenohumeral instability are actually two sides of the same coin, with each condition being to some extent a cause of the other. It is more appropriate to view the shoulder joint as a whole organ, with each component—the bones, articular cartilage, synovial fluid, synovial lining, glenoid labrum, glenohumeral ligaments and joint capsule, rotator cuff muscles and tendons, and the coracoacromial arch—contributing to the functional integrity of the joint. In this whole-organ view of the shoulder, arthritis can be conceptualized as a disease of organ failure, akin to disorders such as heart failure, in which a variety of different causes can lead to a common end point of functional incompetence.

Of all the imaging modalities available for evaluating the shoulder, only MRI has the capability of visualizing all artic-

ular components of this joint simultaneously, and therefore of providing whole-organ evaluation. However, in addition to delineating the anatomy, MRI is also uniquely capable of depicting and quantifying a variety of functional and compositional attributes of articular tissues relevant to the arthritic process. MRI is thus well suited for imaging arthritis. Exactly how best to use MRI in this capacity depends on the specific objectives of imaging, whether the goal is to diagnose arthritis, assess its severity, monitor its progression or its response to treatment, or to identify complications associated with it or with its therapy. Another important consideration is the particular role that the imaging will play, whether it will be purely in service of the clinic or for clinical science or basic science purposes. Each of these roles, while interdependent, place different demands and expectations on MRI.

This chapter reviews this emerging role of MRI in evaluating arthritis, with specific reference to applications in the shoulder.

NEW IMPETUS FOR MAGNETIC RESONANCE IMAGING IN ARTHRITIS

The recent surge in interest in applications of MRI for arthritis stems from a number of factors (Table 10-1). There is growing acknowledgment of the profound human and economic impact that arthritis has on society. Arthritis affects approximately 37 million Americans (15% of the population of the United States) (1), is responsible for 68 million lost

C. G. Peterfy: Department of Radiology, University of California, San Francisco; and Arthritis and MRI Research, Osteoporosis & Arthritis Research Group, San Francisco, California 94143-0628
V. C. Mow: Department of Orthopaedic Surgery, Columbia University, New York, New York 10032
L. U. Bigliani: Department of Orthopaedics, Columbia-Presbyterian Medical Center, New York, New York 10032

TABLE 1. *Reasons for increased impetus for magnetic resonance imaging in arthritis*

Wider acknowledgment of impact of arthritis on society
Increasing prevalence of arthritis in an aging society
New therapies for arthritis on the horizon
Improved magnetic resonance imaging (MRI) techniques for imaging arthritis
Increasing awareness of the utility of MRI for evaluating arthritis

work days per year, and costs approximately $65 billion (for medical care and lost wages) annually in the United States. That value is almost twice the cost of all musculoskeletal trauma and nearly half the total cost of musculoskeletal disease, which is approximately $149 billion, or 2.5% of the gross national product. Moreover, as the first baby-boomers enter their sixth decade and as the elderly sector grows in number, the prevalence of arthritis will increase dramatically. Epidemiologic predictions point to nearly a doubling of the number of individuals with arthritis in the United States by the year 2020.

Balanced against this mounting social concern is a glimmer of light at the end of what was previously a dark and empty tunnel of therapeutic options for these patients. Increased understanding of joint biomechanics, cartilage physiology, and the inflammatory cascade, coupled with advances in molecular engineering, have spawned a host of new therapeutic approaches, including cytokine modulating agents, metalloproteinase inhibitors, chondrocyte transplantation, and osteochondral grafting, renewing the hope of one day curing this disease. These prospects have created a demand in academia and in industry for better ways of diagnosing early arthritis, assessing its severity, and monitoring the progression and response to treatment of structural changes in the joint.

Radiography has been the mainstay of imaging evaluation of arthritis. Even though radiography offers advantages of low cost, wide availability, and extensive experience with its use, the information provided by this modality is fundamentally limited in a number of ways. The projectional viewing perspective of radiography produces morphologic distortion and magnification, which can complicate morphometric analyses. More importantly, however, projectional superimposition can obscure even large structural abnormalities. Tomographic images, such as those of computed tomography (CT) and MRI, although generally providing lower two-point discrimination than radiography, are free of projectional distortion, magnification, and superimposition, so that, in many cases, osseous abnormalities are better visualized. In keeping with this, MRI has been shown to be approximately twice as sensitive as radiography for detecting bone erosions in rheumatoid arthritis (2–4).

In addition to these limitations related to viewing perspective, radiography offers relatively poor contrast for soft tissues that do not contain calcium or fat. Therefore, the articular cartilage, synovium, joint fluid, and labrocapsular structures cannot be directly visualized with radiography. The distance between opposing articular cortices (i.e., joint-space width) on radiographs has been used as an indirect measure for cartilage thickness in many joints (5). However, this is only valid where the articular surfaces are in direct contact with each other. In the knee and hip, this necessitates displacing intervening joint fluid by joint loading. Usually, this is accomplished in the knee or hip by obtaining the images while the patient is standing. Applying an appropriate load to the glenohumeral joint is more difficult. Moreover, beam centering must be tangential to the joint line, which, in the shoulder, requires anterior-oblique positioning, and the clinician must correct for the effects of magnification, which can vary from patient to patient and from time point to time point.

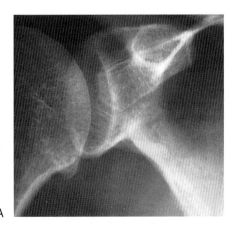 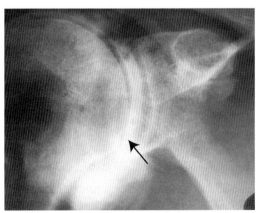

A   B

FIG. 1. Imaging articular cartilage with x-ray arthrography. **A:** Plain radiograph of the shoulder shows only the joint space as an indirect measure of the articular cartilage thickness. **B:** Intraarticular contrast delineates the surfaces of the articular cartilage directly and reveals focal cartilage thinning *(arrow)* over the inferior humeral head. Other portions of the articular surface may be obscured by projectional superimposition.

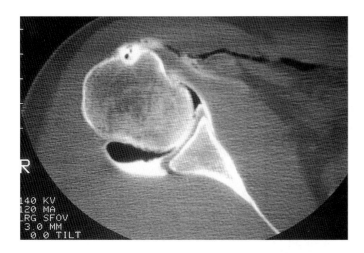

FIG. 2. Computed tomography arthrography of the shoulder. Double-contrast computed tomography arthrogram delineates the surfaces of the articular cartilage, anterior and posterior glenoid labrum, and internal margins of the joint capsule.

Arthrography offers a partial solution by delineating the articular cartilage surfaces in the glenohumeral joint, and it can reveal regions of cartilage loss (Fig. 1). However, projectional superimposition still limits the utility of this approach.

CT offers advantages of tomographic viewing perspective and when combined with intraarticular contrast material provides good images of the bones and the surfaces of glenohumeral articular cartilage and labrocapsular structures (Fig. 2). However, CT arthrography is minimally invasive and cannot visualize intrasubstance changes that may precede morphologic changes in these structures. CT of the shoulder is limited to a direct axial plane of section. Multiplanar reformation is available but results in some degree of image degradation, despite the use of thin sections, which themselves increase imaging time and patient exposure.

Ultrasonography offers direct multiplanar tomography and sufficient soft tissue contrast to visualize the articular cartilage, synovium, joint fluid, and other important articular structures. However, acoustic shadowing from bones can obscure areas, and the technique is highly operator dependent.

MRI is especially well suited to imaging arthritic joints. Not only does it provide direct multiplanar tomography, but it does so with unparalleled soft tissue contrast. This enables all components of the joint to be visualized simultaneously and, therefore, the joint to be evaluated as a whole organ. The following discussion reviews the MRI considerations important to proper imaging of each of these components in patients with arthritis.

IMAGING BONE CHANGES IN ARTHRITIS

Radiography and CT are considered by many researchers to be superior to MRI for evaluating osseous abnormalities. This opinion is based to some extent on the fact that bone tissue lacks sufficient protons to generate any signal with conventional MRI. The phrase "MRI can't see bone" is often used in rhetorical support of this view in that x-ray–based modalities, such as radiography and CT, owe their exceptional contrast for cortical and trabecular bone to the high attenuation coefficient of this tissue. Thus, "x-ray can't see

bone" either, and it is this very deficiency—when phrased in this way—that gives radiography its strength. In reality, depending on the particular sequence used, cortical and trabecular bone can be seen on MR images as linear signal voids silhouetted by signal-rich tissue on either side. And, even though it is true that the two-point resolution of clinical MRI (and CT for that matter) is substantially lower than that of radiography, the tomographic viewing perspective of MRI often gives it a significant advantage in delineating cortical irregularities and abnormal trabecular patterns that may not be visible in the projectional "haystack" of overlapping shadows of a conventional radiograph. In keeping with this, MRI has been shown to be more sensitive than radiography for detecting bone erosions in rheumatoid arthritis (Fig. 3). In a recent study by Palmer et al. (2), only half (65 of 133) of the erosions identified by conventional MRI in the wrists of patients with rheumatoid arthritis were also demonstrable with radiography. Similarly, multiplanar tomography makes MRI extremely effective at delineating marginal and central osteophytes in osteoarthritis (Fig. 4).

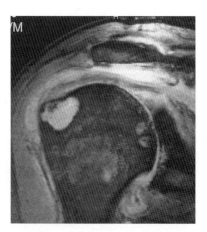

FIG. 3. Imaging bone erosion in rheumatoid arthritis with magnetic resonance imaging. Oblique coronal fat-suppressed T2-weighted fast spin-echo image of the shoulder of a patient with advanced rheumatoid arthritis shows denuding of cartilage and multiple bone erosions.

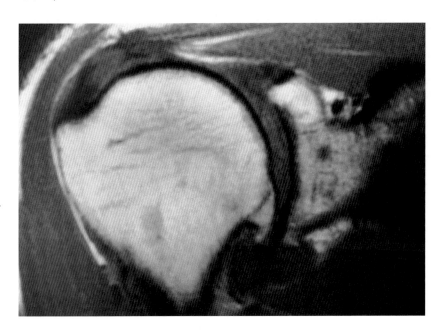

FIG. 4. Imaging osteophytes with magnetic resonance imaging. Oblique coronal T1-weighted spin-echo image of the shoulder of a patient with osteoarthritis shows a salient marginal osteophyte of the inferior humeral head.

However, the greatest strength of MRI in bone imaging comes from its unique ability to directly visualize the soft tissue component of a bone (i.e., the marrow). It is the sensitivity of MRI for even small elevations in marrow water content that makes it the most sensitive technique for detecting bone trauma, osteomyelitis, osteonecrosis, and neoplasia. In arthritic joints, bone marrow edema can sometimes be seen subjacent to areas of articular cartilage loss (Fig. 5). Potential causes of this include (a) pulsion of synovial fluid through cortical defects, (b) subchondral bone trauma or osteonecrosis caused by inadequate stress shielding by an incompetent articular surface or focal overloading of the surface because of joint instability, or (c) intramedullary inflammation caused by underlying systemic disease or the local presence of tissue breakdown products from the synovial cavity. The extent to which each of these may be involved in this finding, however, is not clear. Nor is it known how bone marrow edema correlates with patient symptoms, bone scintigraphy, disease progression, or treatment response. What is clear, however, is that this is a feature of

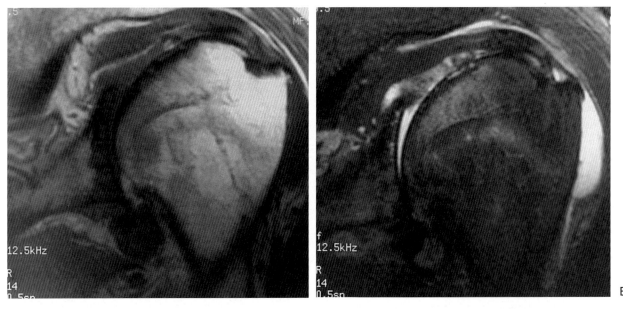

FIG. 5. Marrow edema in osteoarthritis of the shoulder. Oblique coronal T1-weighted spin-echo **(A)** and fat-suppressed T2-weighted fast spin-echo **(B)** images of the shoulder of a patient with osteoarthritis shows complete denuding of glenoid and humeral cartilage, prominent subchondral cyst formation, and extensive subjacent bone marrow edema.

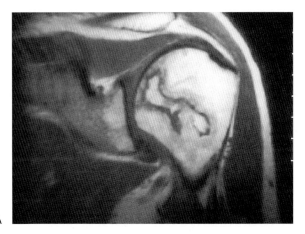
A

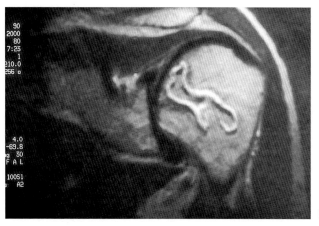
B

FIG. 6. Avascular necrosis of the humeral head. Oblique coronal T1-weighted **(A)** and T2-weighted **(B)** spin-echo images of the shoulder show a lesion in the humeral head with well-defined wavy margins characteristic of avascular necrosis.

arthritis that cannot be seen with radiography, and that MRI is, therefore, uniquely suited to exploring.

These causes of marrow edema associated with arthritis must be distinguished from osteomyelitis, avascular necrosis, or stress fracture complicating treatment with oral steroids or other immunosuppressive agents. This is usually not a problem for avascular necrosis because of its distinctive MRI appearance. Typically, a region of avascular necrosis shows well-defined wavy or jagged margins of reparative tissue and bone delimiting the devitalized vascular territory (Fig. 6). Within these margins are a variable amount of fatty tissue, fibrosis, or liquefactive necrosis. Osteomyelitis, in contrast, usually shows ill-defined margins and diffuse water signal in the marrow. Subacute osteomyelitis (Brodie's abscess) may show well-defined margins, but these are typically smooth rather than wavy and sometimes include a projecting sinus tract, pathognomonic for infection. Linear marrow changes, either transverse or parallel to the cortical surface are consistent with stress fractures (Fig. 7).

Bone marrow edema, regardless of its cause, is most sensitively depicted with short tau inversion recovery (STIR) or fast STIR. Fat-suppressed T2-weighted fast spin-echo is also highly sensitive but offers the added advantage of higher spatial resolution and improved contrast for articular cartilage. As discussed in Chapter 2, fat suppression is necessary when using fast spin-echo to evaluate the marrow because of inherently low fat-water contrast with this sequence. However, spectral fat suppression can be difficult to use in the shoulder because of magnetic field heterogeneities associated with the noncylindrical shape of this part of the anatomy. This usually manifests as increased signal within the greater tuberosity (see Fig. 32 in Chapter 2) and can mimic or mask marrow edema in this region, but the artifact rarely extends to the articular surfaces of the glenohumeral joint, so that subchondral marrow edema can usually be seen. Various options for improving the homogeneity of spectral fat suppression are discussed in Chapter 2; however, none of these are foolproof.

Gradient-echo imaging is relatively insensitive to marrow edema when used at high field strength because of T2* effects within cancellous bone. This is not the case, however, at low field strengths, at which magnetic susceptibility effects are reduced and T2* is dominated by T2. Conventional T2-weighted spin-echo images are relatively sensitive for marrow edema, but are far less so than T1-weighted spin-echo images. When using T1-weighted spin-echo at low magnetic field strength, TR must be shortened appropriately to accommodate the more rapid T1 relaxation.

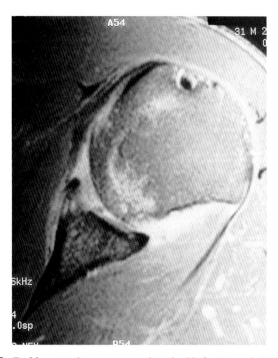

FIG. 7. Marrow changes associated with fracture. Axial fat-suppressed T2-weighted fast spin-echo image shows linear high signal in the humeral head indicative of fracture.

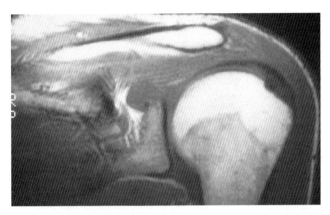

FIG. 8. Residual hematopoietic tissue in the glenohumeral bones. Oblique coronal T1-weighted spin-echo image of a normal shoulder shows intermediate-signal hematopoietic tissue within the glenoid process and the proximal humerus. This tissue is usually restricted to beneath the physeal scar as in this case, but occasionally lines the subchondral marrow. Residual hematopoietic tissue can mimic or obscure mild marrow edema in some cases.

Detecting bone marrow edema in the shoulder can be complicated by the relatively high prevalence of residual hematopoietic tissue in the proximal humerus and glenoid (the scapula, like the spine and pelvis, remains hematopoietic throughout life) (Fig. 8). Although often a sign of chronic anemia in other joints of the body, this can be a normal finding in the shoulder in even normochromic elderly subjects. Residual hematopoietic tissue in the humerus is typically found within the metaphysis but can also be seen along the immediate subchondral marrow where arthritic marrow changes usually occur. Normal hematopoietic tissue usually appears darker than marrow fat but brighter than muscle on T1-weighted spin-echo images, reflecting signal averaging of adjacent adipose and hepatopoietic cells within individual voxels. The degree of elevation of marrow water associated with infection and neoplasia is usually severe enough to lower the signal intensity of affected marrow below that of muscle on T1-weighted spin-echo images, but whether this is also true for the marrow edema associated with arthritis is not known.

IMAGING ARTICULAR CARTILAGE WITH MAGNETIC RESONANCE IMAGING

The MRI appearance of articular cartilage reflects its complex biochemistry and histology (6). To understand these relationships, it is useful to conceptualize the articular cartilage as being composed of two phases: a fluid phase composed of water and dissolved ions and a solid phase of sparse chondrocytes, fibrillar collagen, and aggregated proteoglycans. The collagen fibrils in cartilage radiate from a thin calcified zone at the cartilage–bone interface toward the articular surface in a relatively parallel array of gradually thinning bundles in the so-called radial zone. At the surface is a dense mat of tangentially oriented collagen fibrils that provide tensile resistance and relative impermeability to water. Sandwiched between this superficial tangential zone and the radial zone is the transitional zone of cartilage in which collagen fibrils assume a more random orientation. Embedded within the fibrillar network of collagen are aggregated proteoglycan molecules possessing numerous negatively charged glycosaminogycan (GAG) moieties that attract counter cations, mostly sodium, and with them osmotically water. This Donnan osmotic pressure combined with the electrostatic repulsion of adjacent negatively charged GAGs produces a swelling pressure that keeps the cartilage inflated and the collagen fibrils under tension. The balance between this swelling pressure and the resistance levied against it by the collagen network determines the water content of resting, unloaded cartilage. It is also fundamental to the fluid pressurization mechanism of load bearing by cartilage (7).

It is the presence of hydrogen protons in free water in hyaline articular cartilage that provides the basis for MRI signal. This signal is then modulated by the solid matrix through a variety of mechanisms, including T1 relaxation, T2 relaxation, magnetization transfer, and water diffusion. Each of these factors exert a variable influence on image contrast depending on the particular MRI technique used.

Spin Echo

With conventional spin-echo and fast spin-echo imaging, T2 relaxation is probably the most important factor governing cartilage contrast. As in other fibrous tissues, such as ligaments, tendons, and muscle, collagen in cartilage tends to constrain otherwise mobile water protons and promote dipole–dipole interactions among them, thus lowering T2 (see Fig. 35 in Chapter 2). The T2 of normal cartilage is accordingly relatively short (10–20 ms) (Table 10-2) and varies from zone to zone according to the organization of collagen (6). The marked differences in T2 among the various components in the shoulder joint provides a basis for superb delineation of articular cartilage. On heavily T2-weighted spin-echo images, cartilage appears as a low signal intensity structure in sharp contrast against high signal intensity joint fluid and intermediate signal intensity subchondral bone marrow. Contrast between cartilage and adjacent structures is even greater with fast spin-echo imaging, be-

TABLE 2. *Approximate T2 relaxation times of joint structures*

Articular component	T2 (msec)
Synovial fluid	200
Adipose fat	90
Marrow fat	60
Muscle	50
Articular cartilage	15[a]
Rotator cuff tendons	<1[a]
Glenoid labrum	<1[a]
Glenohumeral ligaments, capsule	<1[a]

[a]Aniostropic

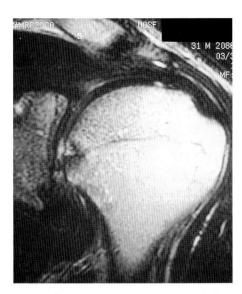

FIG. 9. T2-weighted fast spin-echo imaging of articular cartilage. Oblique coronal T2-weighted fast spin-echo image without fat suppression shows articular cartilage as a low signal intensity band in sharp contrast to adjacent high signal intensity synovial fluid and subchondral bone marrow. Note the focal cartilage loss and subchondral cyst formation in the lower humeral head.

cause this sequence tends to provide heavier T2 weighting and preserves signal intensity in fat (Fig. 9). T2 contrast is not significantly affected by magnetic field strength within the ranges used in clinical imaging.

Another factor affecting the contrast behavior of spin-echo imaging is magnetization transfer (see Chapter 2). Magnetization transfer occurs in multislice imaging because of direct saturation of macromolecular protons and therefore indirectly of any neighboring free water protons by off-resonance irradiation to waiting slices during individual slice selection. This results in loss of signal from hydrated collagen-containing tissues, such as cartilage but not fat or synovial fluid, and therefore greater contrast between cartilage and adjacent synovial fluid and subchondral marrow fat. The effect is augmented as the number of slices is increased and is greater with fast spin-echo imaging because of the additional 180-degree pulses used during each excitation (8).

T2-weighted fast-spin echo images are therefore very useful for examining the articular cartilage in a variety of clinical and research contexts. However, in addition to delineating cartilage morphology, T2-weighted images can detect changes in the compositional and microstructural integrity of this tissue. It is intuitive from the two-phase model of articular cartilage described that degradation of the solid phase of cartilage must be accompanied by an increase in water content if there is no thinning of the cartilage. This is supported by the biophysical literature (7). Therefore, early matrix damage that precedes cartilage loss is associated with increased proton density of cartilage. Additionally, disruption of the solid matrix reduces T2 shortening and magnetization-transfer effects on cartilage water. These three factors com-

bine to elevate signal intensity in the cartilage so that areas of chondromalacia appear as foci of increased signal intensity in otherwise low signal intensity cartilage on T2-weighted images.

By using a multiecho sequence, it is furthermore possible to quantify the T2 of articular cartilage in time frames feasible for clinical imaging. Even though this parameter is multifactorial in terms of its biochemical and biophysical basis, it may serve as a useful, albeit somewhat empirical, marker of disease progression in disorders affecting the cartilage. However, T2 relaxation in cartilage is anisotropic because, as discussed in Chapter 2, collagen constrains water molecules in such a way as to cause them to tumble differently in different directions. As a result, T2 is longest when the collagen fibrils are oriented at 55 degrees relative to the static magnetic field. In cartilage, this occurs where the 55-degree vector is perpendicular to the articular surface, and it can result in artifactually elevated signal intensity on inadequately T2-weighted images. The distribution of "magic-angle" effect in the cartilage of the shoulder can be predicted with knowledge of the patient positioning and the orientation of the static magnetic field (Fig. 10). If sufficiently long TE (>80 ms) is used, magic-angle effects are generally not a problem for subjective assessment of cartilage signal. However, if the objective of the imaging is to quantify and map the T2 of cartilage, consideration of this phenomenon as well as the effects of magnetization transfer (in multislice two-dimensional imaging) becomes critical.

In distinction to T2 relaxation, proton density differences between cartilage and adjacent synovial fluid offer relatively little opportunity to generate image contrast. In normal cartilage, this difference is only 20% to 30% (Fig. 11). More-

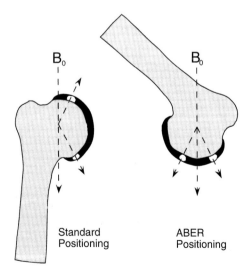

FIG. 10. Magic-angle phenomenon in the articular cartilage of the humeral head. Because of the angular anisotropy of T2 in articular cartilage, certain regions in normal cartilage may show increased signal intensity on T2-weighted images, depending on the TE used and the orientation of the cartilage relative to the static magnetic field (B_0).

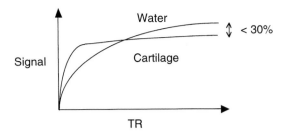

FIG. 11. Effect of TR on proton density contrast. The proton density of articular cartilage is approximately two thirds that of free water in the adjacent synovial fluid. Because of the small magnitude of this difference and the long T1 of synovial fluid, very long TR must be used to generate significant proton-density contrast on MR images.

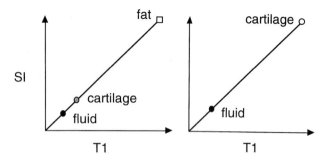

FIG. 13. Augmenting T1 contrast by suppressing fat. Fat normally overshadows cartilage and fluid in terms of gray scale. Suppression of fat results in rescaling of the residual cartilage and fluid signal and, consequently, greater contrast between them.

over, because of the slow T1 relaxation of free water protons in synovial fluid, very long TR (approximately 4000 ms) is necessary to maximize this small difference. To achieve this TR within reasonable imaging times usually necessitates the use of fast spin-echo. Fast spin-echo also adds cartilage-water contrast via magnetization transfer effects. However, as discussed in Chapter 2, care must be taken when using short TE fast spin-echo because of the risk of image blurring unless very short echo spacing can be used.

T1 relaxation offers an additional mechanism for generating contrast between cartilage and adjacent articular structures. T1-weighted spin-echo images provide high contrast between cartilage and subjacent marrow fat, but depict both cartilage and synovial fluid with relatively low signal intensity, making it difficult to delineate the articular surface (Fig. 12). The T1 of cartilage is actually shorter than that of synovial fluid, but this difference is normally overshadowed in gray scale by the much shorter T1 of fat (Fig. 13). Suppres-

sion of fat rescales the remaining signal intensities, augmenting cartilage-fluid contrast. Accordingly, articular cartilage is depicted as a high signal intensity structure flanked on either side by low signal intensity synovial fluid and bone marrow on fat-suppressed T1-weighted images (9,10) (Fig. 14). Even though this method can be used with both spin-echo and gradient-echo technique, the latter is usually preferred because of the higher signal-to-noise (S/N) ratio and possibility of thinner slice thickness.

T1 contrast can also be augmented by differential uptake of intravenous or intraarticular paramagnetic contrast agents that shorten T1. The tissue distribution of these agents depends, among other things, on charge. An anionic agent, such as Gd-DTPA^{2-} for example, is repelled by the negatively charged proteoglycans in normal cartilage and therefore enhances only the synovial fluid, producing an arthrographic effect and sharply delineating the articular surface. Sites of proteoglycan loss, however, allow the Gd-DTPA^{2-} to enter and accumulate, and increases the signal intensity in chondromalacic cartilage on T1-weighted or cartilage-nulled inversion recovery images (11). Cationic agents, such as Mn^{2-} on the other hand, show direct affinity for the fixed negative charges in normal cartilage and decreased enhancement at sites of chondromalacia (12). Unfortunately, toxicity limits the use of Mn^{2-} in humans; however, other cationic agents may one day become available for this purpose. Nonionic agents diffuse freely into articular cartilage without distinction to the fixed negative charge (GAG) density, and therefore show limited potential as markers of chondromalacia.

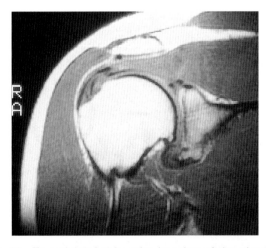

FIG. 12. T1-weighted spin-echo imaging of the shoulder. Oblique coronal T1-weighted spin-echo image of the shoulder shows poor contrast between cartilage and adjacent synovial fluid. Note the marginal osteophyte of the inferior humeral head, the healed Bankart fracture of the inferior glenoid, and the tear of the superior labrum, all well delineated with this technique.

Gradient Echo

Gradient-echo techniques offer the advantage of sufficient speed to allow three-dimensional imaging that combines high in-plain resolution with thinner section thickness and greater S/N ratio than can be achieved with clinically available two-dimensional imaging sequences. One limitation of gradient echo, however, is that it offers little scope for T2 contrast among structures in the millisecond range. Carti-

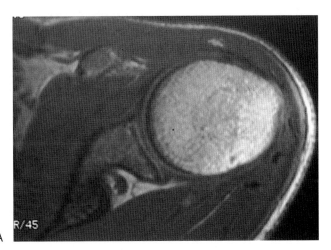
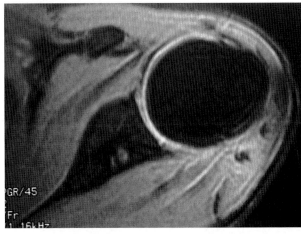

A   B

FIG. 14. Fat-suppressed T1-weighted three-dimensional spoiled gradient echo. Axial image of the shoulder depicts articular cartilage as a high signal intensity structure contrasted against low signal intensity synovial fluid and suppressed marrow fat.

lage-fluid contrast is, therefore, relatively poor on conventional T2*-weighted gradient-echo images. This necessitates harnessing other tissue characteristics, such as magnetization transfer (13,14) or T1, to generate contrast.

Fat-suppressed T1-weighted three-dimensional spoiled gradient-echo (see Fig. 14) is currently the method of choice for delineating articular cartilage anatomy in most joints (6,10,15–18). In a recent study of 41 knees by Recht et al. (15), this technique demonstrated a sensitivity of 81% and specificity of 97% for identifying cartilage surface defects visible on arthroscopy. Other studies have reported similar results (10,19). Moreover, it is widely available and easy to use. Limitations of this technique include poor sensitivity for early matrix changes in cartilage (15,16,20), and vulnerability to magnetic susceptibility effects and field heterogeneity. Frequency shifts near metal, collections of gas, or in association with the shape of the structure being imaged can result not only in signal loss and spatial distortion but also in failure of spectral fat suppression or inadvertent water suppression. This can be particularly problematic in postoperative shoulders or if air is inadvertently injected into the joint during MR arthrography. Although these effects are field-strength dependent, spectral fat suppression becomes more difficult, if not impossible, at low fields. Another limitation of this technique is that it cannot be used in conjunction with MR arthrography with T1 contrast agents. Saline arthrography may be a better alternative in this situation. Indeed, it may be desirable in most cases, because the highly congruent configuration of the glenohumeral joint sometimes makes it difficult to delineate the boundary between contiguous cartilage plates. This problem is lessened by introducing fluid into the joint cavity, or potentially by physically separating the articular surfaces by applying direct traction on the humerus during imaging.

IMAGING SYNOVIAL CHANGES

The synovial lining shows a broad spectrum of involvement in various articular disorders, but in the normal joint it is generally too thin to be delineated with conventional nonenhanced MR imaging. In many cases, the only sign of synovitis is the presence of a joint effusion. Exactly what the appropriate threshold is for defining a quantity of joint fluid as abnormal is not known; however, using three-dimensional reconstruction methods and MRI sequences that provide sufficient contrast between joint fluid and adjacent tissues, it is possible to quantify the amount of free fluid in a joint with extremely high accuracy and precision (21). This may be useful for monitoring treatment response in patients with arthritis or for studying the normal role of synovial fluid in joint physiology in vivo. As for cartilage imaging, however, the critical issue is whether sufficient contrast can be generated between the joint fluid and adjacent tissues, such as cartilage and synovium. Magnetization-transfer techniques may be helpful in this regard (13).

Synovial tissue in the joint can show a variable appearance on MRI. Acutely inflamed, edematous synovium may exhibit slow T2 relaxation because of its high interstitial water content, but as collagen accumulates, the T2 shortens and signal intensity on T2-weighted images decreases. Accordingly, it may be difficult to discriminate some areas of thickened synovial tissue from adjacent joint fluid or cartilage. Hemosiderin deposition or chronic fibrosis lowers the signal intensity of hyperplastic synovial tissue on long TE images and occasionally even short TE images.

Most synovial tissue exhibits a slightly shorter T1 than does joint fluid, but under normal circumstances, the contrast on T1-weighted images is relatively poor. One exception is lipoma arborescens, in which the synovium becomes infil-

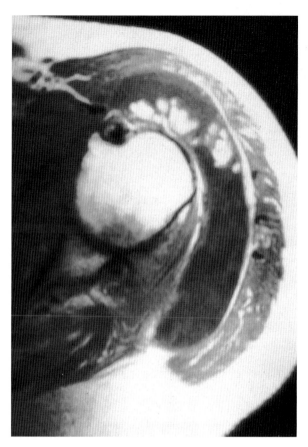

FIG. 15. Lipoma arborescens. Axial T1-weighted image of the shoulder shows villous projections of fat-infiltrated synovial tissue lining the subacromial bursa.

trated with fat and shows high signal intensity villous projections lining the synovial cavity on T1-weighted images (Fig. 15). Lipoma arborescens is a benign disorder but it can be a cause of pain and is often associated with osteoarthritis (22). Intravenous injection of Gd-DTPA can improve synovial contrast by enhancing this highly vascularized tissue on T1-weighted images (23–27) (Fig. 16). Contrast between enhanced synovium and any adjacent high signal intensity adipose tissue can be augmented by applying fat suppression. However, Gd-DTPA is a relatively small molecule, which diffuses rapidly out of even normal capillaries. Accordingly, the Gd-DTPA leaks into the adjacent joint fluid over time (13,28,29). The rate of equilibration of these two compartments depends on a number of factors, including the degree of hyperemia of the synovium, the relative amounts of synovium and joint fluid, and the degree of mechanical mixing in the joint. Whereas this may be a useful property for indirect MR arthrography, it complicates efforts to estimate the amount of synovial tissue using Gd-DTPA.

Gd-DTPA has also been used to grade the severity of synovitis in patients with rheumatoid arthritis (25–27,29,30). Rapid synovial enhancement rate and high maximal enhancement following bolus intravenous injection of Gd-DTPA correlate with severe inflammation and hyperplasia, whereas sluggish enhancement corresponds to chronic fibrotic synovium. This may be useful for monitoring treatment in patients with arthritis.

An unusual synovial condition that presents with monoarticular hemarthrosis is pigmented villonodular synovitis (31–33). This process typically involves large joints, most commonly the knee, and appears as a diffuse, irregular thickening of the synovium with markedly heterogeneous low signal intensity on both long TE and short TE images resulting from extensive hemosiderin deposition from recurrent hemarthrosis. It is indistinguishable on MRI from another cause of recurrent hemarthrosis, hemophilia. These two entities are easily differentiated clinically, but their similarity on MRI emphasizes the importance of hemarthrosis to the MR appearance of pigmented villonodular synovitis.

Another synovial process that may appear low in signal intensity on MR images is synovial osteochondromatosis (33,34) (Fig. 17). In this case, the basis for low signal is the presence of calcification, which typically produces a signal void on MRI. Synovial osteochondromatosis begins as a chondroid metaplasia of the synovium. Small chondroid projections may break loose from the synovium and float freely in the joint, where they can grow nourished by the synovial fluid. These loose intraarticular chondral bodies can reattach to the synovium, develop a vascular supply, and often ossify. Ossified loose bodies may contain fatty marrow and, therefore, show high signal intensity on T1-weighted images. Osteochondral bodies are also readily detectable by conventional radiography and CT, which may additionally show associated bone erosions, but these modalities underestimate the sometimes extensive soft tissue component of these lesions. Moreover, in the absence of any significant calcification, these lesions may be completely occult to x-ray studies. On MRI, noncalcified synovial chondromatosis may be mistaken for loculated fluid collections, such as ganglion cysts or popliteal cysts, unless the fine nodularity of the lesion is identified. There is some speculation that synovial chondromatosis may sometimes undergo malignant transformation to chondrosarcoma (33). However, primary malignancies or even metastatic disease to the synovium, except thorough direct extension, are exceedingly rare. Even synovial cell sarcomas are almost always extraarticular (35).

OTHER ARTICULAR STRUCTURES

Although most of the attention in MRI of arthritis has thus far concentrated on changes in the articular cartilage, synovium, and bone, each of the other components of the shoulder, especially the rotator cuff and labrocapsular structures, is also critical to maintaining the functional integrity of the joint, and each is intimately involved in the arthritic process. MRI evaluation of the rotator cuff and labrocapsular structures is more mature from a clinical standpoint, but it has traditionally focused on implications related to impingement syndrome or glenohumeral instability. Even though these

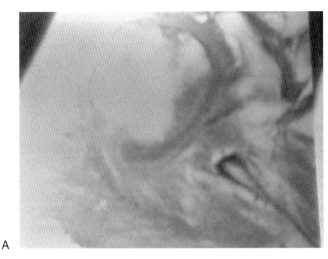
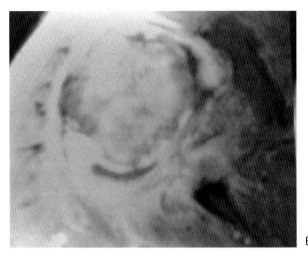

A

B

FIG. 16. Synovial enhancement with Gd-DTPA. **A:** Axial T1-weighted image of a shoulder with rheumatoid arthritis before intravenous administration of Gd-DTPA shows thickened synovium as an intermediate signal intensity structure lining the joint cavity. **B:** Following Gd-DTPA administration, the inflamed synovium enhances intensely and appears thicker than on the pre-Gd-DTPA images because of centripedal diffusion of contrast into the adjacent joint fluid.

conditions are themselves causes of pain and disability, they also lead to further derangement of the shoulder and ultimately osteoarthritis. Excessive tightening of the anterior capsule of the shoulder during surgery in patients with instability can itself promote osteoarthritis by shifting the humeral head posteriorly and disturbing normal glenohumeral contact patterns. In rheumatoid arthritis, disruption of the rotator cuff or labrocapsular structures can add significantly to the disability of this disease. Therefore, as the demand for MRI in this patient population increases, it will be increasingly important to view derangements of these articular components from the perspective of their role in the pathogenesis of arthritis and their immediate and downstream implications to patient symptoms and disability.

In the following sections, the two most common forms of arthritis in the shoulder—osteoarthritis and rheumatoid arthritis—are discussed.

OSTEOARTHRITIS

Osteoarthritis of the glenohumeral joint is a well-documented clinical problem and surgical treatment of this disease is common (36–45). In the United States, glenohumeral joint replacement is the third most frequent total joint replacement procedure (36,43). In 1992, it was reported that from 1985 to 1988, glenohumeral joint replacements accounted for 10.3% of all total joint replacements performed in the United States (43). It is likely that this percentage will continue to increase because of the growing awareness of osteoarthritis in the shoulder, and the recent technical improvements in glenohumeral joint replacement surgery.

The glenohumeral joint has specific characteristics that play important roles in the pathogenesis of osteoarthritis. Some of the functional implications of these are as follows:

1. The normal asymmetry in the duration of load support (i.e., duty cycle), with the cartilage on the smaller glenoid being loaded more frequently and longer than the cartilage on the larger humeral head (1:3 surface area ratio), may lead to different stress and strain fields within the two cartilage layers, even though contact stresses on the opposing surfaces are the same.
2. The size disparity and the shallowness of the glenohumeral joint socket (46–48) compromises the stability of the glenohumeral joint. This instability is a major clinical problem and may often result in secondary osteoarthritis of the glenohumeral joint (44,49–51).
3. Normal glenohumeral joint contact areas and contact stresses are dependent on articulating surface curvatures, joint congruency, and cartilage properties, and thus can also be easily altered (46,47).

Cadaveric studies of osteoarthritis in the glenohumeral joint indicate that cartilage lesions initiate on the glenoid, followed by lesions on both glenoid and humeral head (39,41,42). This progression is a time-dependent process that eventually leads to clinical osteoarthritis. Neer (39) and Petersson (42) found focal articular lesions in 10% to 23% of all cadaveric shoulders. DePalma (43a) noted that changes in the glenoid surface are seen first, occurring as early as the second decade. These consisted of softening, furrowing, and fibrillation in the superficial layers of the central glenoid region. In older specimens, irregular, scalloped, and ulcerated areas were found in the articular cartilage, and the adjacent bony trabeculae were dense and hypertrophied. Osteophyte formation is a classic reactive manifestation of osteoarthritis and is found in the later stages of osteoarthritis in the glenohumeral joint, most commonly along the inferior margin of the humeral head.

Both DePalma and Neer hypothesized that the degenera-

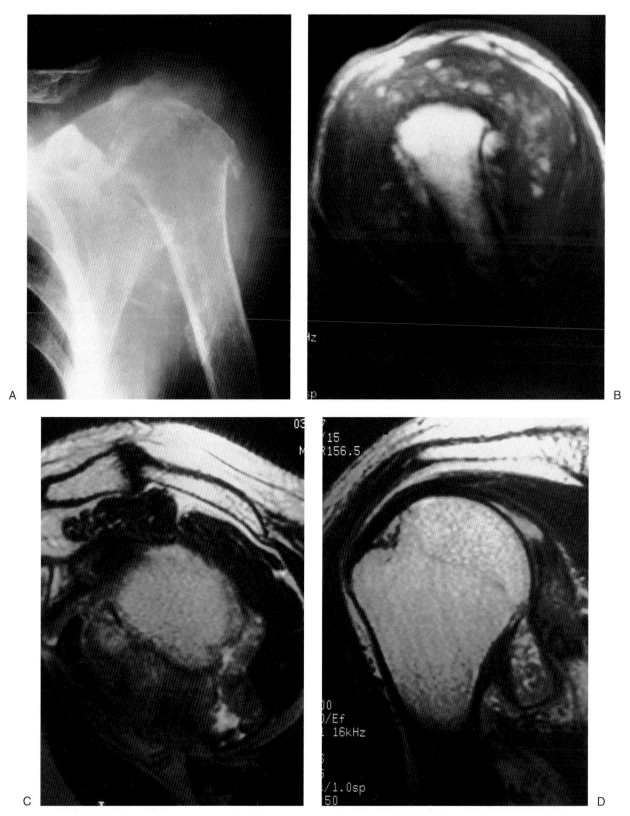

FIG. 17. Synovial osteochondromatosis. **A:** Radiograph of the shoulder of a patient with neuropathic osteoarthropathy shows extensive deformity and erosion of the articular surfaces. **B:** Oblique sagittal T1-weighted image shows numerous osteochondral bodies, some ossified and containing high signal intensity marrow fat thoughout the joint cavity. The findings are consistent with secondary osteochondromatosis. Axial **(C)** and oblique coronal **(D)** T2-weighted fast spin-echo images of a different patient show noncalcified synovial chondromatosis.

tive changes are due to the high contact stresses acting on the smaller glenoid during normal shoulder function. Degenerative lesions of the humeral head especially at the periphery were also noted by DePalma. In 1974, Neer (40) reported that focal areas of wear and sclerosis develop at the point of maximum joint reaction forces when the arm is abducted between 60 and 100 degrees, although contact areas or joint reaction forces were not determined. As the disease progresses, the glenoid surface becomes eburnated and often demonstrates more bone loss posteriorly. This sloping glenoid results in the clinically observed posterior subluxation of the humeral head. Significantly, in most cases, from a radiographic and clinical standpoint, humeral head changes are more readily apparent, even though they may be later reactive changes in the disease process.

Loss of external rotation is an important clinical characteristic of glenohumeral osteoarthritis. Secondary and iatrogenically induced osteoarthritis of the glenohumeral joint has often been reported as sequelae of both traumatic dislocation and the operative treatment of shoulder instability. In 1983, Samilson and Prieto (44) stated that the incidence of arthrosis, following dislocation, is greater than has generally been believed, especially after posterior dislocations. A number of other authors have also reported on the iatrogenic development of arthritis following operative repairs for glenohumeral joint instability (38,44,52,53). One group reported a 72% incidence of moderate to severe osteoarthritis in shoulders treated with the Eden-Hybbinette bone block procedure for anterior dislocations (52). Samilson and Prieto (44) reported that the limitation of external rotation after surgery is correlated with the severity of shoulder osteoarthritis. Neer has postulated that the development of osteoarthritis after an instability repair (the arthritis of dislocations) derives from the performance of a standard unidirectional (anterior) repair on a shoulder that is multidirectionally loose (53,54). The hypothesis is that anterior tightening of an excessively loose glenohumeral joint causes the humeral head to shift posteriorly, thereby causing abnormal joint articulation. Recently, Hawkins and Angelo (38) have reported on the development of osteoarthritis in the glenohumeral joint in 11 shoulders previously treated with a Putti-Platt capsulorrhaphy for recurrent anterior dislocations. They hypothesized that this repair can constitute a restrictive anterior tether, which leads to alterations in shoulder biomechanics. Surgical procedures (open and arthroscopic) that restore external rotation have improved symptomatic osteoarthritis of the shoulder without replacement (45,55). Finally, Friedman et al. (56) reported that glenoid retroversion is significantly correlated with osteoarthritis and observed excessive wear of the posterior rim of the glenoid by CT. Preventing loss of external rotation (caused either by iatrogenic anterior tightening or by excessive retroversion) may be a method of treatment to avoid progression to symptomatic osteoarthritis.

RHEUMATOID ARTHRITIS

Rheumatoid arthritis affects approximately 1% to 2% of the population (57). Most of the clinical attention in this disease has focused on the joints of the hands and wrists. However, the shoulder is affected in as many as 40% to 50% of these patients (57). The earliest MRI finding in rheumatoid arthritis is synovitis and effusion involving the glenohumeral and acromioclavicular joints, as well as the subacromial bursa. Invasive pannus eventually erodes the articular cartilage and bones; however, these destructive changes may not be visible on initial radiographs. MRI shows far greater sensitivity for bone erosion than does radiography (2–4) and may therefore be useful for identifying rheumatoid patients who have synovitis but lack significant structural damage and, therefore, show the greatest opportunity for structural salvage. In keeping with this, Sugimoto et al. (58) found that MRI alone correctly predicted rheumatoid arthritis (based on long-term follow-up evaluations) in 100% of 16 cases while maintaining a specificity of 73%. The sensitivity and specificity of the 1987 American Rheumatism Association revised criteria for rheumatoid arthritis in these patients with negative radiographs were only 69% and 64%, respectively.

Gd-enhanced MRI may also be useful for monitoring treatment in patients with arthritis. Although intravenous Gd-DTPA enhances both the synovium and joint fluid, Palmer et al. (2) demonstrated a strong correlation between changes in the volume of Gd-enhancement in the wrists of patients with rheumatoid arthritis, and the clinical response of these patients to methotrexate. This approach could be refined by including a magnetization transfer pulse to selectively suppress the signal from synovium and cartilage without affecting Gd-enhanced joint fluid (13). This could allow independent quantification of the synovium and joint fluid on delayed Gd-enhanced images.

In addition to quantifying the amount of synovium and joint fluid in arthritic joints, however, Gd-enhanced MRI can also provide objective information about the severity of synovial inflammation. By acquiring rapid serial T1-weighted images following a bolus intravenous injection of Gd-DTPA, the rate of synovial enhancement can be determined (27,29,30,59). Although it is difficult to control for subtle differences in the pharmacokinetics of the Gd-DTPA between examinations, the slope and maxima of synovial enhancement–time curves correlate with the histologic severity of the synovitis (59,60) and can be shown to decrease markedly following therapy. In an examination of ten knees of nine patients with advanced rheumatoid arthritis, Tamai et al. (59) found significant correlations between rapid synovial enhancement rate on preoperative MRI and the presence of high-grade histologic changes of fibrin exudation, polymorphonuclear cell infiltration, villous hypertrophy, vascular proliferation, and granulation formation in biopsy specimens obtained during knee arthroplasty. In contrast, synovial enhancement rate did not correlate with the degree of synovial fibrosis or the degree of multiplication of the synovial lining. The precise relationship between changes in synovial enhancement rate and the progression of clinical and structural changes in arthritic joints has yet to be determined. However, monitoring synovial enhancement with Gd-containing contrast material may provide a more objective measure of therapeutic response and allow drug efficacy to be demonstrated sooner than with radiography. This technique may also enable therapeutic regimens to be optimized for individual patients. Moreover, patients who fail initial therapy could be identified earlier in the course of treatment and be directed to more effective therapy.

Although rheumatoid arthritis is traditionally viewed as a disease of the synovium, as discussed previously, a whole-organ model of joint function that considers all components of the shoulder can provide a richer understanding of the pathogenesis of joint failure in this disease and may help point to additional treatment options in certain patients. Accordingly, in addition to synovitis, joint effusion, and cartilage loss, involvement of other articular and periarticular structures, including the glenoid labrum, joint capsule and glenohumeral ligaments, rotator cuff and biceps tendons, and muscles of the shoulder girdle can contribute significantly to the pain and disability of this disease. Complete rupture of the rotator cuff, for example, is seen in approximately 20% of patients with rheumatoid arthritis (57,61), yet it may go clinically unnoticed because of preexisting pain and immobility. MRI may play a useful role in identifying these patients and directing them to appropriate therapy.

Avascular necrosis, osteomyelitis, or stress fracture may develop as a complication of systemic steroid therapy in some patients with rheumatoid arthritis. Even though the incidence of stress fractures in the shoulder in such patients is not known, the humeral head follows only the hip as the most common site for osteonecrosis. The MRI appearances of these two causes of otherwise nonspecific shoulder pain are very different and usually make possible a specific diagnosis. As discussed, the key differential criteria on MRI are the presence of a characteristic wavy margin (avascular necrosis), linearity of the marrow signal changes (fracture), and the presence of a sinus tract (Brodie's abscess). Whereas infection requires aggressive therapy, treatment of avascular necrosis and stress fracture in the shoulder is generally only supportive.

CONCLUSION

MRI shows great promise as a tool for imaging arthritic joints in ways not possible in the past. To date, most of this development has been based on studies in the knee. Nevertheless, conclusions drawn from this work can be extrapolated to other joints, with certain provisions. Pertinent considerations in the shoulder include the following:

1. Normal residual hematopoietic tissue can mimic or mask marrow edema in the humerus and glenoid.

2. Perturbation of the static magnetic field by the curved shape of the shoulder interferes with spectral fat suppression.

3. Marked congruency of the articular surfaces of the glenohumeral joint makes it more difficult to discern the boundary between contiguous articular surfaces.

4. The glenoid labrum, glenohumeral ligaments, rotator cuff, subacromial bursa, and elements of the coracoacromial arch are important to the functional integrity of the shoulder, but pose technical challenges to evaluation with MRI (see Chapter 2).

The last point is particularly cogent to the emerging view of arthritis as a disease of organ failure and points to the importance of whole-organ evaluation of the shoulder and any other joints affected by this disease. Only MRI can deliver such a comprehensive imaging evaluation in vivo, and, although this application of MRI is still in its infancy and experience in the shoulder is particularly limited, it deserves attention because it will undoubtedly play an increasingly important role in the development of understanding of arthritis as well as of knowledge of how to combat it.

REFERENCES

1. Arthritis and Musculoskeletal Diseases Interagency Coordinating Committee. 1990 Annual Report. Bethesda, MD: Department of Health and Human Services, Public Health Service, National Institutes of Health; 1990:7.
2. Palmer WE, Rosenthal DI, Shoenberg OI, et al. Quantification of inflammation in the wrist with gadolinium-enhanced MR imaging and PET with 2-[F-18]-fluoro-2-deoxy-D-glucose. Radiology 1995;196: 645–655.
3. Adam G, Dammer M, Bohndorf M, et al. Rheumatoid arthritis of the knee: value of gadopentetate dimeglumine-enhanced MR imaging. Am J Roentgenol 1991;156:125–129.
4. Senac M, Deutsch D, Bernstein B, et al. MR imaging in juvenile rheumatoid arthritis. Am J Roentgenol 1988;150:873–878.
5. Buckland-Wright JC, Macfarlane DG, Lynch JA, Jasani MK, Bradshaw CR. Joint space width measures cartilage thickness in osteoarthritis of the knee: high resolution plain film and double contrast macroradiographic investigation. Ann Rheum Dis 1995;54:263–268.
6. Peterfy CG, Genant HK. Emerging applications of magnetic resonance imaging for evaluating the articular cartilage. Radiol Clin North Am 1996;34:195–213.
7. Mow VC, Ratcliffe A, Poole AR. Cartilage and diarthroidial joints as paradigms for hierarchical materials and structures. Biomaterials 1992;13:67–97.
8. Yao L, Gentili A, Thomas A. Incidental magnetization transfer contrast in fast spin-echo imaging of cartilage. JMRI 1996;6:180–184.
9. Chandnani VP, Ho C, Chu P, Trudell P, Resnick D. Knee hyaline cartilage evaluated with MR imaging: a cadaveric study involving multiple imaging sequences and intraarticular injection of gadolinium and saline solution. Radiology 1991;178:557–561.
10. Recht MP, Kramer J, Marcelis S, et al. Abnormalities of articular cartilage in the knee: analysis of available MR techniques. Radiology 1993;187:473–478.
11. Bashir A, Gray ML, Burstein D. Gd-DTPA^{2-} as a measure of cartilage degradation. Magn Reson Med 1996;36:665–673.
12. Kusaka Y, Grunder W, Rumpel H, Dannhauer K-H, Gersone K. MR microimaging of articular cartilage and contrast enhancement by manganese ions. Magn Reson Med 1992;24:137–148.
13. Peterfy CG, Majumdar S, Lang P, van Dijke CF, Sack K, Genant H. MR imaging of the arthritic knee: improved discrimination of cartilage, synovium and effusion with pulsed saturation transfer and fat-suppressed T1-weighted sequences. Radiology 1994;191:413–419.
14. Woolf SD, Chesnick S, Frank JA, Lim KO, Balaban RS. Magnetization transfer contrast: MR imaging of the knee. Radiology 1991; 179:623–628.

15. Recht MP, Pirraino DW, Paletta GA, Schils JP, Belhobek GH. Accuracy of fat-suppressed three-dimensionl spoiled gradient-echo FLASH MR imaging in the detection of patellofemoral articular cartilage abnormalities. *Radiology* 1996;198:209–212.

16. Disler DG, McCauley TR, Kelman CG, et al. Fat-suppressed three-dimensional spoiled gradient-echo MR imaging of hyaline cartilage defects in the knee: comparison with standard MR imaging and arthroscopy. *Am J Roentgenol* 1996;167:127–132.

17. Peterfy CG, van Dijke CF, Janzen DL, et al. Quantification of articular cartilage in the knee by pulsed saturation transfer and fat-suppressed MRI: optimization and validation. *Radiology* 1994;192:485–491.

18. Peterfy CG, van Dijke CF, Lu Y, et al. Quantification of articular cartilage in the metacarpophalangeal joints of the hand: accuracy and precision of 3D MR imaging. *Am J Roentgenol* 1995;165:371–375.

19. Disler DG, McCauley TR, Wirth CR, Fuchs MC. Detection of knee hyaline articular cartilage defects using fat-suppressed three-dimensional spoiled gradient-echo MR imaging: comparison with standard MR imaging and correlation with arthroscopy. *Am J Roentgenol* 1995;165:377–382.

20. Brossmann J, Frank LR, Pauly JM, et al. Short echo time projection reconstruction MR imaging of cartilage: comparison with fat-suppressed spoiled GRASS and magnetization transfer contrast MR imaging. *Radiology* 1997;203:501–507.

21. Heuck AF, Steiger P, Stoller DW, Glüer CC, Genant HK. Quantification of knee joint fluid volume by MR imaging and CT using three-dimensional data processing. *J Comput Assist Tomogr* 1989;13:287–293.

22. Feller JF, Rishi M, Hughes EC. Lipoma arborescens of the knee: MR demonstration. *Am J Roentgenol* 1994;163:162–164.

23. Munk P, Vellet AD, Levin MF, Bell D, Harth M. *Intravenous gadolinium in the evaluation of rheumatoid arthritis of the shoulder.* Berlin, Germany: Society of Magnetic Resonance in Medicine, 1992:457.

24. Björkengren AG, Geborek P, Rydholm U, Holtas S, Petterson H. MR imaging of the knee in acute rheumatoid arthritis: synovial uptake of gadolinium-DOTA. *Am J Roentgenol* 1990;155:329–332.

25. Smith H-J, Larheim TA, Aspestrand F. Rheumatic and nonrheumatic disease in the temporomandibular joint: gadolinium-enhanced MR imaging. *Radiology* 1992;185:229–234.

26. Jevtic V, Watt I, Rozman B, et al. Precontrast and postcontrast (Gd-DTPA) magnetic resonance imaging of hand joints in patients with rheumatoid arthritis. *Clin Radiol* 1993;48:176–181.

27. König H, Sieper J, Wolf KJ. Rheumatoid arthritis: evaluation of hypervascular and fibrous pannus with dynamic MR imaging enhanced with Gd-DTPA. *Radiology* 1990;176:473–477.

28. Winalski CS, Aliabadi P, Wright RJ, Shortkroff S, Sledge CB, Weissman BN. Enhancement of joint fluid with intravenously administered gadopentetate dimeglumine: technique, rationale, and implications. *Radiology* 1993;187:197–185.

29. Drapé J-L, Thelen P, Gay-Depassier P, Silbermann O, Benacerraf R. Intraarticular diffusion of Gd-DOTA after intravenous injection in the knee: MR imaging evaluation. *Radiology* 1993;188:227–234.

30. Yamato M, Tamai K, Yamaguchi T, Ohno W. MRI of the knee in rheumatoid arthritis: Gd-DTPA perfusion dynamics. *J Comput Assist Tomogr* 1993;17:781–785.

31. Jelinek JS, Kransdorf MJ, Utz JA, et al. Imaging of pigmented villonodular synovitis with emphasis on MR imaging. *Am J Roentgenol* 1989;152:337–342.

32. Hughes TH, Sartoris DJ, Schweitzer ME, Resnick DL. Pigmented villonodular synovitis: MRI characteristics. *Skeletal Radiol* 1995;24:7–12.

33. Resnick D. Internal derangements of joints. In: Resnick D, ed. *Diagnosis of bone and joint disorders.* Philadelphia: WB Saunders, 1995:3063–3069.

34. Kramer J, Recht M, Deely DM, et al. MR appearance of idiopathic synovial osteochondromatosis. *J Comput Assist Tomogr* 1993;17:772–776.

35. Resnick D. Soft tissues. In: Resnick D, ed. *Diagnosis of bone and joint disorders.* Philadelphia: WB Saunders, 1995:4548–4548.

36. Cofield RH. Unconstrained total shoulder prostheses. *Clin Orthop* 1983;173:97–108.

37. Cofield RH. Total arthroplasty with the Neer prosthesis. *J Bone Joint Surg* 1984;66A:899–906.

38. Hawkins RJ, Angelo RL. Glenohumeral osteoarthrosis. A late complication of the Putti-Platt repair. *J Bone Joint Surg* 1990;72A:1193–1197.

39. Neer CSI. Degenerative lesions of the proximal humeral articular surface. *Clin Orthop* 1961;20:116–125.

40. Neer CSI. Replacement arthroplasty for glenohumeral arthritis. *J Bone Joint Surg* 1974;56A:1–13.

41. Neer CSI. Recent experience in total shoulder replacement. *J Bone Joint Surg* 1982;64A:319–337.

42. Petersson CJ. Degeneration of the glenohumeral joint. *Acta Orthop Scand* 1983;54:277–283.

43. Praemer A, Furner S, Rice DP. *Musculoskeletal conditions in the United States.* In: Park Ridge, IL: American Academy of Orthopaedic Surgeons, 1992:133.

43a. DePalma AF, White JB, Callery G. Degenerative lesions of the shoulder joint at various age groups which are compatible with good function. *AAOS Inst Course Lect* 1950;Chapter VII:168–180.

44. Samilson RL, Prieto V. Dislocation arthropathy of the shoulder. *J Bone Joint Surg* 1983;65A:456–460.

45. Weinstein DM, Bucchieri JS, Pollock RG, et al. Arthroscopic debridement of the shoulder for OA. *Arthroscopy* 1993;9:366.

46. Soslowsky LJ, Flatow EL, Bigliani LU, Mow VC. Articular geometry of the glenohumeral joint. *Clin Orthop* 1992;285:181–190.

47. Soslowsky LJ, Flatow EL, Bigliani LU, Pawluk RJ, Ateshian GA, Mow VC. Quantitation of in situ contact areas at the glenohumeral joint. A biomechanical study. *J Orthop Res* 1992;10:524–534.

48. Iannotti JP, Gabriel JP, Schneck SL, et al. The normal glenohumeral relationships. *J Bone Joint Surg* 1992;74A:491–500.

49. Harryman DT, Sides JA, Harris SL, Matsen FAI. Laxity of the normal glenohumeral joint: a quantitative in vivio assessment. *J Shoulder Elbow Surg* 1992;1:66–76.

50. Howell SM, Galinat BJ. The glenoid-labral socket. *Clin Orthop* 1989;243:122–125.

51. Kelkar R, Ateshian GA, Pawluk RJ, Flatow EL, Bigliani LU, Mow VC. 3D kinematics of the GHJ during abduction in the scapular plane. *Trans Orthop Res Soc* 1993;18:136.

52. Hindmarsh J, Lindberg A. Eden-Hybbinette's operation for recurrent dislocation of the humero-scapular joint. *Acta Orthop Scand* 1967;38:459–478.

53. Neer CSI. Inferior capsular shift for involuntary inferior and multidirectional instability for the shoulder. *J Bone Joint Surg* 1980;62A:897–908.

54. Neer CSI. *Shoulder reconstruction.* Philadelphia: WB Saunders, 1990.

55. MacDonald PB, Hawkins RJ, Fowler PJ, Miniaci A. Release of the subscapularis after repair for recurrent anterior dislocation of the shoulder. *J Bone Joint Surg* 1992;74A:734–737.

56. Friedman RJ, Hawthorne KB, Genez B. The use of computed tomography in the measurement of glenoid version. *J Bone Joint Surg* 1992;74A:1032–1037.

57. Harris ED. Pathogenesis of rheumatoid arthritis. In: Kelly WN, Harris ED, Ruddy S, et al, eds. *Textbook of rheumatology,* ed 3. Philadelphia: WB Saunders, 1989:905–942.

58. Sugimoto H, Takeda A, Masuyama J, Furuse M. Early-stage rheumatoid arthritis: diagnostic accuracy of MR imaging. *Radiology* 1996;198:185–192.

59. Tamai K, Yamato M, Yamaguchi T, Ohno W. Dynamic magnetic resonance imaging for the evaluation of sunovitis in patients with rheumatoid arthritis. *Arthritis Rheum* 1994;37.

60. Stiskal MA, Neuhold A, Szolar DH, et al. Rheumatoid arthritis of the craniocervical region by MR imaging: detection and characterization. *Am J Roentgenol* 1995;165:585–592.

61. Neer CS. The shoulder. In: Kelly WN, Harris ED, Ruddy S, et al, eds. *Textbook of rheumatology,* ed 3. Philadelphia: WB Saunders, 1989:2013–2026.

Shoulder Magnetic Resonance Imaging,
edited by Lynne S. Steinbach, et al.
Lippincott–Raven Publishers, Philadelphia © 1998.

CHAPTER 11

Miscellaneous Disorders

James H. Welch, Antonio Correa, John F. Feller, and Lynne S. Steinbach

Tumors and Tumor-Like Processes	**Avascular Necrosis/Infarction**
Soft Tissue Tumors	**Trauma**
Osseous Tumors	**Infection**
Marrow Abnormalities	**Paget's Disease**
Lymphoma	**Nerve Entrapment Syndromes**

In addition to evaluating rotator cuff and glenoid labral injuries as well as instability of the glenohumeral joint, magnetic resonance imaging (MRI) provides excellent evaluation of a variety of conditions that can occur in and around the shoulder joint. The excellent soft tissue contrast resolution and multiplanar capabilities make MRI the modality of choice for evaluation of these miscellaneous disorders.

TUMORS AND TUMOR-LIKE PROCESSES

Malignant tumors of the musculoskeletal system account for approximately 0.5% to 0.7% of all malignancies and are more common in children than in adults (1). Secondary malignancies are by far the most common tumors of the musculoskeletal system. Of the primary malignant bone tumors, when all ages are considered, the most common is multiple myeloma followed by osteosarcoma. With musculoskeletal tumors, location within the skeleton and age of the patient are very important in forming differential diagnosis. Most shoulder tumors occur in the proximal humerus (approximately 70%) with other locations being the clavicle (6%–10%) and the scapula (18%–24%) (1). For sarcomas in

general, the shoulder is third in frequency of location following the hip/pelvis and the knee (2). Benign tumors of the musculoskeletal system are most common in the second and third decades of life whereas malignant tumors have a bimodal distribution with peaks occurring in adolescence and middle age (3). In the scapula, the most common primary benign lesion is an osteochondroma and the most common primary malignant lesion is a chondrosarcoma. In the proximal humerus, the most common benign lesions are solitary bone cysts and osteochondromas. Low-grade malignancies in the proximal humerus occur more commonly in older patients and include chondrosarcoma, fibrosarcoma, and giant cell tumors. High grade primary malignancies in the proximal humerus are seen more commonly in younger patients and include osteogenic sarcoma and Ewing's sarcoma.

Clinical presentation usually includes a 3- to 6-month history of symptoms before an accurate diagnosis of musculoskeletal malignancy is made. Not uncommonly, a neoplasm can present with symptoms of rotator cuff injury. The most common presentation of osseous malignant tumors is a history of pain. The distinguishing symptom of a bone malignancy is that of pain at night or at rest. Bone tumors rarely extend into a joint, and findings of joint tenderness, impingement, or weakness suggest an articular process, trauma, degenerative disease, or some other nonneoplastic process. Aggressive bone malignancies typically have an associated soft tissue mass. Regional adenopathy in the presence of a neoplasm commonly represents an inflammatory reaction to the tumor and does not necessarily represent metastatic disease. Nonosseous soft tissue neoplasms present as a palpable mass. In contrast to osseous malignancies, most soft tissue sarcomas have no associated pain. In general, MRI is an extremely sensitive method for evaluating bone tumors. Mar-

J. H. Welch: Department of Radiology, Keesler Medical Center, Keesler Air Force Base, Mississippi 39532

A. Correa: Department of Diagnostic Radiology, Mike O'Callaghan Federal Hospital, Nellis Air Force Base, Las Vegas, Nevada 89191-6601

J. F. Feller: Department of Radiology, Stanford University School of Medicine, Stanford, California 94305; and Desert Medical Imaging, Indian Wells, California 92210

L. S. Steinbach: Department of Radiology, University of California, San Francisco, San Francisco, California 94143

row edema and extent of tumor can be better defined than with conventional radiographs or computed tomography (CT). MRI can also evaluate and characterize any associated soft tissue mass and involvement of the adjacent neurovascular bundle.

MRI can be somewhat limited in assessment of small calcifications and small foci of ossification. Conventional radiographs and CT are superior in arriving at a differential diagnosis of bone lesions in general. When selecting imaging sequences, T1-weighted pulse sequences show anatomic detail and the status of the bone marrow. T2-weighted fast spin-echo fat-suppressed or inversion recovery images usually characterize the tumor mass as increased signal and can evaluate for areas of necrosis and marrow edema, and can characterize areas of hemorrhage. Gradient-recalled flow sensitive sequences evaluate the adjacent vascular structures and simplify differentiation of adenopathy from adjacent vessels with flowing blood. Gadolinium contrast-enhanced images are helpful for evaluation of viable zones within the tumor, which is helpful in directing biopsy, identification of the reactive zone of edema, and assessing tumor vascularity.

SOFT TISSUE TUMORS

MRI may be performed as the initial evaluation of palpable soft tissue masses, but more commonly a soft tissue mass is encountered incidentally when MRI is performed for unrelated symptoms. Most of the tumors encountered in this situation are benign.

Benign soft tissue lesions are typically well marginated with homogeneous signal intensity and do not disrupt adjacent neurovascular or osseous structures (4). In contrast, malignant lesions have irregular margins with heterogeneous signal and tend to encase the neurovascular bundle and invade the adjacent bone (4). Although these characteristics can be used to suggest a benign or malignant process, multiple studies have demonstrated these characteristics to be nonspecific and unreliable in distinguishing between benign and malignant masses (5,6).

The most common soft tissue tumor in an adult is a lipoma (7). It is most frequently found in the extremities, more commonly in females, and is rarely congenital or familial (8). These tumors can occur in any soft tissue that contains fat. Lipomas are composed of a focal collection of mature-appearing fat that may contain other mesenchymal elements such as fibrous or muscular stroma in the form of delicate septa (9). Lipomas are characterized by their anatomic location as either superficial or deep. The superficial lipoma is more common and tends to be smaller in size. The deep lipoma occurs more commonly within the chest wall and the deep soft tissues of the hands and feet and can be intramuscular. In the shoulder, lipomas may occur within the fat planes of the axilla or deep in the anterior deltoid muscle. They also may be found within the subscapular and other perivascular spaces (1). A lipoma typically presents as a slow-growing asymptomatic mass, although it can occasionally be associated with pain in the form of lipoma dolorosa (8). Clinically, the mass is characterized as a palpable, well-circumscribed, soft, freely movable, nontender mass. Those masses in the region of neurovascular bundles may cause nerve compression or entrapment, resulting in weakness, pain, or numbness (10). Lipomas have a typical appearance with MRI, appearing as well-defined lobulated masses paralleling fat signal on all pulse sequences. Lipomas are hyperintense on T1-weighted images with decreasing signal intensity with increasing echo time (TE), as well as, signal loss with fat suppression and no enhancement after contrast administration (9,11,12) (Fig. 1). Delicate fibrous septations

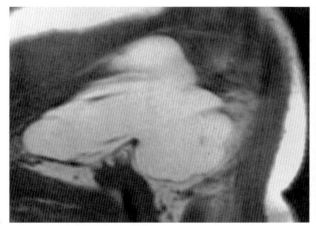
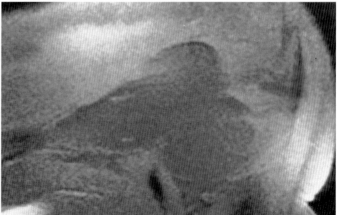

A B

FIG. 1. Lipoma. **A:** T1-weighted coronal image demonstrates a lobulated high signal mass overlying the posterior scapula superficially interposed between fibers of the infraspinatus and teres minor muscles. **B:** T1-weighted coronal fat suppressed image demonstrates signal intensity of the mass to decrease and parallel fat signal.

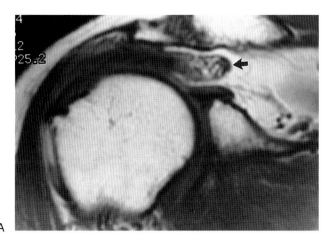 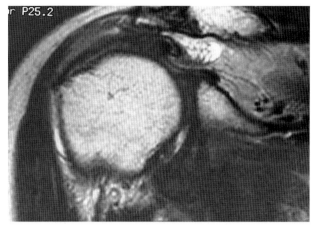

A   B

FIG. 2. Lipoma arborescens. **A:** T1-weighted coronal image shows a heterogeneous fat signal intensity mass anterior and superior to the supraspinatus muscle *(arrow)* **B:** On T2-weighted fast spin-echo image, associated bursal fluid demonstrates increased signal intensity.

may be seen characterized by decreased signal intensity on all pulse sequences, but presence of soft tissue components or thick septations suggest the possibility of liposarcoma (9). Although lipomas do have a characteristic appearance, overlap with well-differentiated liposarcoma can occur.

Other fatty masses include angiolipomas, which represent tumors composed of mature fat cells with focal vascular components that typically occur in the upper extremities of young adults (7). Hibernoma, a rare variant of benign lipoma, represents a vestigial remnant of a fat storage organ and may contain foci of hypervascularity (8). Lipoma arborescens, which is a rare synovial disorder, has been described affecting the subdeltoid bursa (13). Lipoma arborescens may be the result of a nonspecific synovial reaction to trauma and inflammation with consequent infiltration of fat in the subsynovial tissues. It can result in degenerative joint disease and typically presents as a slowly progressive, painless joint swelling. On MRI, lipoma ar-

borescens appears as a villous synovial lesion with signal features that correspond to that of fat with surrounding fluid signal intensity (14) (Fig. 2). Signal loss occurs with fat suppression and chemical shift artifact may be seen resulting from the associated adjacent joint effusion. No enhancement of the lesion is seen after gadolinium administration (15). Lipoblastoma is an uncommon benign tumor that arises from embryonic tissue and tends to occur in the appendages or the superficial tissues of the upper body. Nearly all cases occur before age 3 years, and it has been described in the infant shoulder (16). Except for well differentiated liposarcomas, other variants of liposarcoma demonstrate fatty components in only about 50% of cases (9).

Hemangiomas also have a typical MRI appearance (17–19). On T1-weighted images, the lesions are isointense compared to muscle, with punctate or lace-like foci of increased signal, which parallels that of adjacent fat. On T2-weighted images, hemangiomas are markedly hyperintense

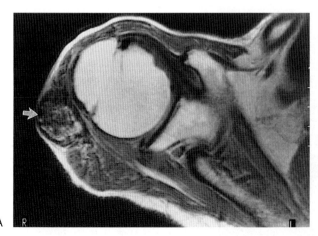 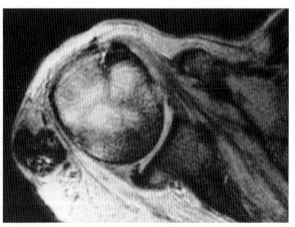

A   B

FIG. 3. Myositis ossificans. **A:** T1-weighted axial image demonstrates a heterogeneous mass within the deltoid muscle posterolaterally *(arrow)*, which is characterized by heterogeneous signal. **B:** Axial gradient recalled image confirms presence of "blooming" artifact with marked signal loss consistent with presence of calcification/ossification.

with globular or serpentine regions of hyperintensity surrounded by low signal fibrous septa. Hemangiomas may have a globular configuration and a well-defined or partially well-defined margin.

Myositis ossificans can also present as a soft tissue mass. Myositis ossificans may occur following trauma, although many cases occur without a history of a definite traumatic event (20). The cause of myositis ossificans is not definitely known. A well-defined progressive change in appearance of the lesion with time has been described. Before visible ossification, new lesions are isointense to muscle on T1-weighted images without definable borders and are recognizable only by their mass effect. T2-weighted images show a focal mass with central high signal intensity greater than fat and diffuse peripheral edema (21). At approximately 6 to 8 weeks, early peripheral ossification occurs, with a low signal intensity border forming on both T1- and T2-weighted images (21). Chronically after several months, the MR features are those of mature bone with marrow signal centrally and a surrounding low signal intensity rim, although atypical appearances have been described (21) (Fig. 3).

Occasionally, multiple masses are seen in a patient with neurofibromatosis. Neurofibromas may occur in any location surrounding the shoulder, but solitary neurofibromas tend to occur in the region of neurovascular bundles. Neurofibromas are characterized by low to intermediate signal on T1 weighting and hyperintense signal on T2-weighted images. A target appearance with central low signal and peripheral hyperintensity with T2 weighting has been described (21a). Enhancement is also seen following gadolinium administration (Fig. 4).

OSSEOUS TUMORS

A variety of benign and malignant osseous neoplasms can be found in the region of the shoulder.

Simple bone cysts are most often discovered in patients younger than 20 years of age and more predominantly in men. The proximal humerus is the most common area of occurrence (22). Simple bone cysts are benign, lytic, expansile tumors of bone, which are usually asymptomatic. Fluid is commonly seen within the cystic cavity. Not uncommonly, patients present with a pathologic fracture. Plain radiographs are characteristic with thinning of the cortex and mild expansion. They most commonly are located in the metaphysis with the fallen fragment sign being characteristic. On MRI, signal characteristics of fluid are seen characterized by low to intermediate signal on T1- and high homogeneous signal on T2-weighted images. Fluid–fluid levels may also be seen, although this is not diagnostic of this process (22).

Aneurysmal bone cyst was originally described as "a peculiar blood containing cyst of large size" (23). At present, most orthopedic pathologists regard aneurysmal bone cyst to be a sequela of a specific pathophysiologic change, which is the result of trauma or a tumor-induced vascular process. In approximately one third of cases, a preexisting lesion is identified, with the most common of these being giant cell tumor, which accounts for 19% to 39% of identified preexisting processes (22). Other precursor lesions include fibrous dysplasia, fibroxanthoma, chrondromyxoid fibroma, solitary bone cyst, fibrous histiocytoma, eosinophilic granuloma, trauma, fibrosarcoma, osteosarcoma, and metastatic carcinoma. Most patients are younger than 20 years old, with

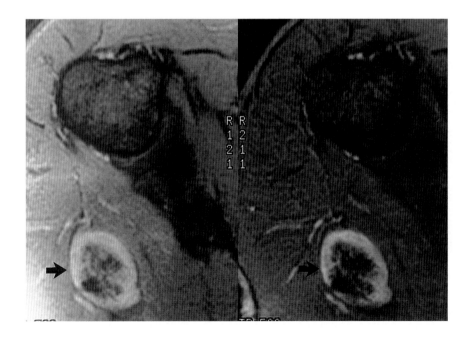

FIG. 4. Neurofibroma. T1-weighted fat-suppressed axial images after contrast administration demonstrate a mass within the quadrilateral space *(arrow)*, which is characterized by central intermediate to low signal and surrounding peripheral enhancement. (Courtesy of Arnold Honick, M.D.)

more than half of such lesions occurring in long bones (23). In relation to the shoulder, approximately 14% of cases occur about the proximal upper extremity, with 9% affecting the humerus, 3% the clavicle, and 2% the scapula (8). Most patients have pain or swelling that has usually been present for 6 months or less (23). Pathologic fracture can also occasionally be seen. Because aneurysmal bone cysts result from a specific pathophysiologic process, identification of the pre-existing lesion is necessary for adequate management. Recurrence occurs in a large number of cases, with 90% recurring within 2 years (24). Conventional radiographs usually demonstrate an eccentric, lytic lesion with an expanded, remodeled, blown-out, or ballooned contour of the host bone. These are usually well defined with geographic borders, although occasionally the cortex is thinned so as not to be identified on conventional radiographs and appears disrupted. CT scanning can better delineate the lesion, with fluid–fluid levels occasionally being seen and the dependent layer showing increased attenuation (25). MRI shows a well-defined lobulated lesion with fluid–fluid levels and internal architecture (Fig. 5). Signal intensity on T1- and T2-weighted

images can be variable because of the presence of multiple phases of blood breakdown products (25).

Giant cell tumors have a slight female predominance and tend to occur in young adults between the ages of 15 and 40 years old, with a peak incidence in the third decade (26–28). Most commonly, giant cell tumors arise about the knee but can be seen in the shoulder, especially within the proximal humerus. On plain radiographs, the lesion appears geographic with an eccentric metaphyseal epicenter, a narrow zone of transition, and extension to the articular surface, but no sclerotic rim (29). Cortical breakthrough and associated soft tissue mass may occasionally be seen. On MRI, low to intermediate signal intensity on T1-weighted images and intermediate to high signal intensity on T2-weighted images is seen (28).

Enchondroma is the second most common benign neoplasm of cartilaginous origin. It consists of discreet islands of hyaline cartilage surrounded by lamellar enchondral bone. With enlargement, endosteal scalloping occurs. Patients are usually between the ages of 10 and 30 years and have nonspecific clinical symptoms (30). Atraumatic pain in an older

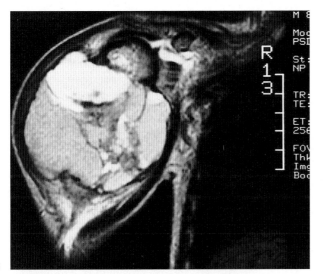

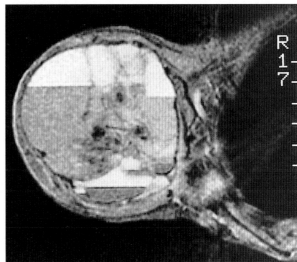

FIG. 5. Aneurysmal bone cyst. **A:** Coronal T2-weighted fast spin-echo image shows prominent expansion of the proximal humeral metaphysis and diaphysis with sparing of the epiphysis and marked heterogeneous signal. **B** and **C:** Gradient echo (GRE) and T2-weighted fast spin-echo fat-suppressed axial images also demonstrate the marked expansion with fluid-fluid levels.

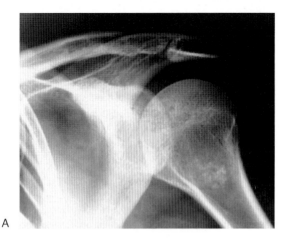

A

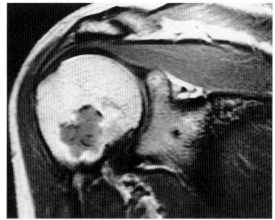

B

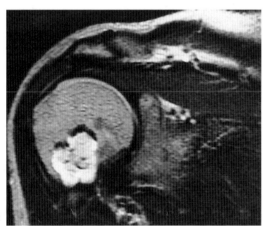

C

FIG. 6. Enchondroma. **A:** Plain film of the shoulder shows a small lesion within the proximal humeral metaphysis, which is characterized by a speckled sclerotic appearance within the medullary cavity. **B** and **C:** Intermediate- and T2-weighted spin-echo coronal images confirm presence of the intramedullary lesion, which demonstrates intermediate signal on first echo and high signal on second echo with small curvilinear low signal foci. Note the prominent chemical shift artifact at the cephalad aspect of the lesion on T2 images.

patient is worrisome for malignant transformation to chondrosarcoma. Although not the most common location for occurrence of enchondroma, the proximal humerus is the most common location within the shoulder and occurs most often within the metadiaphyseal region (30). Plain films demonstrate a geographic lytic lesion with lobulated margins and a cartilaginous matrix consisting of punctate rings and arcs (31). The size of an enchondroma can be underestimated on plain radiographs and CT scan. CT can best evaluate mineralization of the matrix and the integrity of the adjacent cortex. The MR appearance is that of a heterogeneous lobulated mass with high signal intensity on T2-weighted images (32) (Fig. 6). Small low signal rings and arcs may be seen on T1- and T2-weighted images corresponding to foci of calcified matrix.

Malignant bone tumors tend to be symptomatic and are usually apparent on plain radiographs at the time of presentation. In general, MR characteristics include low signal with T1 weighting and heterogeneous hyperintensity with T2 weighting. There is commonly cortical or periosteal disruption and associated soft tissue mass. Primary malignant bone tumors that tend to occur around the shoulder include chondroblastoma, osteosarcoma, and chondrosarcoma, all of which tend to occur in the proximal humerus (1).

MARROW ABNORMALITIES

Bone marrow is the only organ that is imaged on every MRI study performed on the body and should be evaluated on all studies. Two different types of marrow composition can be recognized. Red or hematopoietic marrow consists of 40% water, 40% fat, and 20% protein, whereas fatty or yellow marrow is hematopoietically inactive and is made up of 15% water, 80% fat, and 5% protein (33). Red marrow also tends to be more vascularized than yellow marrow. At birth, red marrow is present throughout the entire skeleton, with a physiologic conversion of red to yellow marrow occurring in a predictable and orderly fashion with advancing age and establishment of an adult pattern by age 25 years (33). In the long bones of the extremities, marrow transformation normally starts in the diaphysis, proceeds to the distal metaphysis, and finally occurs within the proximal metaphysis. In the adult, red marrow persists in the axial skeleton, proximal humerus, and proximal femur (34). Between the ages of 1 and 3 years, the proximal humeral epiphysis ossification center enlarges and fatty marrow deposition occurs. The normal marrow pattern of the shoulder in the adult demonstrates fatty marrow within the proximal humeral epiphysis and diaphysis, although red marrow replacement can occur nor-

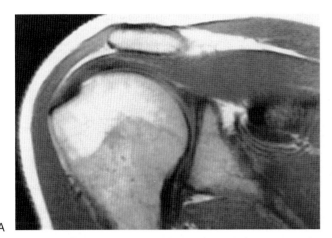
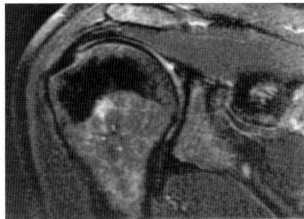

A

B

FIG. 7. Normal variant hematopoietic marrow. **A:** T1-weighted coronal image shows intermediate signal red marrow within the humeral diaphysis and proximal metaphysis as well as a thin rim of intermediate signal replacing the normal fatty marrow of the epiphysis in a subchondral location. **B:** T2-weighted coronal fast spin-echo fat-saturated image also demonstrates this peripheral subchondral epiphyseal intermediate signal consistent with normal variant hematopoietic marrow.

mally within the proximal humeral metaphysis and diaphysis. The acromion is also composed of fatty marrow. The remainder of the scapula behaves like the axial skeleton and transforms at a slower rate than the rest of the shoulder (35). In the adult shoulder, an additional normal variant appearance of the proximal humerus can be seen where a thin band of red marrow replacement is present in the subchondral region of the proximal humeral epiphysis that has been described in adults up to the seventh decade, although the likelihood of this finding does appear to decrease with age (35) (Fig. 7). Demographic predisposition for normal variant subchondral red marrow replacement includes women of menstruating age, cigarette smoking, intense athletic activity such as marathon running, and obesity (36). Reconversion from fatty to red marrow can occur secondary to disease processes that stimulate prominent hematopoiesis. The proximal humeral metaphysis tends to be one of the first portions of the skeleton to respond to this stimulus.

On MRI, superb differentiation between red and yellow marrow on T1-weighted spin-echo images is seen. Yellow marrow on T1-weighted images is hyperintense in contrast to the relatively decreased signal intensity of red marrow. This is a direct reflection of the differences in fat and water content within red and yellow marrow. Both benign and malignant disorders of bone marrow have long T1 values, which results in decreased marrow signal intensity. T2-weighted fast spin-echo fat-suppressed or inversion recovery images demonstrate red marrow replacement and pathologic processes as hyperintense foci.

LYMPHOMA

In patients who have lymphoma, involvement of the bone marrow is an important indicator of disease progression (37,38). Hodgkin's lymphoma demonstrates marrow in-

volvement in approximately 10% of patients whereas non-Hodgkin's lymphoma demonstrates an increased frequency of marrow involvement occurring in up to 45% of patients (39). Primary lymphoma of bone and systemic lymphoma with secondary bone involvement cannot be distinguished radiographically or histologically when a single osseous lesion is present. Primary lymphoma of bone tends to occur in persons between 10 and 30 years of age (40). Patients tend to present with pain, and radiographs demonstrate a permeative lytic process with an indistinct transition zone. Primary lymphoma occurs in the femur, ilium, tibia, and humerus in descending order of frequency (41). MRI demonstrates low signal on T1-weighted images and hyperintensity on T2-weighted images with a variable degree of skeletal destruction (Fig. 8).

AVASCULAR NECROSIS/INFARCTION

The humeral head follows the hip as the second most frequent site for avascular necrosis (42). Avascular necrosis can develop spontaneously or be secondary to a number of conditions to include steroid therapy, sickle cell anemia, trauma, Gaucher's disease, alcoholism, infection, hyperuricemia, radiation therapy, and collagen vascular diseases (42). Common causes of avascular necrosis of the humeral head include fractures of the anatomic neck, which disrupt the blood supply, and steroid therapy. In a series by Neer (42), 40% of the patients evaluated had disease involving both shoulders, and a common association was seen with femoral head disease. The clinical presentation varies from asymptomatic early in the disease to severe pain and limitation of motion as the disease progresses. MRI is the modality of choice for evaluation of avascular necrosis in any body part because radiographs typically appear normal in the early stages. A specificity of 98% and sensitivity of 97% has been reported

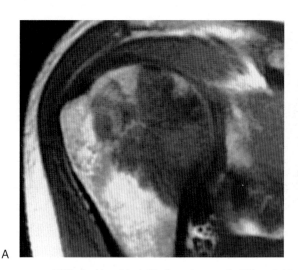
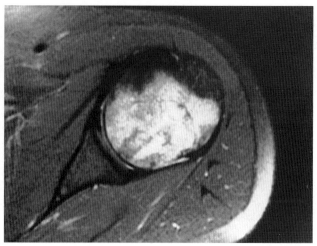

A · B

FIG. 8. Non-Hodgkin lymphoma. **A:** T1-weighted coronal image demonstrates diffuse marrow replacement within the proximal humeral epiphysis with some extension into the metaphysis, with marrow signal being lower in signal than adjacent muscle. No gross cortical disruption is seen. **B:** T2-weighted fast spin-echo fat-suppressed axial image demonstrates marked T2 prolongation corresponding to neoplastic involvement.

(43). In the absence of other conditions such as osteoarthritis, the changes of avascular necrosis in the shoulder are restricted to the subarticular region of the humeral head with sparing of the adjacent glenoid. MRI findings parallel pathologic changes in the subchondral bone. The hallmark of osteonecrosis is the presence of a reactive interface. Early in the course of the disease, the changes can appear as bone marrow edema where decreased signal intensity is seen on T1-weighted images with increased signal on T2-weighted images. Later, the *double-line sign* is appreciated where a well-defined low signal intensity line is seen demarcating the margin of the necrotic segment on T2-weighted sequences (Fig. 9). The necrotic segment may appear relatively bright on T1-weighted sequences. On T2-weighted sequences, the low intensity line demonstrates a bilaminar appearance with

an inner margin of increased signal surrounded by the outer border of low signal intensity. The physiologic basis of this MRI finding is controversial, but current theories suggest that the low signal rim represents fibrosis and sclerosis with the more central high signal line representing reactive granulation tissue (44). Chronic changes are represented by fibrosis characterized by decreased signal on both T1- and T2-weighted images. Imaging techniques include obtaining T1-weighted and T2-weighted sequences with an inversion recovery sequence being very helpful to demonstrate edema within the bone marrow. A variety of staging systems have been described, with the most accepted MR staging system proposed paralleling pathologic changes (44). In class A, the osteonecrotic segment demonstrates characteristics of fat. Class B foci follow characteristics of blood products being

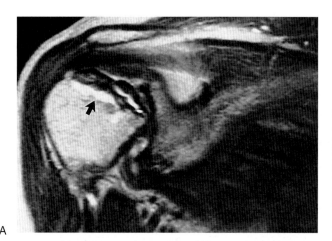
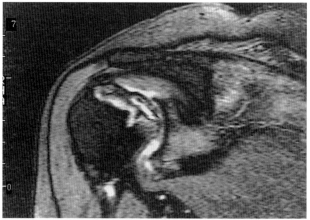

A · B

FIG. 9. Avascular necrosis. **A:** T2-weighted coronal image demonstrates remodeling and flattening of the humeral head with heterogeneous signal as well as presence of a double-line sign *(arrow).* **B:** Inversion recovery coronal image confirms presence of signal alteration within the marrow of the humeral head.

high signal on T1- and T2-weighted sequences. Class C demonstrates increased fluid developing within the necrotic segment with decreased signal on T1-weighted and increased signal on T2-weighted images. Class D shows low signal on T1- and T2-weighted sequences resulting from fibrotic changes.

Bone infarcts can also occur in the shoulder with causes being similar to those of avascular necrosis with the exception of trauma. The term *bone infarct* is reserved for areas of necrosis that are not subchondral in location. Infarction typically occurs in fatty marrow because of its limited vascularity. MRI is again the most sensitive imaging modality when evaluating bone infarction. Bone infarcts tend to be located in the diaphyseal regions and typically have a serpentine low signal border and may demonstrate the aforementioned double-line sign. Bone infarcts may be visualized as foci of marrow edema before progression to the more typical appearance.

TRAUMA

MRI has also emerged as an excellent method to evaluate posttraumatic injuries. Fractures of the proximal humerus comprise up to 5% of all fractures, with 45% of all humeral fractures occurring proximally (45). Eighty percent of proximal humeral fractures have minimal or no displacement because of stabilization by the rotator cuff, joint capsule, and periosteum (46). The most commonly encountered fracture seen during shoulder MRI is a nondisplaced fracture of the greater tuberosity (47). The usual mechanism of injury is related to a fall, commonly a fall on an outstretched hand. Severe trauma with a blow directly to the anterior or anterolateral shoulder appears to be a common cause in younger patients (48). Conventional radiographs are often normal and the referring clinician suspects a rotator cuff injury. When the patient presents acutely, symptoms of pain, swelling, and

limited range of motion are seen. Fracture of the lesser tuberosity can also be seen where it is usually displaced medially by traction from the subscapularis muscle. Malunion of this fracture may result in limited internal rotation of the shoulder. Acromion fractures are also important because they can reduce the subacromial space resulting in impingement with limited motion and pain (49). MRI is an excellent method for evaluating these fractures and can evaluate number, size, and extent of displacement or angulation of fracture fragments and evaluate associated soft tissue injuries. The not uncommon occurrence of avascular necrosis associated with trauma can also be well evaluated with MRI. T1-weighted images demonstrate excellent anatomic detail with T2 fast spin-echo or inversion recovery sequences, providing high sensitivity for associated marrow edema. Bone contusion is characterized by low signal intensity on T1-weighted images with hyperintensity with T2 weighting. Signal alteration is representative of blood, edema, hyperemia, and microfracture of the trabeculae (50). Acute nondisplaced fractures are characterized by marrow edema as described previously with the additional appearance of a visualized fracture line. This appears as a linear focus of decreased signal intensity on T1-weighted images, which can also be seen as a low signal line surrounded by hyperintensity on T2-weighted images (Fig. 10). Anecdotal reports have suggested increased visualization of the fracture line with T1-weighted fat saturation gadolinium-enhanced images, which result in surrounding enhancement with better visualization of the fracture line.

Acromioclavicular joint injuries are usually seen in individuals between the ages of 15 and 40 years of age, most commonly secondary to athletic activities. Acromioclavicular joint separations make up approximately 10% of all dislocations involving the shoulder (8). Most commonly, a direct downward blow to the lateral aspect of the shoulder forces the acromion inferiorly. The clavicle and scapula are

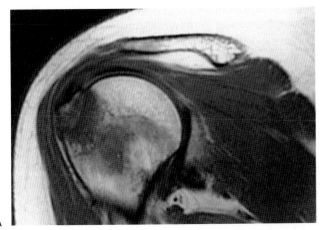
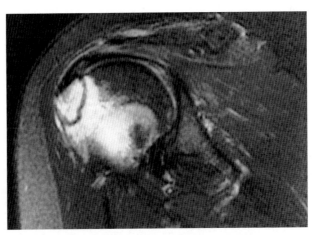

A   B

FIG. 10. Nondisplaced greater tuberosity fracture. **A:** T1-weighted coronal image demonstrates marrow edema involving the greater tuberosity near the insertion of the rotator cuff. **B:** T2-weighted fast spin-echo fat-suppressed coronal image demonstrates marked marrow edema as well as visualization of a nondisplaced fracture line through the greater tuberosity.

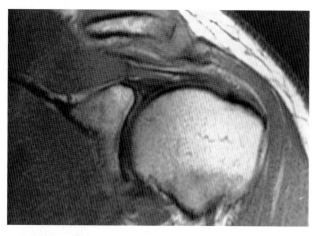

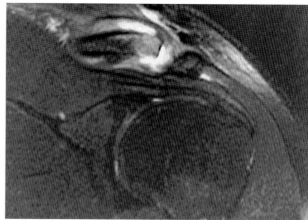

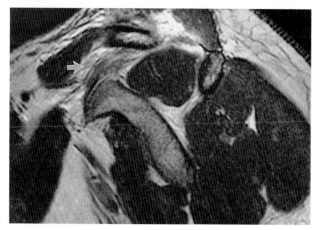

FIG. 11. First degree acromioclavicular joint separation. **A:** T1-weighted coronal image demonstrates marrow edema of the acromion and clavicle at the acromioclavicular joint as well as intermediate signal surrounding the joint. **B:** T2-weighted fast spin-echo fat-suppressed image demonstrates marrow edema as well as fluid signal and inflammatory changes surrounding the acromioclavicular joint. **C:** T2-weighted fast spin-echo sagittal image demonstrates marked thickening and edema of the coracoclavicular ligament *(arrow)*.

driven downward, but inferior motion of the clavicle is limited by the first rib, resulting in the acromioclavicular joint injury and an occasional first rib fracture. Additional mechanisms of injury are traction on the arm and falling on an outstretched hand or a flexed elbow (51). A radiographic grading system for acromioclavicular joint injuries is used, with type 1 representing a mild sprain of the acromioclavicular ligament, type 2 representing a tear of the acromioclavicular ligament and sprain of the coracoclavicular ligament, and type 3 representing tears of both acromioclavicular and coracoclavicular ligaments. Clinically, the patient complains of pain, swelling, and limitation of motion. Plain film radiographs with and without weights are commonly performed for evaluation and can characterize the three types of injuries. Coronal MR images demonstrate marrow edema of the clavicle and acromion with fluid signal seen filling and surrounding the acromioclavicular joint, which is characterized by a bright signal on T2 fast spin-echo fat-suppressed images or inversion recovery images (Fig. 11). Edema can also be seen in the surrounding soft tissues. Sagittal images can evaluate the coracoclavicular ligament, which should normally be low signal on all sequences, and either demonstrate disruption or thickening with increased signal on T1- and T2-weighted images following injury.

Osteolysis of the distal clavicle is seen as a posttraumatic process or as occurring after activities involving repetitive strain of the acromioclavicular joint (8,52). Conventional radiographs show extensive bony destruction involving the distal clavicle and acromion with widening of the acromioclavicular joint space. MRI findings include signal changes within the distal clavicle consistent with diffuse bone marrow edema most conspicuous on inversion recovery sequences, cortical thinning, irregularity of the distal clavicle, and tiny subchondral cysts (52).

INFECTION

The pathogenesis of infection of the shoulder follows that of all intraarticular infections. Three fundamental pathways for infection to enter a joint occur—spontaneous hematogenous seeding from the synovial blood supply, contiguous spread from adjacent metaphyseal osteomyelitis, and penetration of the joint by trauma, therapy, or surgery (1). A variety of infectious processes can arise around the shoulder, including cellulitis/myositis, septic arthritis, abscess, and osteomyelitis, which can all present with similar clinical findings. Because these different processes may affect the appropriate therapy, MRI is helpful for differentiation. Age-dependent presentations of hematogenous osteomyelitis and septic arthritis of the shoulder are related to the vascular development about the growth plate and epiphysis. In patients younger than 8 months of age, direct vascular communications across the growth plate and epiphyseal involvement with subsequent joint sepsis is common. At approximately 1 year of age, the growth plate becomes a barrier to vascular communication between the metaphysis and epiphysis. Nutrient arteries develop slow flow adjacent to the growth plate and create an ideal medium for infection in the metaphyseal region. With obliteration of the growth plate in a mature skeleton, a connection between the metaphysis and epiphysis is again established and infection can extend into the joint from the adjacent bone. Communications between the multiple bursa surrounding the shoulder as well as communication with the synovial covering of the tendon of the long head of the biceps also provide a pathway for spread of infection.

Septic arthritis of the shoulder represents up to 14% of all septic arthritis cases in adults and only 4% in children (1,53). *Staphylococcus aureus* is the most common infectious source overall, with a variety of other agents being implicated. Hematogenous osteomyelitis accounts for up to 90% of osteomyelitis in children whereas contiguous osteomyelitis secondary to surgery or direct inoculation is more common in adults (1). Of the bones of the shoulder, the humerus is most frequently involved. Infection of the clavicle is seen occasionally in drug addicts. Early signs of infection include pain, loss of motion, and joint effusion.

Radiographs are insensitive, with findings ranging from a normal appearance early in infection to a widened or narrow joint space in septic arthritis and gross bony destruction with periosteal reaction in advanced osteomyelitis. Chronic osteomyelitis can result in draining sinuses and Brodie's abscesses. Nuclear medicine scintigraphy using bone imaging agents as well as gallium and tagged white blood cells has been the favored imaging modality in the past with relatively high sensitivity but poor specificity. Spatial resolution is limited in nuclear medicine studies and anatomic definition as well as identification of focal abnormalities within the soft tissues are poor. For example, associated soft tissue abscesses are not reliably diagnosed with a nuclear medicine bone scan. MRI unquestionably yields greater spatial resolution with high sensitivity. Recent series have reported very high sensitivity of 89% to 100% with low specificity of 46% to 88% (54). Inflammation from infection prolongs T1 and T2 relaxation times secondary to increased presence of water, which appear as a bright signal on T2-weighted images and loss of the normal fatty marrow signal on T1-weighted images. These findings are nonspecific and can be seen in a variety of noninfectious processes. Gadolinium enhancement of bone marrow is a highly sensitive sign for osteomyelitis, but again is not specific for infectious lesions. Synovial enhancement in septic arthritis is nonspecific and can also be seen with sterile inflammatory synovitis, but the absence of joint effusion with enhancing synovium can be

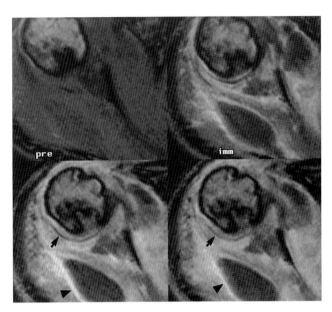

FIG. 12. Pseudomonas osteomyelitis. Spoiled gradient recalled axial images before and after contrast through the proximal humerus. Precontrast images demonstrate erosive changes of the proximal humerus as well as disruption on the surrounding tissue planes. Contrast-enhanced images show enhancement of the involved bone as well as the periosteum *(arrow)* and surrounding soft tissues. Abscess cavities within the surrounding soft tissues are also better demonstrated *(arrowhead)*.

used to exclude pyarthrosis (54). Cellulitis appears as gadolinium enhancement of the surrounding soft tissues as well as bright signal on T2-weighted images. Abscess cavities within the soft tissues appear as rim-enhancing fluid collections (Fig. 12). The ability of MRI to demonstrate fluid collections and abscess cavities appears to be particularly useful to direct surgical drainage.

PAGET'S DISEASE

Paget's disease is a disorder of bone architecture resulting from an imbalance between bone resorption and formation. The cause is unknown, but current theory suggests a viral agent. A definite racial and age-related distribution is seen with an incidence of 3% in populations of European descent. Prevalence of Paget's disease increases in persons older than 40 years of age and is uncommon in persons of Asian or African descent. Men are also affected two to three times more commonly than women (55). Paget's disease occurs in decreasing order in the pelvis, skull, lumbar/cervical spine, and femur. Involvement of the shoulder most commonly affects the proximal humerus, although involvement of the clavicle and scapula can be seen. Pathophysiologically, the process is characterized by a lytic phase early in the disease, followed by a more prominent osteoblastic phase. The result is a structurally weakened and deformed bone. The most common presentation is pain, although up to 20% of patients

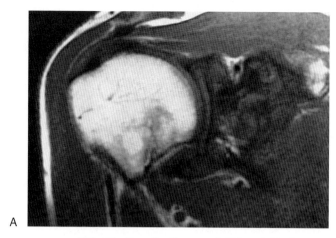
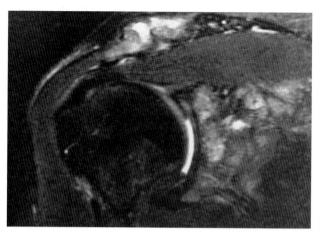

A

B

FIG. 13. Paget's disease. **A:** T1-weighted coronal image demonstrates expansion and decreased signal involving the glenoid. **B:** T2-weighted fast spin-echo fat-suppressed coronal image demonstrates presence of expansion and increased signal within the glenoid as well as the acromion and clavicle.

are asymptomatic (56). Other clinical presentations can include skull deformities, pathologic fractures, and symptoms related to nerve compression. Malignant degeneration to multiple sarcomas has been described with an overall incidence of 1% (55). In general, the sites of sarcomatous transformation are in direct proportion to the frequency of distribution of uncomplicated Paget's disease with higher degree of malignant transformation than expected seen in the humerus (55).

Plain film findings have been well described and MRI is rarely performed for evaluation of Paget's disease. MR findings are variable, but cortical thickening, increased size of the bone, and coarse thickened trabeculae are seen. On both T1- and T2-weighted images, trabecular thickening is seen as linear or oval areas of low signal intensity against a background of normal, although often reduced in size, fatty marrow (57). Active disease may have additional findings of high signal foci on T2-weighted images representing fibrovascular marrow (Fig. 13). In general, some normal fatty marrow signal appears to be preserved in all stages of Paget's disease unless a complication such as acute fracture or malignant degeneration is present (58). Other signs of malignant degeneration can include a soft tissue mass associated with loss of intramedullary marrow signal.

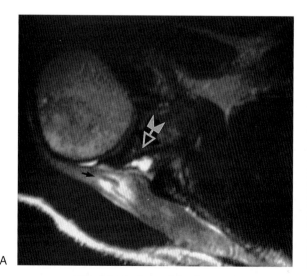
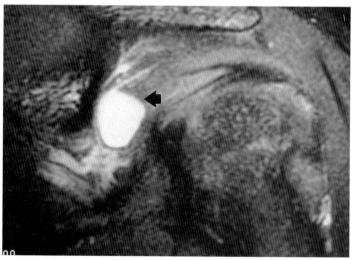

A

B

FIG. 14. **A:** A paralabral cyst extends into the spinoglenoid notch *(white arrow)*. Notice the denervation of the infraspinatus muscle producing high signal intensity *(black arrow)* on this axial T2-weighted MR image. **B:** A large paralabral cyst lies behind the spinoglenoid notch on this oblique coronal fat-saturated fast spin-echo MR image *(arrow)*. The surrounding infraspinatus muscle is high signal intensity related to subacute denervation.

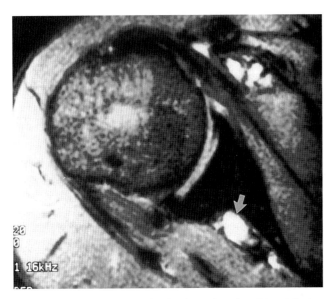

FIG. 15. A varicose vein lies in the spinoglenoid notch *(arrow)* on this axial gradient echo MR image. This patient had shoulder pain related to the compressed suprascapular nerve.

NERVE ENTRAPMENT SYNDROMES

The suprascapular nerve is derived from the upper trunk of the brachial plexus. It passes deep to the trapezius and omohyoid muscles before entering the supraspinatus fossa through the suprascapular notch. In the supraspinatus fossa, it gives off two motor branches to the supraspinatus muscle and receives sensory branches from the capsular and ligamentous structures of the shoulder and acromioclavicular joint. The nerve then runs deep to the supraspinatus muscle, entering the infraspinatus fossa through the spinoglenoid notch. In the infraspinatus fossa, the suprascapular nerve gives off motor branches to the infraspinatus muscle, as well as to the shoulder joint and capsule. The nerve can become compressed along its path by masses such as cysts, ganglions, and neuromas. These masses are well seen on MRI (59). The most common presentation that we have seen is compression of the nerve by a paralabral cyst in the suprascapular or spinoglenoid notch, related to superior or posterior labral tears, respectively (60) (Fig. 14). This usually occurs in men and is common in weight lifters. Other causes of injury or entrapment of the suprascapular nerve include humeral and scapular fractures, anterior shoulder dislocation, traction or kinking of the nerve, and anomalous or thickened transverse scapular ligaments. Denervation changes such as atrophy and edema are often seen in the affected supraspinatus or infraspinatus muscles (Fig. 14). MRI can allow for earlier diagnosis of suprascapular nerve entrapment and it can localize and characterize masses causing the syndrome. Varicose veins may be seen in the spinoglenoid notch and can cause the syndrome (Fig. 15).

It is also important to check for signs of axillary neuropathy in patients who have dislocated anteriorly or following

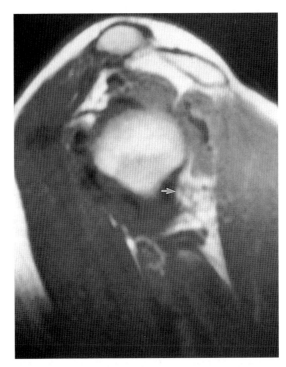

FIG. 16. There is chronic denervation in the form of fatty infiltration of the teres minor *(arrow)* related to axillary neuropathy on this oblique sagittal T1-weighted MR image.

shoulder surgery. An axillary neuropathy develops in approximately 10% of patients if the shoulder has been dislocated for more than an 1 hour. With chronic axillary neuropathy, denervative changes may be seen in the deltoid and teres minor muscles on MRI (61,62) (Fig. 16).

REFERENCES

1. Rockwood CA, Matsen FA. *The shoulder.* Philadelphia: WB Saunders, 1990.
2. Rosenberg SA, Suit FD, Baker LH. Sarcoma of soft tissue. In: Devita VT, Hellman S, Rosenberg SA, eds. *Cancer: principles and practice of oncology,* 2nd ed. Philadelphia: JB Lippincott Co, 1985.
3. Conrad EU. Tumors and related conditions. In: Rockwood CA, Matsen FA, eds. *The shoulder.* Philadelphia: WB Saunders, 1990.
4. Berquist TH, Ehman RL, King BF, et al. Value of MR imaging in differentiating benign from malignant soft tissue masses: study of 95 lesions. *Am J Roentgenol* 1990;155:1251–1255.
5. Crim JR, Seeger LL, Yao L, et al. Diagnosis of soft tissue masses with MR imaging: Can benign masses be differentiated from malignant ones? *Radiology* 1992;185:581–586.
6. Sundaram M, Mcguire MH, Herbold DR. Magnetic resonance imaging of soft tissue masses: an evaluation of 53 histologically proven tumors. *Magn Reson Imaging* 1988;6:237–248.
7. Damjanov I, James L. *Anderson's pathology.* St Louis: Mosby–Year Book, 1996.
8. Resnick D, Niwayama G. *Diagnosis of bone and joint disorders,* 2nd ed. Philadelphia: WB Saunders, 1988.
9. Kransdorf MJ, Jelinek JS, Moser RP. Imaging of soft tissue tumors. *Radiol Clin North Am* 1993;31 (2):359–372.
10. Higgs PE, Young L, Schuster R, Weeks PM. Giant lipomas of the hand and forearm. *South Med J* 1993;86 (8):887–890.
11. Logan PM, Janzen DL, O'Connell JX, et al. MRI and histopathologic appearances of benign soft-tissue masses of the foot. *Can Assoc Radiol*

J 1996;47 (1):36–43.

12. Peh WC, Troung NP, Totty WG, Gilula LA. Pictorial review: magnetic resonance imaging of benign soft tissue masses of the hand and wrist. *Clin Radiol* 1995;50 (8):519–525.

13. Dawson JS, Dowling F, Preston BJ, Neumann L. Case report: lipoma arborescens of the sub-deltoid bursa. *Br J Radiol* 1995;68 (806):197–199.

14. Feller JF, Rishi M, Hughes EC. Lipoma arborescens of the knee: MR demonstration. *Am J Roentgenol* 1994;163 (1):162–164.

15. Chaljub G, Johnson PR. In vivo MRI characteristics of lipoma arborescens utilizing fat suppression and contrast administration. *J Comp Assist Tomogr* 1996;20 (1):85–87.

16. Letourneau L, Dufour M, Deschenes J. Shoulder lipoblastoma: MRI characteristics. *Can Assoc Radiol J* 1993;44 (3):211–214.

17. Buetow PC, Kransdorf MJ, Moser RPJ, et al. Radiologic appearance of intramuscular hemangioma with emphasis on MR imaging. *Am J Roentgenol* 1990;154:563–567.

18. Cohen EK, Kressel HY, Dalinka MK, et al. MR imaging of soft-tissue hemangiomas: correlation with pathologic findings. *Am J Roentgenol* 1988;150:1079–1081.

19. Nelson MC, Stull MA, Teitelbaum GP, et al. Magnetic resonance imaging of peripheral soft tissue hemangiomas. *Skeletal Radiol* 1990;19: 477–482.

20. Kransdorf MJ, Meis JM, Jelinek JS. Myositis ossificans: MR appearance with radiologic-pathologic correlation. *Am J Roentgenol* 1991;157 :1243–1248.

21. De Smet AA, Norris MA, Fisher DR. Magnetic resonance imaging of myositis ossificans: analysis of seven cases. *Skeletal Radiol* 1992;21: 503–507.

21a. Suh JS, Abenoza P, Galloway HR, et al. Peripheral (extracranial) nerve tumors: correlation of MR imaging and histologic findings. *Radiology* 1992;183:341–346.

22. Burr BA, Resnick D, Syklawer R, Haghighi P. Case report: fluid-fluid levels in a unicameral bone cyst: CT and MR findings. *J Comp Assist Tomogr* 1993;17 (1):134–136.

23. Kransdorf MJ, Sweet DE. Aneurysmal bone cyst: concept, controversy, clinical presentation, and imaging. *Am J Roentgenol* 1995;164 (3):573–580.

24. Vergel De Dios AM, Bond JR, Shives TC, Mcleod RA, Unni KK. Aneurysmal bone cyst: a clinicopathologic study of 238 cases. *Cancer* 1992;69:2921–2931.

25. Cory DA, Fritsch SA, Cohen MD, et al. Aneurysmal bone cysts: imaging findings and embolotherapy. *Am J Roentgenol* 1989;153:369–373.

26. Dahlin DC. Giant cell tumor (osteoclastoma). In: *Bone tumors,* 3rd ed. Springfield, IL: Charles C. Thomas Publisher, 1978.

27. Goldenberg RR, Campbell CJ, Bonfiglio M. Giant cell tumor of bone. An analysis of 218 cases. *J Bone Joint Surg* 1970;52:619–664.

28. Moser RP, Kransdorg MJ, Gilkey FW, et al. Giant cell tumor of the upper extremity. *Radiographics* 1990;10:83–102.

29. McInerney DP, Middlemiss JH. Giant cell tumor of bone. *Skeletal Radiol* 1978;2:195–204.

30. Moser RP. *Cartilaginous tumors of the skeleton.* Philadelphia: Hanley and Belfus, 1990.

31. Sweet DE, Madewell JE, Ragsdale BD. Radiologic and pathologic analysis of solitary bone lesions: Part III. Matrix patterns. *Radiol Clin North Am* 1981;19:785.

32. Cohen EK, Kressel HY, Frank TS, et al. Hyaline cartilage-origin bone and soft tissue neoplasms: MR appearance and histologic correlation. *Radiology* 1988;167:477–481.

33. Vogler JB III, Murphy WA. Bone marrow imaging. *Radiology* 1988;168:679–693.

34. Taccone A, Oddone M, Dell'Acqua AD, Occhi M, Ciccone MA. MRI "road-map" of normal age-related bone marrow. II. Thorax, pelvis and extremities. *Pediatr Radiol* 1995;25 (8):596–606.

35. Richardson ML, Patten RM. Age-related changes in marrow distribution in the shoulder: MR imaging findings. *Radiology* 1994;192 (1):209–215.

36. Steiner RM, Mitchell DG, Rao VM, Schweitser ME. MRI of diffuse bone marrow disease. *Radiol Clin North Am* 1993;31 (2):383–409.

37. Negedank WG, Al-Katib AM, Karanes C, et al. Lymphomas: MR imaging contrast characteristics. *Radiology* 1990;177:209.

38. Shields AF, Porter BA, Churchley S, et al. The detection of bone marrow involvement by lymphoma using magnetic resonance imaging. *J Clin Oncol* 1987;5:225.

39. Linden A, Lankovich R, Theissen P, et al. Malignant lymphoma: bone marrow imaging versus biopsy. *Radiology* 1988;173:335.

40. Coles WC, Schulz MD. Bone involvement in malignant lymphona. *Radiology* 1948;50:458–462.

41. Edeiken-Monroe B, Edeiken J, Kim EE. Radiologic concepts of lymphoma of bone. *Radiol Clin North Am* 1990;28 (4):841–864.

42. Neer CS. *Shoulder reconstruction.* Philadelphia: WB Saunders, 1990.

43. Sebes JI. Diagnostic imaging of bone and joint abnormalities associated with sickle cell hemoglobinopathies. *Am J Roentgenol* 1989;152 (2):1153–1159.

44. Mitchell DG, Kressel HY. MR imaging of early avascular necrosis. *Radiology* 1988;169:281–282.

45. Brien H, Noftall F, MacMaster S, Cummings T, Landells C, Rockwood P. Neer's classification system: a critical appraisal. *J Trauma* 1995;38 (2):257–260.

46. Stoller DW. *MRI in orthopaedics and sports medicine.* Philadelphia: JB Lippincott Co, 1993.

47. Deutsch AL, Mink JH. Magnetic resonance imaging of miscellaneous disorders of the shoulder. *MRI Clin North Am* 1993;1 (1):171–183.

48. Pettrone FA. *Athletic injuries of the shoulder.* New York: McGraw-Hill, 1995.

49. Kuhn JE, Blasier RB, Carpenter JE. Fractures of the acromion process: a proposed classification system. *J Orthop Trauma* 1994;8 (1):6–13.

50. Newberg AH, Wetzner SM. Bone bruises: their patterns and significance. *Semin Ultrasound CT MR* 1994;15 (5):396–409.

51. Greenspan A. *Orthopedic radiology: a practical approach.* Philadelphia: JB Lippincott Co, 1988.

52. Patten RM. Atraumatic osteolysis of the distal clavicle: MR findings. *J Comput Assist Tomogr* 1995;19 (1):92–95.

53. Deleted in proof.

54. Hopkins KL, King CPL, Bergman G. Gadolinium-DTPA-enhanced magnetic resonance imaging of musculoskeletal infectious processes. *Skeletal Radiol* 1995;24:325.

55. Mirra JM, Brien EW, Tehranzadeh J. Paget's disease of bone: review with emphasis on radiologic features, part I and II. *Skeletal Radiol* 1995;24:163–171.

56. Merkow RL, Lane JM. Paget's disease of bone. *Orthop Clin North Am* 1990;21 (1):171–189.

57. Roberts MC, Kressel HY, Fallon MD, et al. Paget disease: MR imaging findings. *Radiology* 1989;173:341–345.

58. Kaufmann GA, Sundaran M, Mcdonald DJ. Magnetic resonance imaging in symptomatic Paget's disease. *Skeletal Radiol* 1991;20:413–418.

59. Fritz R, Helms CA, Steinbach LS, et al. MR imaging of suprascapular nerve entrapment. *Radiology* 1992;182:437–444.

60. Tirman PFJ, Feller JFF, Janzen DL, Peterfy CG, Bergman G. Association of glenoid labral cysts with labral tears and glenohumeral instability: radiologic findings and clinical significance. *Radiology* 1994;190: 653–658.

61. Linker CS, Helms CA, Fritz RC. Quadrilateral space syndrome: findings at MR imaging. *Radiology* 1993;188:675–676.

62. Tuckman GA, Devlin TC. Axillary nerve injury after anterior glenohumeral dislocation: MR findings in three patients. *Am J Roentgenol* 1996;167:695–697.

Subject Index

Page references followed by t or f indicate tables or figures, respectively.

A

Abduction and external rotation positioning. *See* ABER (abduction and external rotation) positioning

ABER (abduction and external rotation) positioning, 42, 42f, 47–48, 48f
  imaging in, 1, 15f, 16f
    oblique axial plane, 47–48, 48f
    protocol for, 60t, 61
    structures delineated by, 43t
  in magic angle phenomenon elimination, 59, 59f
  in MR arthrography, 64–65, 65f
    of ALPSA lesion, 152, 154f
    anatomy of, 69f, 70, 70f
    of Bankart lesion, 150, 152f
    of glenohumeral instability, 137, 137f, 138f
    of Perthes lesion, 155f, 156
    of rotator cuff, 106, 107f

Abscess, Brodie's, 225

Abscess cavities, in infection, 247, 247f

Acromial decompression, in rotator cuff repair, 197, 199

Acromioclavicular joint
  abnormalities of, in impingement syndrome, 107–111, 107–112f, 107t
  alignment of, 19, 19f
  arthritis of, in rotator cuff disease, 91
  cyst of, in rotator cuff tear, 125, 125f
  dislocation of, mechanism of, 82t
  imaging of
    oblique coronal, 7f
    oblique sagittal, 4f
  os acromiale vs., 111, 112f
  osteophytes of, and recurrent impingement syndrome, 194, 196f
  palpation of, 84
  surgical absence of, after acromioplasty, 192, 194f
  traumatic injury of, 245–246, 246f

Acromiohumeral articulation, in full-thickness rotator cuff tear, 122, 124f

Acromion
  abnormalities of, in impingement syndrome, 107–111, 107–112f, 107t
  fracture of, 245
  imaging of
    in ABER positioning, 15f, 16f
    magnetic resonance, 104, 105f
    oblique coronal, 6–9f
    oblique sagittal, 2–5f
  os acromiale attachment to, 110, 111f

Paget's disease of, 111, 112f
shapes of, 107–109, 108f, 109f
  anatomic classification of, 17, 18f
  in impingement syndrome, 79, 109–110, 109f, 110f
  magnetic resonance imaging of, 109, 109f
  prevalence of, 17, 17t
slant of, 19, 19f

Acromionectomy, total, for impingement, 189

Acromioplasty
  anterior, for impingement, 189–190, 189f
    scar tissue after, 190f, 191
  magnetic resonance imaging findings after, 191–192, 192–194f
  recurrent impingement syndrome after, causes of, 194–195, 196f, 197f
  in rotator cuff repair, 197

Adhesive capsulitis, clinical evaluation of, 96f, 97

Adson's test, 88

Air bubble artifact, in MR arthrography, 66–67, 67f

Allografts, in rotator cuff repair, 199

ALPSA (anterior labroligamentous periosteal sleeve avulsion) lesion, 148f, 152, 153–155f, 156
  chronic, 152, 153f, 155f
  imaging of, in ABER position, 152, 154f
  recurrent, 215f

AMBRI (atraumatic, multidirectional, bilateral recurrent instability), 92, 135

Aneurysmal bone cyst, 240–241, 241f

Angliolipoma, 239

Anterior band, of inferior glenohumeral ligament, 142f
  insertion of, 138, 140f

Anterior capsule, imaging of
  in ABER positioning, 15f, 16f
  axial, 13f
  oblique sagittal, 5f

Anterior glenoid labrum
  hyaline joint cartilage of, 26, 33f
  imaging of
    in ABER positioning, 16f
    axial, 10–13f
    oblique coronal, 6f, 7f

Anterior glenoid recess, imaging of
  axial, 12f, 13f
  oblique sagittal, 5f

Anterior joint space, oblique sagittal imaging of, 4f

Anterior labroligamentous periosteal sleeve avulsion (ALPSA) lesion, 148f, 152, 153–155f, 156
  chronic, 152, 153f, 155f
  imaging of, in ABER position, 152, 154f
  recurrent, 215f

Anterior labrum
  appearance of, variations in, 26, 31f, 142, 143f
  normal, arthrographic imaging of, 68, 68f
  oblique sagittal imaging of, 4f, 5f
  shape of, 139
    variations in, 35t
  tear of

ALPSA. *See* ALPSA (anterior labroligamentous periosteal sleeve avulsion lesion)
  in Bankart lesion, 149, 151f
  dilute gadolinium arthrography in, ABER positioning for, 65, 65f
  MR arthrography in, 71, 72f
  partial, diagnosis of, 149

Perthes. *See* Perthes lesion

Anterosuperior labrum
  absence of, 142, 145f
  detachment of, 142, 144f
  tear of, 143, 146f

Apprehension test, 94, 94f

Arthritis
  acromioclavicular, in rotator cuff disease, 91
  arthrography in, 222–223, 222f
  bone changes in, 223–226, 223–226f
  magnetic resonance imaging in, 221–234
    reasons for, 221–223, 222f, 222t, 223f
  radiography in, limitations of, 222
  rheumatoid, 233–234
  septic, 247
  ultrasonography in, 223

Arthrography
  in arthritis, 222–223, 222f
  computed tomography
    in arthritis, 223, 223f
    in glenohumeral instability, 71
    in impingement syndrome, 101
  magnetic resonance. *See* MR arthrography
  in rotator cuff tear, 101

Arthrography injection technique, of MR arthrography, 63

Arthroscopic decompression, for impingement, 189f, 190
  complications of, 190

Arthroscopy
  for recurrent glenohumeral instability
    anterior, 206, 207f

251